Health Issues Confronting Minority Men Who Have Sex with Men

Sana Loue

Editor

Health Issues Confronting Minority Men Who Have Sex with Men

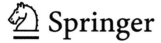 Springer

Editor
Sana Loue
Department of Epidemiology and
Biostatistics, School of Medicine
Case Western Reserve University
Cleveland, OH 44106-4945, USA
sana.loue@case.edu

Library of Congress Control Number: 2007936600

ISBN: 978-0-387-74538-1   e-ISBN: 978-0-387-74539-8

Printed on acid-free paper

9 8 7 6 5 4 3 2 1

springer.com

Preface

Much of what we know about men who have sex with men—not just gay men, but all men who have sex with men—comes to us through research related to HIV and HIV risk. Although we as health researchers, health care providers, and community advocates know and understand more than we once did as a result of this approach, knowledge garnered through this single lens often remains, not surprisingly, uni-dimensional and devoid of depth. Just as in the story of the blind men attempting to "see" and describe the elephant, an understanding of reality requires that we amalgamate and integrate diverse perspectives.

Accordingly, this text is an effort to look beyond the issues that arise in the context of HIV risk and prevention. The initial chapter defines who is a "MSM," comparing self-definition with other-definition, a distinction that almost invariably triggers issues relating to stigma, exclusion, and compensatory mechanisms in both individuals and communities to address these assaults on one's integrity and validity.

The chapters that follow present a seeming avalanche of health issues and effects. Arreola Grant presents her findings relating to childhood sexual abuse of Latino MSM and its resulting emotional pain and behavioral sequelae, including unprotected sex, depression, dissociation, and shame. These same themes inhabit the chapters that follow in discussions of body image disorder (Heinberg and Kraft), substance use and abuse (Loue and Romaniuk), homelessness (chapters by Holbrook and by Walters and colleagues), HIV and sexually transmitted disease (chapters by O'Shea and by Bruckman), and HIV-related stigma (chapters by Kang and Rapkin and by Zea). Each such chapter provides an overview of the current relevant literature and findings from one or more studies conducted in whole or part by each of the authors.

These writings underscore in many ways our tremendous dearth of knowledge and understanding of even the most basic aspects of the daily lives of these men—how they cope with rejection by and exclusion from their families and communities, how they choose and build families and communities of choice, how they formulate and achieve goals and dreams despite the adverse circumstances that many of them endure. What is abundantly clear from these scholarly contributions is the interwoven nature of many of these inherently complex issues. The observation by His Holiness the Dalai Lama, albeit in another context, is relevant here:

> First, all conditioned things and events in the world come into being only as a result of the interaction of causes and conditions. They don't just arise from nowhere, fully formed. Second, there is mutual dependence between parts and the whole; without parts there can be no whole, without a whole it makes no sense to speak of parts. This interdependence of parts and the whole applies in both spatial and temporal terms. Third, anything that exists and has an identity does so only within the total network of everything that as a possible or potential relation to it. No phenomenon exists with an independent or intrinsic identity.
>
> And the world is made up of a network of complex interrelationships. We cannot speak of the reality of a discrete entity outside the context of its range of interrelations with its environment and other phenomena, including language, concepts, and other conventions (His Holiness the Dalai Lama, 2006: 64).

Each of these chapters provides what most would term an "objective" perspective, one that is rooted in numbers and statistical analyses and theory, seemingly untouched by emotion, its complications, and its resulting subjectivity. They permit the reader to maintain his or her distance from the events described, to remain insulated from the emotional experience of the events and circumstances they encounter.

The contributions from the MSM themselves, who come from diverse geographical regions of this country, and from almost every socioeconomic strata and educational level, shatter this protective shield. Their experiences speak of a search for themselves, of mental illness, abuse, stigma, HIV infection, and often a daily struggle to survive through the world around them. Their voices do not permit us the luxury of distance, of "objectivity" but, instead, challenge us to feel their pain with them, to contemplate existence as a Latino gay man, as an African American transgender male-to-female-to-male, living at the juncture at these multiple assaults on their authenticity.

Throughout the scholarly chapters and personal writings are woven yet other threads: strength, courage, the ability to flourish despite seemingly overwhelming adversities. The individuals who contributed their personal accounts of their own journeys and/or their photos are truly courageous in their willingness to self-disclose so that we may begin to learn and understand. We acknowledge and give gratitude here for these efforts. The concluding chapter by Jones and Pike describes the building of a community which, in the truest sense of the word, came together as a unified force following the murder of one of its members. Indeed, the growth that Jones and Pike describe is, in essence, a journey of growth of individuals and community alike.

Many of the contributors to this volume were surprised, shocked, dismayed by the paths that their writings revealed. One man, re-traumatized by painful memories of family abuse that haunted him as he wrote, took a three-month leave of absence from his work to travel to his hometown in an attempt to resolve the bitterness that characterized his relations with his birth family. Yet another was finally able to express to his partner for the first time the depth of his commitment and his gratitude for the life that they have been able to build together.

So, too, has this volume shown me a path I would not have contemplated. That path has been variously marked by pain, engendered by the anger of one would-be contributor who, unable to resolve his emotional pain caused by his family's rejection of him, severed his friendship with me, hopefully only temporarily; joy, as a witness to individuals' reconciliations with themselves and others, prompted through their writing experiences; and, finally, an endless sense of gratitude, appreciation, and privilege at being accepted as a witness to individuals' lives and to their growth.

These contributions challenge us to learn more, to know more, to understand the strengths as well as the adversities, and to work with minority men who have sex with men, their families, and their communities, towards the successful amelioration of these intersecting inequities and injustices. This book begins a discussion of health and health-related issues that confront minority men who have sex with men. It is not a complete discussion. It does not address all existing issues or their innumerable permutations. It is, however, a beginning, one that has been long-needed and too long neglected.

References

His Holiness the Dalai Lama. (2006). *The universe in a single atom: The convergence of science and spirituality*. New York: Morgan Road Books.

Contents

PART I. IDENTITIES

1. Defining Men who have Sex with Men (MSM)   3
   Sana Loue
   Portrait One: Rebirth: Evolution of a Gender   25
   Travis A. Garry
   Portrait Two: ¿De Donde?   29
   Hank Ramírez
   Portrait Three: Untitled   35
   Cristina Caruth

PART II. SEXUAL ABUSE

2. Childhood Sexual Abuse and its Sequelae Among Latino Gay
   and Bisexual Men   41
   Sonya Grant Arreola
   Portrait Four: May and December: Dangerous Intimacies   57
   L. Michael Gipson

PART III. MENTAL ILLNESS AND SUBSTANCE USE

3. Body Image Disturbance and its Related Disorders   67
   Leslie J. Heinberg and Chris Kraft
   Portrait Five: Cutting   83
   Anonymous

4. Substance Use among Minority Men who have Sex with Men   87
   Sana Loue and Jaroslaw Richard Romaniuk

PART IV. HOMELESSNESS

5. Homelessness among Substance-Using Minority Men who have Sex
   with Men   109
   James M. Holbrook

6. "My Body and My Spirit Took Care of Me": Homelessness,
   Violence, and Resilience Among American Indian
   Two-Spirit Men... 125
      Karina L. Walters, David H. Chae, A. Tyler Perry, Antony
      Stately, Roy Old Person and Jane M. Simoni

PART V. HIV/AIDS

7. National Trends in HIV Transmission Among Minority Men
   who have Sex with Men 157
      Daniel J. O'Shea

8. HIV/AIDS in Cleveland: A Case Study of One Community........ 177
      David Bruckman

PART VI. HIV, MULTIPLE MINORITY STATUS, AND STIGMA

9. Why Tell? Serostatus Disclosure and HIV Stigma among HIV
   Seropositive Asians and Pacific Islander Men who have Sex
   with Men in New York City................................. 197
      Ezer Kang and Bruce D. Rapkin

10. Disclosure of HIV Status and Mental Health among Latino Men
    who have Sex with Men 219
      Maria Cecilia Zea

PART VII. BUILDING COMMUNITY

11. The Beyond Identities Community Center: A Community-
    Focused, Rights-Based Program to Address HIV/AIDS and Sexual
    Health Among Young Men Who have Sex with Men of Color in
    Cleveland, Ohio 233
      Tracy Jones and Earl Pike
    Portrait Six: For Jayla 245
      L. Michael Gipson
    Portrait Seven: Rage of Betrayal 249
      Erik Bradford
    Portrait Eight: Community Commitment 251
      Various

Index... 255

Contributors

Sonya Grant Arreola, Ph.D., M.P.H
San Francisco Department of Public
Health, San Francisco, CA

David Bruckman, MS, MT (ASCP)
Cleveland Department of Public
Health, Cleveland, OH

Cristina Caruth
San Diego, CA

David H. Chae, Sc.D
University of California Berkeley
and University of California San
Francisco, CA

Erik Bradford
Cleveland, OH

L. Michael Gipson
LMG Consulting Partnerships, Ltd.,
Washington, DC

Leslie J. Heinberg, Ph.D
Case Western Reserve University
School of Medicine, Cleveland, OH

James M. Holbrook
Cleveland, OH

Tracy Jones
MNO, AIDS Taskforce of Greater
Cleveland, Cleveland, OH

Ezer Kang, Ph.D
Columbia-Presbyterian Center
of New York Presbyterian
Hospital; Harlem Hospital Center;
New York State Psychiatric Institute,
New York, NY

Chris Kraft, Ph.D
Johns Hopkins University School
of Medicine, Baltimore, MD

Sana Loue, J.D., Ph.D., M.P.H
Case Western Reserve University,
School of Medicine, Cleveland, OH

Roy Old Person, M.S.W
University of Washington School
of Social Work, Seattle, WA

Daniel J. O'Shea
County of San Diego Health and
Human Services Agency, San
Diego, CA

A. Tyler Perry, M.S.W
University of Washington School
of Social Work, Seattle, WA

Earl Pike
AIDS Taskforce of Greater
Cleveland, Cleveland, OH

Hank Ramírez
San Diego, CA

Bruce D. Rapkin, Ph.D
Memorial Sloan-Kettering Cancer
Center, New York, NY

Jaroslaw Richard Romaniuk, Ph.D
Case Western Reserve University,
Mandel School of Applied Social
Sciences, Cleveland, OH

Jane M. Simoni, Ph.D
University of Washington,
Seattle, WA

Antony Stately, Ph.D
Center on Translational Research,
Indigenous Wellness Research
Institute, University of Washington,
Seattle, WA

Karina L. Walters, Ph.D
University of Washington School of
Social Work, Seattle, WA

Maria Cecilia Zea, Ph.D
George Washington University,
Washington, D.C.

The majority of individuals who contributed their photos to this volume asked to remain unnamed and we have honored their request.

Tables and Figures

1.1 Selected studies related to sexual identity and behavior among minority MSM 10

4.1 Substance Use... 96

6.1 Socio-demographic characteristics of male and transgender sexual minority participants by housing status 132

9.1 Means and standard deviations of predictor and outcomes variables for participants who self-identified as MSM or heterosexual 206

9.2 Hierarchical forward stepwise regression predicting non-disclosure due to difficulty accepting HIV serostatus 207

P1.1 Photo of Meokah Diamond 26

P1.2 Photo of Travis A. Garry 28

2.1 Preliminary Model of Childhood Sexual Abuse and HIV Risk 51

P5.1 Photograph 84

8.1 Black/African American Population Distribution across Statistical Planning Areas of Cleveland, 2000 178

8.2 Age Distribution (Percent) of White Non-Hispanic, Black/African American Non-Hispanic and Hispanic Persons from Cleveland at Time of Initial Diagnosis. Cases Reported in 2004, 2005, and 2006 182

P8.1 Community Commitment 252

P8.2 Photograph 254

Part I
Identities

Chapter One
Defining Men who have Sex with Men (MSM)

Sana Loue

Who are MSMs?

The term "men who have sex with men," or MSM, came into being in the 1980s in the context of public health efforts to understand men's sexual behavior as it relates to HIV transmission and prevention (Mays, Cochran, & Zamudio, 2004; Woodyard, Peterson, & Stokes, 2000). The term is used to refer to a wide range of distinct groups of men: those who self-identify as gay, bisexual, or transgender; incarcerated self-identified heterosexual men who, due to their circumstances, engage in voluntary sex with other men; self-identified heterosexual men who engage in sex with other men as a means of survival during incarceration, periods of homelessness, or for economic gain; men who have sex with females and/or with male-to-female transgender persons but also have sex with males; men who self-identify as "same-gender loving" or "sexual freaks;" and men who self-identify as "questioning" (Goldbaum, Perdue, & Higgins, 1996; Mays et al., 2004).

The subject of how and why individuals who seemingly engage in similar behavior self-identify in such diverse ways is too vast an undertaking for one chapter. Consequently, this chapter provides a brief discussion of how sexual identity, gender identity, and sexual orientation are formed and examines the various factors that may affect the development of individuals' self-identity in these realms. This chapter is intended to serve as a basic introduction to this topic and to provide a foundation for the chapters that follow.

Sana Loue
Case Western Reserve University, School of Medicine, Cleveland, OH, USA

S. Loue (ed.), *Health Issues Confronting Minority Men Who Have Sex with Men.*
© Springer 2008

Gender Identity and Gender Role

Defining Gender Identity and Gender Role

Gender identity and gender role are distinct concepts:

> Gender identity has been defined as the private experience of gender role: the experience of one's sameness, unity, and the persistence of one's individuality as male, female, or androgynous, expressed in both self-awareness and behavior. Gender role is everything that a person says and does to indicate to others or to self the degree to which one is either male, female, or androgynous. Gender role would thus include public presentations of self in dress and verbal and nonverbal communication; the economic and family roles one plays; the sexual feelings (desires) one has and the persons to whom such feelings are directed; the sexual role one plays and emotions one experiences and displays; and the experiencing of one's body, as it is defined as masculine or feminine in any particular society. Gender identity and gender role are said to have a unity, like two sides of a coin (Nanda, 1994: 395–396).

Money and Erhardt (1972) similarly distinguished between the concept of gender and that of gender identity:

> Gender Identity: The sameness, unity, and persistence of one's individuality as male, female, or ambivalent, in greater or lesser degree, especially as it is experienced in self awareness and behaviour; gender identity is the private experience of gender role, and gender role is the public expression of gender identity.

Stoller also discusses gender identity and gender role as they relate to the public—private distinction:

> I am using the word *identity* to mean one's own awareness (whether one is conscious of it or not) of one's existence or purpose in this world or, to put it a bit differently, the organization of those psychic components that are to preserve one's awareness of existing (Stoller, 1968: x).

The concept of gender identity is also distinguishable from that of core gender identity, which represents a "person's unquestioning certainty that he belongs to one of only two sexes" (Stoller, 1968: 39):

> This essentially unalterable core of gender identity [I am a male] is to be distinguished from the related but different belief, I am manly (or masculine). The latter attitude is a more subtle and complicated development. It emerges only after a child learned how his parents expect him to express masculinity (Stoller, 1968: 40).

In contrast to core gender identity, which signifies the feeling that "I am a male" or "I am a female," gender role represents "a masculine or feminine way of behaving" (Walinder, 1967: 74). "Thus, of a patient who says 'I am not a very masculine man,' it is possible to say that his gender identity is male although he recognizes his lack of so-called masculinity" (Stoller, 1964: 220).

One's apparent biological sex, which results from the appearance of the external genitalia, the morphology of the gonads (ovaries or testes), the chromosomal structure, and hormonal levels (Dreger, 1998), is not invariably synchronous with one's gender identity, as in the case of transgenderism, or one's sexual identity, as in the case of transsexuality.

Transgenderism

The term *transgender* can be used to refer to (1) all those "who challenge the boundaries of sex and gender" (Feinberg, 1996: x), (2) those who modify their sex with which they were labeled or identified with at birth, and (3) those individuals whose expressed gender is considered inappropriate for their apparent sex (Feinberg, 1996). Transgender individuals may be distinguished from transsexuals, who change/modify or wish to change/modify the sex that they were assigned at birth. In contrast to transsexuals, transgender individuals have been defined as those who "blur the [boundaries] of the *gender expression*" that is traditionally associated with the biological sexes (Feinberg, 1996). It has been asserted that "the guide principle of this [transgender] movement is that people should be free to change, either temporarily or permanently, the sex type to which they were assigned since infancy" (Rothblatt, 1995: 16).

Cross-dressing represents one such form of blurring (Garber, 1992). Cross-dressing, or wearing the clothing that is most frequently associated with the opposite biological sex, occurs for various reasons in numerous contexts; in fact, it may not be associated with transgenderism, depending upon its purpose and the context in which it occurs. Women may assume "an imitation man look" in order to succeed in business (Molloy, 1977). Males, regardless of their sexual orientation, may don women's clothing to perform as female impersonators. Gay men may cross-dress as a means of self-assertion or activism (Garber, 1992). Cross-dressing has been central in theater (Heriot, 1975) and, to a lesser degree, in religion (Barrett, 1931; Garber, 1992).

Transsexuality

Transsexuals have been described as "individuals with a cross-sex identity," regardless of their surgical status or apparent biological sex (Bolin, 1992: 14). Alternatively, the term has been used to refer to "individuals who desire to live... permanently in the social role of the opposite gender" and who desire sexual reassignment surgery in order to effectuate this intent (Cohen-Kettenis & Gooren, 1999: 316). The psychiatric profession continues to classify transsexuality as a disorder within the larger diagnostic category of gender identity disorders (American Psychiatric Association, 2000; Reid & Wise, 1995). In the USA, absent a medical diagnosis, it may be impossible to obtain health care insurance benefits to finance sex reassignment surgery in the relatively few circumstances in which health care insurance policies will cover such procedures. With such a diagnosis, individuals may be perceived as ill and/or deviant (Bayer, 1981; Luchetta, 1999; Szasz, 1970).

The Formation of Sexual Orientation

Sexual orientation has been defined as "the preponderance of sexual or erotic feelings, thoughts, fantasies, and/or behaviors one has for members of one sex or the other, both, or neither" (Savan-Williams, 1998: 3). The development of one's sexual orientation is often a process, rather than an event. In the context of same-sex orientation, scholars have conceived of it in a stage fashion, whereby an individual first becomes aware of one's same-sex attraction, then begins to experiment, and ultimately accepts one's same-sex orientation and discloses it publicly (Cass, 1979; Coleman, 1982; Troiden, 1989).

The behavioral view of sexual orientation asserts that one determines sexual orientation by reference to the sex of the individual with whom one is involved sexually: if it is an individual of the same sex, then one is a homosexual, while if the person is of the opposite sex, one is heterosexual (Stein, 1999). However, this viewpoint suffers from a number of limitations. First, it equates behavior with orientation, despite the possibility that there may be multiple explanations for the same behaviors. Second, it assumes that only two sexual orientations exist. Third, the theory is concerned with whether the sexual partner is of the same or opposite sex, rather than whether the sexual partner is a man or woman. Additionally, it is unclear as to the exact point in time at which this assessment is to be made: is it premised on the sex of the first person with whom one has sexual relations, the sex of the most recent partner, or the sex of the majority of partners during one's lifetime? If the latter, at what point in an individual's lifetime can "majority of partners" be determined with accuracy, short of one's death?

The self-identification view asserts that individuals' sexual orientation is identifiable based on their beliefs about themselves; if someone believes, for instance, that one is heterosexual, then one is heterosexual. This view fails to consider instances in which an individual may experience attraction toward a member of the same sex, but not to classify such feelings as homoerotic (Stein, 1999).

The dispositional view seemingly melds the basic tenets of the behavioral and self-identification perspectives. According to this view, an individual's sexual orientation is a function of both one's sexual desires and fantasies about sexual relations with members of a specific sex and one's choice of sexual partner under ideal conditions. This perspective allows for the possibility that an individual may have a sexual orientation before one actually ever has sexual relations. This perspective is not, however, without its difficulties, in that it may not be possible to know what an individual's choice of partner would be under circumstances that do not exist.

The Kinsey scale of sexual orientation has been termed a dispositional one because it simultaneously considers an individual's sexual behavior, desires, and fantasies in determining sexual orientation and also recognizes that these features may be discordant within the same individual (Stein, 1999). Kinsey and colleagues explained:

The rating which an individual receives has a dual basis. It takes account of his overt sexual experience and/or his psychosexual reactions. In the majority of instances, the two aspects of the history parallel, but sometimes they are not in accord. In the latter case, the rating of an individual must be based upon an evaluation of the relative importance of the overt and the psychic in his history.... The position of an individual on this scale is always based upon the relation of the heterosexual to the homosexual in his history, rather than upon the actual amount of overt experience or psychic reaction (Kinsey, Pomeroy, & Martin, 1948: 647).

Sexual orientation has traditionally been viewed as a binary phenomenon: hetero- and homosexual (Stein, 1999). This construction of sexual orientation does not permit the existence, for instance, of bisexuality and is unable to explain situational same-sex behaviors, such as male—male sex during imprisonment or periods of homelessness for the purpose of self-protection or due to force (Greenberg, 1988; Seal et al., 2004; Trexler, 1995). As an example, many African American prison inmates may view same-sex sexual encounters as situational in nature and not as a reflection of their sexual orientation or identity (Braithwaite & Arriola, 2003).

In contrast, the bipolar construction views sexual orientation along a continuum, with exclusive heterosexuality at one end and exclusive homosexuality at the other (Kinsey et al., 1948). The Kinsey seven-point scale reflects this polarity with respect to sexual experience and desires:

0 = exclusively heterosexual, no homosexual
1 = predominately heterosexual, only incidental homosexual
2 = predominately heterosexual, but more than incidental homosexual
3 = equally heterosexual and homosexual
4 = predominately homosexual but more than incidental heterosexual
5 = predominately homosexual, but only incidental heterosexual
6 = exclusively homosexual with no heterosexual
X = no social-sexual contacts or reactions (Kinsey et al., 1948).

However, Kinsey's conceptualization of sexuality as a heterosexual—homosexual continuum has been challenged by a number of researchers. Stein (1999) has criticized this schema, noting that the classification of bisexuals as equally hetero- and homosexual fails to consider the diversity that exists within bisexuality. For instance, individuals may be strongly attracted to individuals of both the same sex and the opposite sex, or moderately attracted to individuals of both sexes, or they may be weakly attracted to individuals of both sexes (cf. McKirnan, Stokes, Doll, & Burzette, 1995).

Storms (1979, 1980, 1981) has argued that sexual orientation may be conceived of along two axes: one axis represents the degree of attraction to individuals of the same sex—gender and the second axis refers to the degree of attraction to those of a different sex—gender. Individuals are mapped on this grid irrespective of their own physical sex, i.e., irrespective of whether they are male or female, but only with reference to the sameness or differentness of their partner's sex. Consequently, a male and a female may share the same position on the grid, despite the difference in their sex.

Stein (1999) has advocated a variation of this grid, which would utilize the y-axis to indicate the degree of attraction to women and the x-axis to represent the degree of attraction to men. The resulting grid would group together those who are attracted to men or women. He has further suggested the addition of a third axis to represent the degree of attraction to members of a third sex—gender and a fourth axis to depict the sexual object choice, such as heterosexual women, homosexual men, etc. Shively and De Cecco (1977) asserted that sexual orientation reflects two different continua, one of which represents the degree of heterosexuality and the other represents that of homosexuality. In addition, sexual orientation is composed of two different aspects, the physical and the affectional preferences, each of which consists of hetero- and homosexual continua. The Sell scale of sexual orientation, developed by Gonsiorek, Sell, and Weinrich (1995), assesses the frequency and strength of sexual interests, the frequency of sexual contacts, and self-identity in degrees of hetero-, homo-, and bisexuality. Klein (1978) characterized both hetero- and homosexuality as limited, whereas bisexuality was perceived of as tolerating ambiguity.

> Divergent perspectives have been voiced in an attempt to understand bisexuality. Arguments have been made to the effect that bisexuality does not exist (Altshuler, 1984), while other scholars have asserted that the concept of bisexuality, as it is commonly used, represents a cultural construct (Paul, 2000). Indeed, personal views about sexuality in the abstract reflect wider cultural understandings, and affect, in turn, the concrete constructions people place on their own feelings and experiences and thereby affect their behavior. So it is essential to accept cultural understandings of sexuality as crucial data, while at the same time rejecting the scientific validity of their underlying premise (Blumstein & Schwartz, 1977: 31).

The conflict theory of bisexuality posits that sexual orientation is a dichotomous construct consisting of hetero- and homosexuality in opposition (Zinik, 2000). According to this theory, a bisexual individual must therefore be (1) experiencing confusion or identity conflict, (2) in a transitional phase that is masking the individual's true sexual orientation, and (3) self-identifying as bisexual in order to consciously deny or subconsciously defend against one's true (homosexual) orientation. Zinik (2000) has noted that this theory implicitly assumes that homosexuality must cancel out heterosexuality, i.e., that they cannot co-exist in the same individual. Further, this perspective suggests that because no individual would choose homosexuality voluntarily, given the tremendous social costs associated with this orientation, any homosexual behavior is indicative of a homosexual orientation.

In contrast, the flexibility theory views bisexuality as the integration of hetero- and homosexual identities. Unlike the conflict theory, the flexibility theory does not view bisexuality as inherently problematic (Zinik, 2000).

Researchers have attempted to distinguish between various categories of bisexuality, often differentiating such groupings based upon the duration of bisexual activity, the nature of the bisexual relationship, and/or the context in which the bisexual behavior occurs. Klein (1978, 1993), for instance, delineated four types of bisexuality: transitional, historical, sequential, and concurrent. *Transitional bisexuality* refers to a phase that some individuals pass through in their evolution from heterosexuality to homosexuality. An *historical bisexual* is an individual who has had both male and female partners during one's lifetime. *Sequential bisexuality* refers to individuals who have had relationships with both men and women, but with only one sex at a time, while *concurrent bisexuality* refers to individuals who have sexual relations with a male and a female partner during the same period of time. However, others' characterization of individuals or their behavior as bisexual may not reflect or be consonant with an individual's self-definition and self-identity.

A Comparison of Identity, Orientation, and Behavior

The apparent sex of one's sexual or romantic partner is often equated with one's sexual orientation. However, data indicate that homosexuality and homosexual behavior are not synonymous. One study of male sexual behavior in the USA found that 2% of the respondents of age 20–39 reported having had any same-sex sexual activity during the preceding 10 years, but only 1% reported exclusively same-sex sexual activity during the same time period (Billy, Tanfer, Grady, & Keplinger, 1993). An ethnographic study of men having sex with men found that although only 14% of the individuals were primarily interested in homosexual relationships, over one-half of the men were married, and many of the married men engaged in sex with other men due to family planning concerns stemming from their observance of Catholic tenets relating to birth control (Humphreys, 1970).

In yet another study conducted in Sweden with 244 males of varying nationalities who had engaged in cybersex, it was found that 76.2% were heterosexual in both orientation and behavior, 15.6% were gay or bisexual and reported male or both male and female sexual contact on the Internet, and 8.2% were self-identified heterosexuals who reported sex with other men (Ross, Månsson, Daneback, & Tikkanen, 2005). Of the MSM who were not gay- or bisexual-identified 36.8% reported that sexual thoughts and behaviors were causing a problem in their lives and 26.3% reported that their desire to have sex created problems in their everyday lives.

Clearly, sexual identity may not be congruent with the behavior that is stereotypically associated with a specified identity. The sample of studies included in Table 1.1 pertaining to minority MSM underscores the discordance that may exist between identity and behavior.

Table 1.1 Selected studies related to sexual identity and behavior among minority MSM

Study	Sample	Critical findings
Absalon et al., 2006	Of 590 men, of whom 97.5% were of minority status The majority self-identified as heterosexual	11% reported sex with other men 50% of the MSM reported sex with both men and women
Carballo-Diéguez & Dolezal, 1994	Of a sample of Latino MSM: • 20% self-identified as bisexual or *hombres modernos* ("modern men") • 10% self-identified as heterosexual • 65% self-identified as gay • 4% self-identified as drag queens	80% of bisexual men had had sex with a woman during the previous year, compared with 63% of heterosexual-identified men Almost three out of five of the self-identified gay men had ever had sexual relations with a woman 8% of the self-identified gay men had had sexual relations with a woman during the previous year
Finlinson, Colón, Robles, & Soto, 2006	Of 20 MSM in Puerto Rico, 8 indicated NGI; of these, 2 self-identified as bisexual	All reported hearing pejorative remarks about gay men during childhood All had lifetime histories of sex with women Same sex debut between ages of 13 and 15 All engaged in same-sex relations to support drug habits, but also maintained long-term relationships with primary male partners as a central focus of their emotional lives Heterosexual relationships less important than same-sex relationships, even among those who had fathered children
Goldbaum et al., 1998	Of 1,369 minority and nonminority MSM from public environments in four US cities, 50% self-identified as gay, 40% as bisexual, and 10% as straight	• Of 52 African American MSM, 44.2% self-identified as straight • 38.8% of Latino MSM self-identified as straight • 35.3% of 17 "other" MSM self-identified as straight
Heckman, Kelly, Bogart, Kalichman, & Rompa, 1999	In a sample of 79 African American MSM and 174 White MSM, African American men were more likely to have sexual relations with both men and women	

Table 1.1 (continued)

Study	Sample	Critical findings
Irwin & Morgenstern 2005	Of 198 MSM, 60.1% were minority	• 34% of African Americans, 33% of Latinos, and 12% of "other" self-identified as gay, compared with 83.5% of non-Hispanic Whites • 38.2% of African Americans, 31.2% of Latinos, and 4% of other self-identified as bisexual or heterosexual
Jimenez, 2003	Of 110 self-identified minority MSM: • 29% self-identified as bisexual • 16% self-identified as mostly or completely straight • 52% self-identified as gay	40% reported current or previous legal marriage to a woman 19% had sex mostly with men but occasionally with women 11% reported sex with equal numbers of men and woman 18% had sex mostly with women but occasionally with men
Kral et al., 2005	Of 357 MSM who were injecting drug users (IDU) of whom 37% were of minority status: 34.5% self-identified as gay 43.7% self-identified as bisexual 21.9% self-identified as heterosexual	35% of heterosexual-identified men had had anal sex with a man 88% of heterosexual-identified men had had oral sex with a man 3% of gay-identified men had had sex with a woman
Martinez & Hosek, 2005	Of six African American NGI-MSM, all self-identified as heterosexual	Classification of their sexual orientation using the Kinsey scale to categorize according to the behavior: • 33.3% were mostly heterosexual and infrequently homosexual • 33.3% were often heterosexual, sometimes homosexual • 33.3% were equally hetero- and homosexual
Millet, Malebranche, Mason, & Spikes, 2005	18–35% of heterosexual-identified Latino men, 18–46.5% of heterosexual-identified non-Hispanic White men reported having had anal or oral sex with a man	
Montgomery, Mokotoff, Gentry, & Blair, 2003	5,156 MSM of whom 48% were non-Hispanic White, 31% non-Hispanic Black, 19% Hispanic, 2% American Indian/Alaskan Native, and 1% Asian Pacific Islander	• Among who had only sex with men, (MSM): Among African American men, 3% self-identified as heterosexual and 11% as bisexual

Table 1.1 (continued)

Study	Sample	Critical findings
		• Among Hispanic MSM, 1% self-identified as heterosexual and 10% as bisexual • Among White MSM, <1% self-identified as heterosexual and 5% self-identified as bisexual Among those who had sex with both men and women: • Among African American men, 12% self-identified as heterosexual, 22% as homosexual, and 61% as bisexual • Among Hispanic men, 10% self-identified as heterosexual, 28% as homosexual, and 59% as bisexual • Among White men, 9% self-identified as heterosexual, 31% as homosexual, and 56% as bisexual
Rietmeijer, Wolitski, Fishbein, Corby, & Cohn, 1998	Of 1,290 MSM respondents to a questionnaire administered in Denver and Long Beach, 417 (32%) were NGI • Of the 417 NGI, 10% straight-identified • Of the NGI-MSM, 65.3% were White, 10.3% were Black, 18.6% were Latino, and 6.7% were "other"	Hispanic and "other" ethnicity were associated with NGI
Ross, Essien, Williams, & Fernandez-Esquer, 2003	Of self-identified heterosexual men, 49% of African American men, 17.3% of Asian men, 18.3% of Latino men, and 46.5% of non-Hispanic White men reported sexual contact with both males and females during the preceding 3 months	
Solorio, Swendeman, & Rotheram-Borus, 2003	Of 231 HIV+ youth (MSM) of whom 69.3% were of minority status: • 75.3% self-identified as gay • 12.6% self-identified as bisexual • 8.7% self-identified as straight	Based on the behavior (sex with males only or both males and females), investigators classified • 50% of gay-identified youth as bisexual and 50% as gay • 89.7% of bisexual-identified youth as bisexual and 10.3%

Table 1.1 (continued)

Study	Sample	Critical findings
		of bisexual-identified youth as gay
		• 90% of straight-identified youth as bisexual and 10% as gay
Waldo, McFarland, Katz, MacKellar, & Valleroy, 2000	719 MSM between the ages of 15 and 22, of whom 498 (69.3%) were of minority status	63.3% self-identified as gay 27.3% self-identified as bisexual 3.4% self-identified as heterosexual
Williams, Wyatt, Resell, Peterson & Asuan-O'Brien, 2004	Of 23 minority MSM, 5 AA reported identity as gay, 5 AA reported NGI; of 11 Latinos, 5 reported gay identity, 6 reported NGI	NGI more likely to have sex with women in order to maintain masculine identity NGI more likely to report that sex with women was more emotionally satisfying, but sex with men was more sexually satisfying
Wohl et al., 2002	362 self-identified heterosexual African American men in Los Angeles County	19.6% had had anal sex with a man during the previous year Of the men who had had anal sex with a man during the preceding year, 95.8% had also had vaginal sex with a female partner during the same time period

Factors Affecting Self-Identification

It is critical to recognize not only an individual's internal processes relating to the development of one's self-awareness, but also the external processes that may influence the development of relationships, disclosure, and community involvement (Parks, Hughes, & Matthews, 2004). An individual's self-definition may vary depending on one's level of self-awareness, as well as both the external environment and the interactive dynamic between the individual and the larger environment.

Societal Environment and Response

The extent to which society does or does not sanction specific behaviors may impact on how an individual chooses to identify himself to others and/or to his own self. Behavior that may lead to societal repercussions may inhibit individuals' disclosure of their sexual identity and/or sexual behaviors.

As an example of the potential consequences that may come of self-identification as homo- or bisexual, consider the various meanings that have been attributed to same-sex orientation. Homosexuality has been conceived of as an innate, relatively stable condition (Murray, 1987); a congenital, but not hereditary, condition (Heller, 1981); a form of congenital degeneracy (Gindorf, 1977); an earlier evolutionary form of the human race, i.e., bisexual or hermaphroditic (Krafft-Ebing, 1965); a perverse and immature orientation resulting from family interactions during childhood development (Dynes, 1987; Freud, 1920); and the result of psychological processes similar to those that lead to heterosexuality, modifiable through various forms of therapy (Akers, 1977). Prior to 1973, the American Psychiatric Association classified homosexuality as a form of mental illness (Greenberg, 1988). And, until relatively recently, same-sex sexual relations were punishable by imprisonment in various jurisdictions within the USA (*Lawrence v. Texas*, 2003) and continue to be punishable, sometimes by death, in other countries (International Lesbian and Gay Association, 1999).

Even in the absence of legal prohibitions, individuals identifying as nonheterosexuals or admitting to nonheterosexual behaviors may face stigmatization and loss of opportunities, such as employment. This may be particularly true for bisexuals, who may be regarded as homosexuals by heterosexuals and resented for "passing" as heterosexuals by homosexuals. Indeed, bisexuals are often viewed simultaneously as homosexual within heterosexual communities and as "double agents" within homosexual and lesbian communities, suffering stigmatization from both (Hemmings, 1993; Ochs, 1996). In the context of sexual behavior, any nonheterosexual liaison may be deemed sufficient to justify classification of an individual by heterosexuals as homosexual, while any heterosexual behavior justifies for homosexuals the classification of an individual as heterosexual or "passing."

Third, the manner and context in which individuals are asked to self-identify may affect how they choose to respond. Responses may differ depending upon the time frame for the behavior in the question (e.g., lifetime, last 5 years, previous year), the focus of the question (sexual orientation, sexual identity, sexual attraction, or sexual activities), and the format of the question.

Cultural Expectations of Men and Masculinity

The construction of maleness and masculinity are inextricably intertwined (Whitehead & Barrett, 2001); how they are constructed within a specific culture provides a reference point for that culture's view of same-sex orientation and sexual relations. Consider, for example, the elements that are believed to comprise masculinity and the condition of "being a man" with "mainstream" USA. Masculine man, that is, a "man's man," is often depicted as excelling in sports and being in control of not only his own emotions, but also every situation (Kimmel, 2003). Consequently, men who do not display these traits may be perceived as effeminate and less than "real men" and, as a consequence, may be relegated to a lower rung on the positional hierarchy within larger society (Whitehead & Barrett, 2001).

In a number of societies, sexual relations between younger and older men were structured by age (Greenberg, 1988). The older male often assumed the active role in a relationship, while the younger male the passive role. The sexual act could include masturbation, anal intercourse, and/or fellatio. The motivation for these relationships varied depending on the culture, but could derive from any of various beliefs that: the older male could transmit special healing powers to the younger male through these acts; physical maturation of the younger male required the implantation of semen in his body by an older adult; and/or heterosexual intercourse would deplete one's vitality and/or harm men as a result of women's polluting qualities (Greenberg, 1988). Additionally, sex with other men may be a means of satisfying one's sexual needs in the absence of an adequate number of women.

The status of Native American berdache and Asian Indian hijra has often mistakenly been equated with homosexuality. A berdache has been defined as "a morphological male who does not fit society's standard man's role, who has a nonmasculine character" (Williams, 1992: 2). Native Americans often referred to berdaches as "halfmen—halfwomen," although they were neither transsexuals nor hermaphrodites. Berdaches, now more commonly referred to as "two-spirit people" (Lang, 1996), existed within a number of Native American tribes, including the Cheyenne, Creek, Klamath, Mohave, Navaho, Pima, Sioux, and Zuni (Greenberg, 1988; Roscoe, 1991; Williams, 1992). The two-spirit people have been described as androgynous and have been perceived as being of an alternative gender due to their use of the behaviors, social roles, and dress of both men and women. Although some individuals assumed the passive/receptive role in a sexual relationship with another man, the sexual relationship was a secondary component of one's status as a berdache (Callender & Kochens, 1983; Williams, 1992). Similarly, some two-spirit women adopted some male roles and dress and had sexual relations with women (Schaeffer, 1965). The berdache tradition, however, has declined due to missionary and US government efforts. Additionally, younger Native Americans may have rejected the role of the berdache and self-identify, instead, as gay males (Williams, 1992).

The hijras of India have been called "neither man nor woman and woman and man" (Nanda, 1990, 1994). They are biologically males who may or may not have been castrated, but live as women and have assumed the dress and mannerisms of women (Asthana & Osstvogels, 2001; Khan, 2001). In the past, hijras have played a religious role, derived from Hinduism, by blessing newborn male children and performing at wedding ceremonies (Nanda, 1990). Hijras are defined as such by their lack of sexual desire for and sexual impotence with women, rather than by their sexual relations with men. Their impotence with women has been attributed to a defect in or absence of male sexual organs from birth or through their surgical removal (Nanda, 1990). Hijras self-define as "not men" due to their impotence with women and as "not women" because of their inability to bear children; as such, they collapse sex and gender into one category. They incorporate various aspects of the female role, such as dress, gendered erotic fantasies, a desire for male sexual partner, and a gender identity of a woman or hijra, with those of a male role, which include coarse speech and the use of the hookah for smoking (Nanda, 1994). Despite their sexual relations with other men, hijras do not self-define as homosexuals.

Observations across diverse Latino cultures suggest that many Latino men who engage in sexual relations with other men may continue to self-identify as heterosexual (Aliaga & Cortes, 1997; Caceres & Rosasco, 1999; Diaz, 1998; Gonzalez & Espin, 1996; Ramirez, 1999; Rodriguéz Rust, 2000). Homosexuals/ gays are believed to be effeminate and, like woman, assume a receptive and passive (*pasivo*) role, allowing themselves to be penetrated by men. Accordingly, self-identification as homosexual/gay signifies femininity and womanliness. In contrast, assumption of the active (*activo*), i.e., the insertive role during sex, even with another man, preserves one's maleness and masculinity (Diaz, 1998). The concurrent fulfillment of culturally imposed family obligations—the maintenance of close family ties, marriage, and fathering of children—while performing as *activos* in male—male sexual relations permits both public and private self-identification as a heterosexual male (Gonzalez & Espin, 1996; Rodriguéz Rust, 2000).

In contrast, the overt acknowledgement or public disclosure of one's homosexuality or same-sex relations may meet with severe disapproval (Morales, 1992) and may be considered as an act of treason against one's family. As a result, the same-sex relationships of many Latino men may remain clandestine, and those men who self-identify as gay or bisexual may remain "closeted" (Morales, 1992).

As in Latino culture, Asian American men may have sexual relations with other men and those relationships are not necessarily seen as being gay (Greene, 1994). Open disclosure of same-sex orientation, however, would bring shame to the family (Chan, 1992) and signify a rejection and violation of cultural expectations of marriage, propagation of children, and continuation of the family line (Chan, 1992; Wooden, Kawasaki, & Mayeda, 1983). Indeed, research suggests that Asian American men may feel pressured to choose between a "gay" identity and an identity within the Asian community and may suffer more discrimination in response to their sexual orientation than their Asian ethnicity (Chan, 1989).

Reported high rates of nondisclosure of male—male sexual encounters (being on the "down-low") and same-sex sexual orientation in African American communities (Ostrow et al., 1991) have been attributed to extremely homophobic and rejecting attitudes within those communities (Icard, 1986). These responses may be associated with the strong presence and influence of Christian religiosity and strict construction of Biblical passages (Claybourne, 1978), a legacy of sexual racism that portrayed African Americans as promiscuous and immoral (cf. Walker, 1997), and the perceived shortage of marriageable African American men (Dyne, 1980).

Disparate Meanings

Definitional issues may also be critical in the formulation of the questions. As an example, a question that is framed in terms of "sexual contact" may refer to any sexual contact, including kissing, or to only relations involving genital contact. The word "intercourse" is similarly ambiguous, as it can refer to vaginal intercourse, anal intercourse, and oral intercourse. It is also unclear whether this term encompasses the use of sex toys, such as dildos and vibrators, for penetrative sex. The use of the word "gay," for instance, may convey a significantly different meaning than the word "homosexual," which differs in meaning from the term "men who have sex with men." Individuals may self-identify as gay and/or as homosexual and/or as a man who has sex with men:

> Homosexual was the label that was applied to Gay people as a device for separating us from the rest of the population.... Gay is a descriptive label we have assigned to ourselves as a way of reminding ourselves and others that awareness of our sexuality facilitates a capability rather than creating a restriction. It means that we are capable of fully loving a person of the same gender.... But the label does not limit us (Clark, 1977: 103–106).

The term "gay," unlike the term "homosexual," evolved through the Gay Liberation Movement to embody political connotations. Gays were redefined as a stigmatized minority, and the concept of the gay community emerged (Paul, 2000). Accordingly, the choice of the term to be used may differ depending upon the information sought and may be critical to respondents' understanding of the question.

Finally, the context of the question may affect the response. As an example, men may have sexual encounters with other men while in prison (Kang, Deren, Andia, Colón, Robles, & Oliver-Velez, 2005), but may not view the activity as homosexual in nature (Braithwaite & Arriola, 2003), particularly if it occurred through force, coercion, or violence (cf. Seal et al., 2004).

Summary

There are several noteworthy messages that can be derived from the findings of existing research:

- Individuals can display homo- or heterosexuality in any one or more of three domains: sexual attraction, sexual behavior, and sexual identity.

- The incidence of hetero-, homo-, or bisexual behavior, attraction, and/or identity depends on the point in time and length of the time period during which the behavior, attraction, or identity is being assessed.
- Responses regarding lifetime sexual experience vary depending on whether respondents are permitted to use their own definitions and terms to refer to their behavior or whether they are forced to choose from a preformulated listing.
- Sexual behavior (the sex of an individual and of their partner), sexual attraction (the sex of the individual to whom someone is attracted), sexual identity (as male, female, or transsexual), and gender (masculine, feminine, or androgynous) are not necessarily congruent.
- Self-identity does not predict sexual behavior (Rodríguez Rust, 2000).

The potential implications of these findings are enormous. The contributions that follow this chapter testify to the complexity inherent in self-identity and the consequences that may result to individuals' mental health, relationships with others, safety, and risk of disease from an inability to express and live their identity safely.

Acknowledgments The author thanks the Grossman Trust for its partial support of this research, through the Cleveland Foundation (Bipolar Disorder as a Predictor of HIV Risk in African American Men).

References

Absalon, J., Fuller, C. M., Ompad, D. C., Blaney, S., Koblin, B., & Galea, S. et al. (2006). Gender differences in sexual behaviors, sexual partnerships, and HIV drug users in New York City. *AIDS Behavior, 10*, 707–715.

Akers, R. L. (1977). *Deviant behavior: A social learning approach*. Belmont, California: Wadsworth.

Aliaga, J., & Cortés, J. M. G. (1997). *Identidad y diferencia: Sobre la cultura gay en España*. Barcelona, Spain: Editorial Gay y Lesbiana (EAGLES).

Altshuler, K. Z. (1984). On the question of bisexuality. *American Journal of Psychotherapy 38*(4), 484–493.

American Psychiatric Association. (2000). *Diagnostic and statistical manual, fourth edition-text revision (DSM-IV-TR)*. Washington, D.C.: Author.

Asthana, S., & Osstvogels, R. (2001). The social construction of male 'homosexuality' in India: Implications for HIV transmission and prevention. *Social Science and Medicine, 52*(5), 707–721.

Barrett, W. P. (Trans.). (1931). *The trial of Jeanne d"Arc*. London: Routledge.

Bayer, R. (1981). *Homosexuality and American psychiatry: The politics of diagnosis*. New York: Basic Books, Inc.

Billy, J. O. G., Tanfer, K., Grady, W. R., & Klepinger, D. H. (1993). The sexual behavior of men in the United States. *Family Planning Perspectives 25*, 52–60.

Blumstein, P. W., & Schwartz, P. (1977). Bisexuality: Some social-psychological issues. *Journal of Social Issues 33*, 30–45.

Bolin, A. (1992). Coming of age among transsexuals. In T. L. Whitehead, B. V. Reid (Eds.), *Gender constructs and social issues* (pp. 13–39). Chicago: University of Chicago Press.

Braithwaite, R. L., & Arriola, K. R. J. (2003). Male prisoners and HIV prevention: A call for action ignored. *American Journal of Public Health, 93*(5), 759–763.

Caceres, C. F., & Rosasco, A. M. (1999). The margin has many sides: Diversity among gay and homosexually active men in Lima. *Culture, Health, and Sexuality, 1*(3), 261–275.

Callender, C., & Kochens, L. (1983). The North American berdache. *Cultural Anthropology, 24*(4).

Cass, V. (1979). Homosexual identity formation: A theoretical model. *Journal of Homosexuality 4*(3), 219–235.

Chan, C. (1992). Cultural considerations in counseling Asian American lesbian and gay men. In S. Dworkin & F. Gutierrez (Eds.), *Counseling gay men and lesbians* (pp. 115–124). Alexandria, Virginia: American Association for Counseling and development.

Chan, C. (1989). Issues of identity development among Asian American lesbians and gay men. *Journal of Counseling and Development, 68*, 16–20.

Clark, D. (1977). *Loving someone gay*. Millbrae, California: Celestial Arts.

Cohen-Kettenis, R. P., & Gooren, L. J. G. (1999). Transsexualism: A review of etiology, diagnosis and treatment. *Journal of Psychosomatic Research, 46*(4), 315–333.

Claybourne, J. (1978). Blacks and gay liberation. In K. Jay & A. Young (Eds.), *Lavender culture* (pp. 458–465). New York: Harcourt, Brace, Jovanovich.

Coleman, E. (1982). Developmental stages in the coming-out process. In W. Paul, J. D. Weinrich, J. C. Gonsiorek, & M. E. Hotvedt (Eds.), *Homosexuality: Social, psychological, and biological issues* (pp. 144–158). Beverly Hills, California: Sage.

Diaz, R. M. (1998). *Latino gay men and HIV: Culture, sexuality, and risk behavior*. New York: Routledge Press.

Dreger, A. D. (1998). *Hermaphrodites and the medical invention of sex*. Cambridge, Massachusetts: Harvard University Press.

Dyne, L. (1980). Is D. C. becoming the gay capitol of America? *The Washingtonian, Sept.*, 96–101, 133–141.

Dynes, W. (1987). *Homosexuality: A research guide*. New York: Garland.

Feinberg, L. (1996). *Transgender warriors*. Boston: Beacon Press.

Finlinson, H. A., Colón, H. M., Robles, R. R., & Soto, M. (2006). Sexual identity formation and AIDS prevention: An exploratory study of non-gay-identified Puerto Rican MSM from working class neighborhoods. *AIDS Behavior, 10*, 531–539.

Freud, S. (1920). The psychogenesis of a case of homosexuality in a woman. In P. Rieff (Ed.). (1963). *Sexuality and the psychology of love* (pp. 133–159). New York: Collier.

Garber, M. (1992). *Vested interests: Cross-Dressing and cultural anxiety*. New York: HarperCollins.

Gindorf, R. (1977). Wissenschaftliche Ideologien im Wandel: Die Angst von der Homosexualitat als intellektuelles Ereignis. In J. S. Hohmann (Ed.). *Der underdruckte Sexus* (pp. 129–144). Berlin: Andreas Achenbach Lollar. Cited in D. F. Greenberg. (1988). *The construction of homosexuality*. Chicago: University of Chicago Press.

Goldbaum, G., Perdue, T., & Higgins, D. (1996). Non-gay-identifying men who have sex with men: Formative research results from Seattle, Washington. *Public Health Reports, 111* (Suppl. 1), 36–40.

Goldbaum, G., Perdue, T., Wolitski, R. et al. (1998). Differences in risk behavior and sources of AIDS information among gay, bisexual and straight-identified men who have sex with men. *AIDS Behavior, 2*, 13–21.

Gonsiorek, J. C., Sell, R. L., & Weinrich, J. D. (1995). Definition and measurement of sexual orientation. *Suicide and Life-Threatening Behavior 25*(1), 40–51.

Gonzalez, F. J., & Espin, O. M. (1996). Latino men, Latina women, and homosexuality. In R. P. Cabaj & T. S. Stein (Eds.), *Textbook of homosexuality and mental health* (pp. 583–601). Washington, D. C.: American Psychiatric Press.

Greenberg, D. F. (1988). *The construction of homosexuality*. Chicago: University of Chicago Press.

Greene, B. (1994). Ethnic-minority lesbians and gay men: Mental health and treatment issues. *Journal of Counseling and Clinical Psychology, 62*(2), 243–251.

Heckman, T. G., Kelly, J. A., Bogart, L. M., Kalichman, S. C., & Rompa, D. J. (1999). HIV risk differences between African-American and white men who have sex with men. *Journal of the National Medical Association, 91*, 92–100.

Heller, P. (1981). A quarrel over bisexuality. In G. Chapple, & H. H. Schulte (Eds.). *The turn of the century: German literature and art, 1890–1915* (pp. 87–115). Bonn: Bouvier Verlag Herbert Grundmann.

Hemmings, C. (1993). Resituating the bisexual body: From identity to difference. In J. Bristow, & A. R. Wilson (Eds.), *Activating theory: Lesbian, gay, & bisexual politics* (pp. 118–138). London: Lawrence and Wishart.

Heriot, A. (1975). *The castrati in opera*. New York: Da Capo Press.

Humphreys, L. (1970). *Tearoom trade: Impersonal sex in public places*. Chicago: Aldine.

Icard, L. (1986). Black gay men and conflicting social identities: Sexual orientation versus racial identity. *Journal of Social Work and Human Sexuality, 4*, 83–93.

International Lesbian and Gay Association. (1999). World Legal Survey. Last accessed September 21, 2005; Available at http://www.ilga.info/Information/Legal_survey/Summary%20information/ death_penalty_for homosexual_act.htm

Irwin, T. W., & Morgenstern, J. (2005). Drug-use patterns among men who have sex with men presenting for alcohol treatment: Differences in ethnic and sexual identity. *Journal of Urban Health, 82*(Suppl. 1), 127–133.

Jimenez, A. D. (2003). Triple jeopardy: Targeting older men of color who have sex with men. *Journal of Acquired Immune Deficiency Syndromes, 33*, S222–S225.

Kang, S-Y., Deren, S., Andia, J., Colón, H. M., Robles, R., & Oliver-Velez, D. (2005). HIV transmission behaviors in jail/prison among Puerto Rican injectors in New York and Puerto Rico. *AIDS and Behavior, 9(3)*, 377–386.

Khan, S. (2001). Culture, sexualities, and identities: Men who have sex with men in India. *Journal of Homosexuality, 40*(3–4), 99–115.

Kimmel, M. S. (2003). Masculinity as homophobia. In E. Disch (Ed.). *Reconstructing gender: A multicultural anthology*. Boston: McGraw Hill.

Kinsey, A., Pomeroy, W., & Martin, C. (1948). *Sexual behavior in the human male*. Philadelphia: W. B. Saunders.

Klein, F. (1993). *The Bisexual option*, 2nd ed. New York: Harrington Park.

Klein, F. (1978). *The Bisexual option: A concept of one-hundred percent intimacy*. New York: Arbor House.

Krafft-Ebing, R. V. (1965). *Psychopathia sexualis: A medico-forensic study* (H. E. Wedeck, Trans.). New York: G. P. Putnam's Sons [original work pub. 1886].

Kral, A. H. Lorvik, J., Ciccarone, D., Wenger, L., Gee, L., & Martinez, A. et al. (2005). HIV prevalence and risk behaviors among men who have sex with men and inject drugs in San Francisco. *Journal of Urban Health, 82*(1, Supp. 1), 43–50.

Lang, S. (1996). There is more than just women and men: Gender variance in North American Indian cultures. In S. P. Ramer (Ed.), *Gender reversals and gender cultures*. London: Routledge.

Lawrence v. Texas. (2003). 539 U.S. 558.

Luchetta, Y. (1999). Relationships between homophobia, HIV/AIDS stigma, and HIV/AIDS knowledge. In L. Pardie, & T. Luchetta (Eds.), *The construction of attitudes towards lesbians and gay men* (pp. 1–18). Binghamton, NY: Harrington Park Press.

Martinez, J., & Hoselk, S. G. (2005). An exploration of the down-low identity: Nongay identified young African-American men who have sex with men. *Journal of the National Medical Association, 97*(8), 1103–1112.

Mays, V. M., Cochran, S. D., & Zamudio, A. (2004). HIV prevention research: Are we meeting the needs of African American men who have sex with men? *Journal of Black Psychology, 30,* 78–103.

McKirnan, D., Stokes, J., Doll, L. et al. (1995). Bisexually active men: Social characteristics and sexual behavior. *Journal of Sex Research, 32,* 65–76.

Millet, G., Malebranche, D., Mason, B., & Spikes, P. (2005). Focusing "down low": Bisexual black men, HIV risk and heterosexual transmission. *Journal of the National Medical Association, 97*(7), 52S–59S.

Molloy, J. T. (1977). *The woman's dress for success book.* New York: Warner Books.

Money, J., & Erhardt, A. (1972). *Man and woman, boy and girl.* Baltimore, Maryland: Johns Hopkins University Press.

Montgomery, J. P., Mokotoff, E. D., Gentry, A. C., & Blair, J. M. (2003). The extent of bisexual behaviour in HIV-infected men and implications for transmission to their female sex partners. *AIDS Care, 15(6),* 829–837.

Morales, E. (1992). Latino gays and Latina lesbians. In S. Dworkin & F. Gutierrez (Eds.), *Counseling gay men and lesbians: Journey to the end of the rainbow* (pp. 125–139). Alexandria, Virginia: American Association for Counseling and Development.

Murray, S. O. (1987). Homosexual acts and selves in early modern Europe. *Journal of Homosexuality, 15,* 421–439.

Nanda, S. (1994). Hijras: An alternative sex and gender role in India. In G. Herdt (Ed.), *Third sex, third gender: Beyond sexual dimorphism in culture and history* (pp. 373–417). New York: Zone Books.

Nanda, S. (1990). *Neither man nor woman: The hijras of India.* Belmont, California: Wadsworth Publishing Company.

Ochs, R. (1996). Biphobia: It goes more than two ways. In B. A. Firestein (Ed.), *Bisexuality: The psychology of an invisible minority* (pp. 217–239). Thousand Oaks, California:

Ostrow, D.G., Whitaker, R. E., Frasier, K. et al. (1991). Racial differences in social support and mental health in men with HIV infection: A pilot study. *AIDS Care, 3(1),* 55–62.

Seal, D. W., Belcher, L., Morrow, K. et al. (2004). A qualitative study of substance use and sexual behavior among 18- to 29-year-old men while incarcerated in the United States. *Health Education & Behavior, 31(6),* 775–789.

Parks, C. A., Hughes, T. L., & Matthews, A. K. (2004). Race/ethnicity and sexual orientation: Intersecting identities. *Cultural Diversity and Ethnic Minority Psychology, 10*(3), 241–254.

Paul, J. P. (2000). Bisexuality: Reassessing our paradigms of sexuality. In P. C. Rodríguez Rust (Ed.), *Bisexuality in the United States* (pp. 11–23). New York: Columbia University Press.

Ramirez, R. L. (1999). *What it means to be a man: Reflections on Puerto Rican masculinity.* New Brunswick, NJ: Rutgers University Press.

Reid, W. H., & Wise, M. G. (1995). *DSM-IV training guide.* New York: Brunner Mazel.

Rietmeijer, C. A., Wolitski, R. J., Fishbein, M, Corby, N., & Cohn, D. L. (1998). Sex hustling, injection drug use, and non-gay identification by men who have sex with men: Associations with high-risk sexual behaviors and condom use. *Sexually Transmitted Diseases, 25*(7), 353–360.

Rodríguez Rust, P. C. (2000). Alternatives to binary sexuality: Modeling bisexuality. In P. C. Rodríguez Rust (Ed.), *Bisexuality in the United States* (pp. 33–54). New York: Columbia University Press.

Rodriguéz Rust, P. C. (2000). Bisexuality in HIV research. In P. C. Rodriguéz Rust (Ed.), *Bisexuality in the United States* (pp. 356–399). New York: Columbia University Press

Roscoe, W. (1991). *The Zuni man-woman.* Albuquerque, New Mexico: University of New Mexico Press.

Ross, M. W., Essien, E. J., Williams, M. L., & Fernandez-Esquer, M. E. (2003). Concordance between sexual behavior and sexual identity in street outreach samples of four racial/ ethnic groups. *Sexually Transmitted Diseases, 30(2)*, 110–113.

Ross, M. W., Månsson, S-A., Daneback, K., & Tikkanen, R. (2005). Characteristics of men who have sex with men on the internet but identify as heterosexual, compared with heterosexually identified men who have sex with women. *Cyberpsychology & Behavior, 8(2)*, 131–139.

Rothblatt, M. (1995). *The apartheid of sex: A manifesto in the freedom of gender*. New York: Crown Publishers.

Savan-Williams, R. C. (1998). *". . . And then I became gay": Young men's stories*. New York City: Routledge Press.

Schaeffer, C. E. (1965). The Kutenai female berdache. *Ethnohistory, 12*(3), 193–236.

Seal, D. W., Belcher, L., Morrow, K., Eldridge, G., Binson, D., & Kacanek, D. et al. (2004). A qualitative study of substance use and sexual behavior among 18- to 29-year old men while incarcerated in the United States. *Health Education and Behavior, 31*(6), 775–789.

Shively, M. G., & De Cecco, J. P. (1977). Components of sexual identity. *Journal of Homosexuality, 3*(1), 41–48.

Solorio, R., Swenderman, D., & Rotheram-Borus, M. J. (2003). Risk among young gay and bisexual men living with HIV. *AIDS Education and Prevention, 15*(Suppl. A), 80–89.

Stein, E. (1999). *The mismeasure of desire: The science, theory, and ethics of sexual orientation*. Oxford, U.K.: Oxford University Press.

Stoller, R. J. (1964). A contribution to the study of gender identity. *Journal of the American Medical Association, 45*, 220–226.

Stoller, R. J. (1968). *Sex and gender: On the development of masculinity and femininity*. New York: Science House.

Storms, M. (1979). Sex-role identity and its relationship to sex-role attributes and sex-role stereotypes. *Journal of Personality and Social Psychology, 37*, 1779–1789.

Storms, M. (1980). Theories of sexual orientation. *Journal of Personality and Social Psychology, 38*, 783–792.

Storms, M. (1981). A theory of erotic orientation development. *Psychological Review, 88*, 340–353.

Szasz, T. (1970). *The manufacture of madness*. New York: Delta Books.

Trexler, R. C. (1995). *Sex and conquest: Gendered violence, political order, and the European conquest of the Americas*. Ithaca, NY: Cornell University Press.

Troiden, R. R. (1989). The formation of homosexual identities. *Journal of Homosexuality, 17*(1/2), 43–73.

Vance, C. S. (1995). Social construction theory and sexuality. In M. Berger, B. Wallis, & S. Watson (Eds.). *Constructing masculinity* (pp. 37–48). New York: Routledge.

Waldo, C. R., McFarland, W., Katz, M. H., MacKellar, D., & Valleroy, L. A. (2000). Very young gay and bisexual men are at risk for HIV infection: The San Francisco Bay Area Young Men's Survey II. *Journal of Acquired Immune Deficiency Syndromes, 24*, 168–174.

Walinder, J. (1967). *Transsexualism: A study of forty-three cases* (H. Fry, Trans.). Stockholm: Scandinavian University Books.

Walker, A. (1997). Legislating virtue: How segregationists disguised racial discrimination as moral reform following *Brown v. Board of Education, Duke Law Journal, 47*, 399–424.

Whitehead, S. M., & Barrett, F. J. (2001). The sociology of masculinity. In S. M. Whitehead, & F. J. Barrett (Eds.), *The masculinities reader* (pp. 1–26). Malden, MA: Blackwell Publishers Inc.

Williams, J. K., Wyatt, G. E., Resell, J., Peterson, J., & Asuan-O'Brien, A. (2004). Psychosocial issues among gay- and non-gay-identifying HIV-seropositive African American and Latino MSM. *Cultural Diversity and Ethnic Minority Psychology, 10*(3), 268–286.

Williams, W. L. (1992). *The spirit and the flesh: Sexual diversity in American Indian culture.* Boston: Beacon Press.

Wooden, W. S., Kawasaki, H., & Mayeda, R. (1983). Lifestyles and identity maintenance among gay Japanese-American males. *Alternative Lifestyles, 5*, 236–243.

Woodyard, J. L., Peterson, J. L., & Stokes, J. P. (2000). "Let us go into the house of the Lord": Participation in African American churches among young African American men who have sex with men. *Journal of Pastoral Care, 54(4)*, 451–60.

Wohl, A. R., Johnson, D. F., Lu, S. et al. (2002). HIV risk behaviors among African American men in Los Angeles County who self-identify as heterosexual. *Journal of Acquired Immune Deficiency Syndromes, 31,* 354–360.

Zinik, G. (2000). Identity conflict or adaptive flexibility? Bisexuality reconsidered. In P. C. Rodríguez Rust (Ed.), *Bisexuality in the United States* (pp. 55–60). New York: Columbia University Press.

Portrait One
Rebirth: Evolution of a Gender

Travis A. Garry

As a child, I often struggled to identify my sexuality and furthermore my masculine and feminine characteristics. This included experimenting with hair lengths, color, and texture. Straight versus curly, long versus short and a variety of colors from midnight blue to blonde highlights. Some styles of which were condoned and assisted by my own mother.

Growing up, I was also intrigued by other males and how they viewed me. Having feminine facial features like long eye lashes, smooth skin, and full lips as well as a high-pitched voice garnered a lot of attention from older as well as younger males. Not to mention overall being mistaken for a girl. At times, this was frustrating and confusing.

I did not know if this was a defect or if it was simply the way God intended me to be. Either way as I began to mature into a questioning teenager, I decided to explore different looks and embrace my feminine traits. Eventually, it became flattering to me to be mistaken for a woman, especially from handsome older men. To be able to mystify men and be flattered by their flirtatious advances was like a high for me. By the time I was 18, I began to do drag.

Becoming a young adult came with a new outlook on life including my sexuality and how I chose to express myself as a gender. I felt more comfortable looking and dressing as a woman. I also began working in society as a woman. This had now become my life (which early on I had said was something I'd never do). I realized that this was bigger than me. It was more than dressing like a woman; it was fun, exciting, and most of all liberating. Just knowing that I could exhibit my gender to the rest of the world any way, I so chose in a society where people were classified as male or female and not transgender was one of the most amazing discoveries I had ever experienced.

Defying social and religious norms was never my intent, but knowing that I set the tone for how I wished to be addressed was absolutely thrilling to me, so much that I also considered becoming a woman permanently. However, before

Travis A. Garry
Cleveland, Ohio

S. Loue (ed.), *Health Issues Confronting Minority Men Who Have Sex with Men.*
© Springer 2008

Fig. P1.1 Photo of
Meokah Diamond

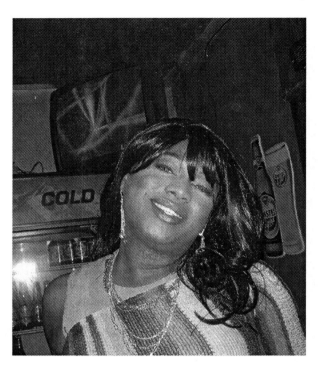

making that decision I continued over the next few years and well into my early 20s to live life 24 hours a day, 7 days a week as a woman. This was a key determining factor in making such a lifelong decision.

Mastering how to make myself appear more and more like a "passable" woman was my favorite pastime. This was everything from hair, make up, clothing, accessories, posture, and overall demeanor. I was inspired by many influences like TV, magazines, and the overall observation of everyday women. I also began tapping into ways to alter my body. I viewed it as realigning my exterior to match the way I felt within.

While exploring these options through research, conversations with transgenders, and even my own doctor, I began hormone therapy. This was a drastic step that was daunting and exhilarating to me at the same time. "So here goes," I said to myself as I swallowed my first hormone pill. Knowing that over a period of time this little blue pill would begin to transform my body was something I thought about every waking moment, yet at the same time I was thinking "I JUST WANNA BE A GIRL"! After a period of about 45 days or so (give or take), I began to notice that my chest was getting bigger, my arms and legs were becoming more soft, shapely, and feminine; all that in conjunction with other trivial changes that I noticed as the days went on.

I continued this regimen on and off before I came to the realization that most people that knew me thought was just a phase which was the fact that I no longer had the desire to become a woman. To this day, I still can't isolate what exactly made me have a change of heart. I still liked embodying most aspects of being a woman, but at this point, I thought maybe this was just a stage. To change the physical appearance of my body permanently was something I no longer had the desire to do. I continued dressing as a woman for quite a while, although at this point I was living what seemed to have become a character I had created.

This character that I created who was now known as Meokah (MEE-A-KAH) Diamond would go on to win pageants and become an entertainer, she also co-wrote and co-starred in a movie titled "Destinies Fulfilled" and almost instantly became a local celebrity. However, along the way something happened that I never fathomed in a million years. I had started to become more of an image and less of a person. It now seemed like most people just saw me as a pretty face but didn't quite take me seriously. I also began to adopt this mentality of being only a shell of my former self. This female counterpart that I had created was robbing me of who I was as an individual. I knew then that I had to find a happy medium to express my sexuality, gender, as well as to afford society the opportunity to know me as a whole; thus I began my rebirth.

This reinvention was a chance to reclaim my life on my terms. There were minor things I would have to sacrifice for this transition to take place. One of which was the type of men I would attract and/or date (being that most of the men I dated previously liked the fact that I dressed as a woman, and those were the men I was attracted to) as well as growing facial hair and wearing men's clothing. I knew this transition would not be as seamless as I would have liked for it to have been, nonetheless it was a challenge I looked forward to.

I felt like a chameleon of sorts and it also gave me the option of exploring new style and fashion realms on a more masculine spectrum and still keep a hint of effeminate flavor that was still a part of me. I must admit the change was not as picture perfect as I had anticipated, but the payoff was well worth it. People began to sit up and take notice and I also gained a new found level of respect and admiration for still being me and overcoming all obstacles and barriers. I did admire past parts of myself both masculine and feminine and I also realized that I was perfectly content with being a Black gay man without being a woman or emulating one. I also gained a new skill in being able to navigate through different demographics as a person rather than a self-made idol. This was a breath of fresh air and it was breathed through the lungs of a new existence. . .his name?

Fig. P1.2 Photo of
Travis A. Garry

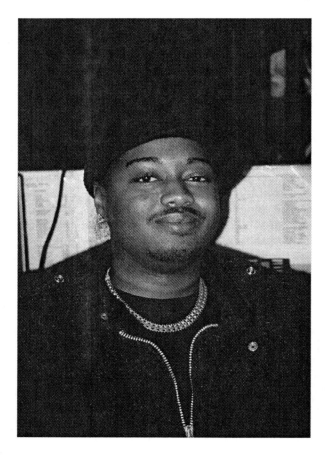

Portrait Two
¿De Donde?

Hank Ramírez

Who am I? The answer to this question has eluded me for the 53 years of my existence on this earth. While growing up, I heard the phrase "*Órale, ese. ¿De donde?*" uttered many times. In the *barrio* where I grew up, this said "What the fuck are you doing here?" although it really means "Hey you – where you from?" For me, the quest to find the answer to this question became personal.

I grew up in the barrio of a small town in California, the oldest of five children in a Latino Catholic family. My father is a first generation Californian, his parents having emigrated from Mexico to the United States to find a better life. My mother was raised by her grandparents in Pueblo, Colorado and later moved to California at the age of 16 with her mother. After her first disastrous marriage ended in divorce, my parents met in a bar and were married within a year.

I was born in 1953 and discovered my attraction to men at around the age of three. Something told me that this was not normal, that little boys shouldn't feel this way. I instinctively knew, perhaps out of a sense of survival, that this wasn't something I could safely share with my parents. I began to build walls and harbor secrets.

My attraction to men hit full force in sixth grade when I met my first male teacher. He was tall with deep blue eyes and light brown hair. I remember thinking "Oh, please God, let him call on me," and at the same time feeling terrified that he might. For Valentine's Day, I wanted to give him my home-made card.

The other boys at school sensed this difference and began to pick on me, calling me names—*joto*, sissy, *mariposa*. Since we lived in the same *barrio*, I couldn't escape the name calling. I wasn't invited to play with them unless our mothers forced us to play with each other. When I entered my teens, I tried to find myself by diving into schoolwork and the church, both which became my sanctuary from not only being around my *Latino* peers, but also from my father's abusive alcoholism. I began to believe that if I could excel in these

Hank Ramírez
San Diego, CA

S. Loue (ed.), *Health Issues Confronting Minority Men Who Have Sex with Men.*   29
© Springer 2008

two areas, be perfect in every way, it would make up for my attraction to men, not being like the other boys, and keep my secret hidden.

I excelled in school, hung around with the *gringos* who I felt accepted me, and was very involved in my church. However, despite my new friends, my scholastic achievements and stellar attendance at church, I still felt different. "What if they find out? What if they don't like me anymore?" I would constantly think to myself. I went out of my way to fit in at school and at church, always careful to hide my attraction to men, but still no clearer as to my identity. The walls I began building as a young child became thicker and higher.

College opened a whole new world for me. I found myself in an environment in which I felt free to question what had been my life for 18 years. Although still closeted, I questioned my religious upbringing and the cultural constraints imposed on me as the eldest child in a *Latino* family. Out of the *barrio* and in an environment where students were encouraged to question and search, I looked at the world and my presence in it with new eyes. Although still involved with my church, I explored other faiths, eager to find a home where God accepted me unconditionally. But, how could that be? I had convinced myself that I was damaged goods, and how could God accept, much less love, me?

It was while I was in college that I had my first sexual encounter with a man. I met him through my church and we quickly became good friends. I was very attracted to his handsome blonde looks and deep blue eyes. Our friendship continued to develop, and one day, he asked me to be his best man. After he was married, our feelings for each other surfaced and we began to meet to have sex. However, my Catholic guilt overwhelmed me and I couldn't handle what was going on. No matter how much I tried praying away my "deviancy," I couldn't bring myself to accept what I was doing.

It was during my third year in college a young priest was assigned to my parish. His spirituality and holiness inspired me, touching something deep within me. I began to spend time with him and, after about a year into our friendship, he asked if I ever considered being a priest. At first, I strongly opposed the idea. Not because I didn't think it wasn't a noble profession, but because I thought I would be the last person that God would want leading His people. However, as we spent more time with each other and the yearning for something deeper in my life grew, I began to open myself to the possibility that this might be my calling, my identity. Did I, after all these years, finally find the path to myself and be able to finally have my answer?

At 27 years of age, I entered seminary to study for the Roman Catholic priesthood. As part of my development as a seminarian, I was assigned to a spiritual director who was a priest on the faculty of the seminary. I made a promise to myself that, if I was going to find out if I was indeed destined to be a priest, I needed to be totally honest about my sexuality. So, I told my spiritual director everything. He didn't seem to have a problem with my sharing, and actually encouraged me to share more details with him. I found out later that he was living in his own fortress of denial regarding his own sexuality and felt that he was living vicariously through my experiences. I felt violated and betrayed.

Changing spiritual directors, I finished college and continued on to study theology in graduate school.

I blossomed! The time I spent in graduate school is the most life defining of my life thus far. I not only had more opportunities for intellectual and spiritual growth, but the priest I chose as my spiritual director encouraged me to become serious in my search for my identity, and once finding it, to embrace it. After 6 months of spiritual direction, he arranged for me to meet with a therapist off campus who had extensive experience and knowledge in working with individuals grappling with their sexual identity.

This decision was monumental. I finally found myself working with an individual who not only accepted me for who I am, but also encouraged and guided me on the path to self-acceptance. We met weekly, sometimes twice a week, for 1–3 hours as I worked my way through the secrets, lies, and pains of my life. I began the long road to acceptance of my sexuality and, more importantly, of myself. I finally began to believe that not only could God love me, but that others could love and accept me for who I am and what I choose to do with my life. I began the process of tearing down the walls that I had been building for more than 25 years.

While in graduate school, I grappled with becoming a priest. Aside from the Church's view on homosexuality, I also had difficulty accepting its positions on abortion, marriage, and the role of women in the church. I had seen the impact of these positions on the lives of those important to me, and increasingly felt that I could not, with good conscience, represent a belief system that embraced these as values at all costs to others. After much time spent in soul searching, I decided to take time off from my priesthood studies to further explore my path.

While in school, my family went through many changes. My parents divorced, my mother began drinking, my sister and one of my brothers became heroin addicts, another brother was discharged from the military for alcoholism, and my youngest brother got lost in the divorce and the dysfunction of my family. Although I felt "called" to help people, I didn't feel that I could help my own family. How could I help when I didn't know them? The walls I had built not only protected me, but it also kept them out. I was carrying too much pain tied to my family and knew that I would only get sucked down into the mess, if I was around them. Even though I experienced a lot of pain and guilt watching my family's spiraling descent into hell, I decided not to move back home and to make a new life for myself elsewhere.

I moved to San Diego in 1981 and it has been my home ever since. I found a job, made a new home, and began to make new friends. I began going to gay bars to express my acceptance of my sexuality. I was like a little kid in a candy store whose parents had told him "Help yourself!" The experience was a heady one. I was new in town, newly out of the closet, and riding the wave of sexual expression and freedom. I still nurtured my spiritual side as a member of Dignity, an organization of gay and lesbian Catholics. It seemed like a safe place where I could keep in touch with my religious upbringing, but maintain that I did not support the institutional hierarchy of the church and its old world views.

Not long after moving to San Diego, I began to read about G.R.I.D.— Gay-Related Immune Disorder. It seemed that this "disease" was impacting the big cities—San Francisco, New York, Los Angeles—but I didn't pay too much attention to it because it wasn't part of my world. I was having fun, but I was careful. I knew the guys I dated were nice and wouldn't be the type to *not* tell me that they had some kind of infection, much less G.R.I.D. Why should I worry? Plus, I finally met the man I thought, I would spend my life with. I loved him and he loved me. What could go wrong?

Well, in the summer of 1986, the good times came to a screeching halt. Although my lover and I felt relatively healthy, the gay newspapers and the local news carried more and more stories about the "gay disease" that was mysteriously killing gay men. We also had lost a couple of friends to the disease by this time. Gay men were being encouraged to get tested, but there were so many false positives that it took us a while before we decided to get tested.

I went to get my HIV test in June 1986. The 2-week waiting period was the most horrendously, agonizingly long two weeks of my life. I remember so many things running through my head—would I die soon after finding out, will it be a horrible death, how would I explain this to my family. I knew as I walked down the very long hallway to the testing area that my test would come back positive.

I felt nothing when I received the results. I was prepared for the worst, and I got it. Although I had been working hard to accept and love myself over the years, all the old familiar tapes came back in a rush. "I told you God didn't love you. How could he love a fag, a *joto*? You will die the death you deserve." As I left, I felt like one of the walking dead and that everyone knew.

My lover also tested positive. Although we tried to remain upbeat about our situation, we couldn't handle the stress and soon broke up. It was a difficult time for me. Once again, the old familiar tapes came back to reinforce that I didn't deserve to be loved. I didn't know how to handle what I perceived to be the death sentence and the rejection, so I buried my feelings and starting rebuilding the old familiar walls.

However, a small voice came through all the pain and numbness, and I decided to volunteer for an AIDS organization. I told myself that even if I couldn't do anything for myself, I could at least try to help someone else. My volunteer commitment led to a job with that same organization, followed by 15 years of service to the HIV/AIDS community. I've volunteered and worked with many HIV/AIDS community organizations in providing necessary services to the marginalized and stigmatized segment of our society. My 15 years with community-based organizations led to my current position with the County of San Diego where I oversee the procurement process for services for the Health and Human Services Agency. In my own way, I am still helping others by ensuring that the most qualified agencies are selected to provide the best possible services to those who need them the most. And, in this way, I continue to nourish my spiritual side.

As for my personal life, I have been in wonderful and, at times, challenging relationship with a fantastic man whom I love deeply for the past 17 years. He is also HIV positive and we both have ridden the roller coast of life living with HIV. It wasn't until about 5 years into our relationship that we both began thinking that, maybe, we were going to live a long life, and better start planning for retirement. Through his example, my partner has taught me to see the world through different eyes and given me experiences that I never would have had. I know that I face many more challenges for my life, but I feel comforted knowing that he will be by my side through it all.

As for my family, my mom passed away in 1989, having experienced more than her share of pain and grief. I pray that she has found the peace and rest that eluded her most of her life. My sister also died at a young age, continuing to support her heroin addiction through prostitution. I still feel the pain of her absence in my life, and can only imagine what her own inner demons might have been as she futilely tried to find herself. The one blessing is that she brought a beautiful daughter into this world. I have watched my niece and godchild grow and experience the pains and joys of this life. I've seen her triumph over many obstacles to become a wonderful mother and role model for others.

Two of my brothers continue their search for themselves. One is living in prison, the other from job to job, hotel to hotel. Not lives I would have chosen for myself, but I fully understand how they both arrived where they are. My remaining brother married and has two daughters. Reconnecting our lives wasn't easy at first. He and his wife are Christian fundamentalists and I am a gay. Not a good combination for a reunion. However, over the years, the fundamentalism has relaxed and now my partner and I are welcomed into their home as members of the family. Blood, many times, overcomes division.

My father is also back in my life. Although, never very close while I was growing up, we now have a relationship of sorts. It's not exactly a chummy Father/Son relationship, but it is one in which I've realized the importance of some of the lessons and values he tried to instill in us as kids, and he respects the life I am living, even if it isn't what he would have chosen for me.

So, what of my search, my identity? Well, so far, I'm:

- a Latino
- a man
- a spiritual being
- gay
- intelligent
- stubborn
- successful
- a son
- a *tío* (uncle)
- a lover
- a brother
- a former seminarian

- a person committed to helping others
- opinionated
- a person who has made a difference in the world
- a long-term survivor living with HIV (over 20 years)
- a volunteer
- a conscientious worker
- a good citizen
- someone who can have a temper
- someone, I believe, who is respected by others; and ultimately,
- someone still searching

I am none of the above and all of the above. I am what I've kept of each experience, of each person who has passed through my life, of each obstacle and triumph, of each pain and joy. At 53 years of age, I have come to realize, especially, since committing my thoughts to paper, that I will always be searching and that I am to embrace and love myself for who I believe I am at any point in my life. I am to embrace the search for I *am* the search.

Portrait Three
Untitled

Cristina Caruth

This is an essay by Cristina Caruth. She speaks about her life as an Asian male-to-female transgender person who has been diagnosed with bipolar disorder. All of the names used here are fictitious, with the exception of Cristina Caruth, in order to protect the privacy of others.

My name is Cristina Caruth.

There are struggles between transgenderism and depression. Moving out and coming out to my family was difficult because of what an Asian family should be. Macho, tough, etc. My brother can be supportive, but at times he can be critical about transgender issues. He shares the same interests as myself. I know that I am a girl since I was 5 years old and I couldn't let anyone know.

Being in school was a challenge because my teachers didn't understand why my mom dresses me up like a girl, because she didn't wash my boy's clothes. My teacher screams because they themselves have personality issues. I guess being a transgender person, is like being a mirror to somebody's soul. A lot of people don't like to see their flaws, shortcomings, and insecurity.

As I grow older, validation was more important in the process. Being accepted by peers was important to my personal happiness. During the fourth grade, my depression hit very hard. I wasn't aware of any type of medication of treating my personal illness. There were many hours in personal counseling.

The relief for my depression during my elementary school years was going to the beach or up to Greenwich Village with my dad. Just to entertain my mind with happiness was to daydream. Being someplace far like going to Toronto, Canada, or Santa Barbara because reality was too hard for my emotions. Biking was a hobby that I love. Escapism was a substitute instead of me on medication. Living in New York can be stressful and it caused a lot of depression because the winters are grey and we get socked in with 3–5 ft snow drifts. I never got any light therapy so nights were long and depressing.

Cristina Caruth
San Diego, CA

S. Loue (ed.), *Health Issues Confronting Minority Men Who Have Sex with Men.*   35
© Springer 2008

There seems to be mixed signals when I come out with my parents because I
don't know how I should be like it was. Sure, my dad wanted to give me girl
jeans because I just have to guess. There seems to be a shift in attitude of being
androgynous in my parents' decision.

I think the way of my parents was to be protective and it leads me into
depression.

When I was in my 20s, I dressed up a lot going to transgender support
meetings and learning a lot from my friends Paula and Babette because they
were into dressing up. We experimented with panty hose and make-up. Usually,
the meeting was at night. It felt like I was living a double life. There were shows
at the Limelight, performers who dressed like Rusty Barrel or Polly Esther
Slacks. There was a sense of division amongst the clubbers and the transgender
group because of the age difference. I learned to embrace the two groups
because I was young.

Oh! my love life. I was dating a girl named Carmela, back then. I was dating a
girl believe it or not. She was very very keen about me being my androgynous
side of me and accepted me as a girl totally. I'm bisexual. Right, I'm definitely
bisexual because the fact of the matter is that I like boys, I like girls and when I
feel so I'm bisexual.

Personally, I have bipolar disorder. There is hope in the process. Finding a
personal sanctuary and lots of prayer to be on a rigid medication routine is
important. Aromatherapy helps me a whole lot because smelling the fragrances
of gardens brings a sense of joy. Going on short trips to the Getty Museum in
Los Angeles helps me out in the process.

Listening to music was an important way to cope with the insanity of the
sickness especially to quiet the storm, which is modern jazz. Venting out is
another process of dealing with emotions. Going to a tanning booth was
another way I dealt with my depression. Eating chocolate was another coping
mechanism.

My life experience is like a spectrum. I mean some days it's really, really
good that people are very accepting and very, very loving to you and there are
some days that they're very hostile and very, very territorial. People like step
into your boundaries and what I feel encroach into your personal boundaries
because you're like a transgender person. Another big challenge is like when
you're brought up in a Christian church and what I feel that can be a major
challenge because say, for instance, the pastor doesn't like you because you're
transgender and they can't accept that, you know. At this specific time [life
feels like] a very mixed bag, because there's some times when I feel very, very
comfortable with myself, when I feel I would be kind of like a mirror to
someone else's soul, kind of like a reflective mirror, like someone's walk
through and just look at themselves. What I feel, they can see their real self
if they're at all secure, are they wealthy enough, are they poor enough, they
just look at me.

Well, being a bipolar person is the same perspective as being a transgender
person because I would have like a disability. I would say that my bipolarism is

more of a disability than anything else, everything else, because it causes me not to function correctly, not to focus, one billion percent onto any logic in my feel in my life, you know. If I want to write, you know, it just stops me from being motivated. It stops me from getting out of my bed, so on and so forth, doing the things I like to do you know.

Part II
Sexual Abuse

Chapter Two
Childhood Sexual Abuse and its Sequelae Among Latino Gay and Bisexual Men

Sonya Grant Arreola

Introduction

Childhood sexual abuse is strongly associated with increased risk for HIV, particularly among Latino gay/bisexual men (Carballo-Dieguez & Dolezal, 1995; Jinich et al., 1998; Paul, Catania, Pollack, & Stall, 2001). Latino gay/bisexual men comprise one of the most vulnerable groups in the United States for transmission of HIV (Anon., 2005; Centers for Disease Control and Prevention, 2001a, 2001b, 2002a, 2002c, 2004, 2005, 2006a, 2006b). Compared with non-Latino gay/bisexual men, Latino gay/bisexual men are twice as likely to have a history of childhood sexual abuse (Arreola, Neilands, Pollack, Paul, & Catania, 2005) and the abuse is more severe (Jinich et al., 1998; Moisan, Sanders-Phillips, & Moisan, 1997).

It is important to research childhood sexual abuse specifically among Latinos for several reasons. As Fontes has noted, "cultural issues are relevant to childhood sexual abuse in three major ways: how cultural beliefs or attitudes contribute to family climates in which children can be abused; how cultural organization prohibits or hinders disclosure; and how culture plays a role in seeking or accepting social service or mental health assistance" (Fontes, 1995: xiii). However, insufficient childhood sexual abuse research has been conducted, which is specific to Latinos. Nor is there an existing theoretical model that explains the relationship between childhood sexual abuse and HIV risk.

The present chapter presents a review of some findings from research on sociocultural, psychological, and contextual determinants of HIV risk to propose a preliminary model that explains the relationship between childhood sexual abuse and HIV risk among Latino gay and bisexual men.

Sonya Grant Arreola
San Francisco Department of Public Health, San Francisco, CA

S. Loue (ed.), *Health Issues Confronting Minority Men Who Have Sex with Men.*   41
© Springer 2008

HIV and Latino Gay and Bisexual Men

Men who have sex with men (MSM) continue to carry the burden of HIV infection in the United States. Recent evidence suggests a resurgence of HIV transmission among MSM. During the period from 2001 to 2004, an estimated 44% of new HIV infections were in MSM, predominantly among African Americans and Latinos, who together account for 69% of all reported HIV/AIDS cases (Anon., 2005; Centers for Disease Control and Prevention, 2005, 2006b). Additionally, while the estimated annual percentage change for all other transmission categories indicated a substantial decrease, among MSM the trend in HIV/AIDS cases remained stable between 2001 and 2004 (Centers for Disease Control and Prevention, 2005).

Latino MSM have disproportionately high rates of HIV in United States (Anon., 2005; Centers for Disease Control and Prevention, 2001a, 2001b, 2002a, 2002c; 2004; 2005; 2006a; 2006c). The Young Men's Survey, a cross-sectional, multisite, venue-based survey of MSM, conducted from 1994 through 1998, found a high prevalence of HIV infection (7.2% overall) that increased with age, from 0% among 15-year-olds to 9.7% among 22-year olds (Valleroy et al., 2000). Compared with Whites, the multivariate-adjusted HIV infection prevalence was even higher among Latinos (OR = 2.3; 95% CI = 1.5–3.4). Although more recent reports indicate a decrease in overall AIDS incidence in the USA, they also show continued disparities among racial/ethnic minority populations (Anon., 2005; Centers for Disease Control and Prevention, 2006a, 2006c). For example, from 1981 to 1995, Whites were the predominant racial/ethnic group among persons who had AIDS diagnoses (47%). However, in 2004, estimated HIV/AIDS case rates for Latinos (29.5 per 100,000) were 3.3 times higher than rates for Whites (9.0 per 100,000) and from 2001 to 2004 Latinos accounted for 20% of AIDS cases (Centers for Disease Control and Prevention, 2006a), while the 2000 US census found that they made up 12.5% of the US population (Guzman, 2001). The high rates of HIV infection among Latinos, particularly among MSM, point to the need to broaden and intensify AIDS prevention efforts for Latino gay and bisexual men.

As high as the reported rates of HIV infection and AIDS among Latino gay and bisexual men are, they probably underestimate the actual prevalence and incidence, due to low rates of testing among ethnic minorities who engage in high-risk behaviors. Thirty-five percent of Latinos with perceived risk or reported HIV risk behavior report never having been tested for HIV infection (Centers for Disease Control and Prevention, 2001). Nonetheless, the high rate of infection is consistent with the finding that Latino men report the highest rates of unprotected anal intercourse, compared with men from other ethnic minority groups (Diaz, 1998).

More than 50% of Latino gay and bisexual men report unprotected anal sex within a year of being asked despite their substantial knowledge about HIV, accurate perceptions of personal risk, and strong intentions to practice safer sex (Diaz, 1998). These findings indicate that knowledge and intentions to practice safer sex alone may not be sufficient to encourage the actual practice of safer sex. Nonetheless, most HIV prevention studies have focused on demographic and individual behavioral predictors of HIV risk. Although important, this approach has provided only a partial understanding of how HIV risk patterns are maintained among gay and bisexual men generally and among Latino gay and bisexual men particularly.

In an attempt to expand our knowledge of how to appropriately guide HIV-reduction intervention efforts for Latinos, scientists have recently emphasized the need for a more comprehensive HIV risk research agenda that incorporates an investigation of the contextual, sociocultural, and structural determinants of HIV-risky sexual behaviors (Diaz, 1997, 1998; Diaz & Ayala, 1999; Diaz, Ayala, Bein, Henne, & Marin, 2001; Diaz, Ayala, & Marin, 2000). Because of its strong association with HIV infection, childhood sexual abuse has become an important component of this research agenda (Arreola, 2001, 2006; Arreola & Diaz, 2001; Arreola et al., 2005).

Historically, most research on childhood sexual abuse concentrates on the sexual abuse of girls. However, efforts to explain the high incidence of HIV among gay and bisexual men have led investigators to identify determinants of increased risky sexual behavior; they have found that a history of childhood sexual abuse increases the risk for HIV (Carballo-Dieguez & Dolezal, 1995; Jinich et al., 1998; Paul et al., 2001). This has fostered interest in research on the prevalence of childhood sexual abuse among MSM, including Latino gay and bisexual men. Notably, much of this research is derived from probability-based data and has begun to contend with the issue of defining childhood sexual abuse using empirical data.

Childhood Sexual Abuse

Defining Childhood Sexual Abuse

In general, childhood sexual abuse has been dichotomized into those who have and those who have not experienced childhood sexual abuse. Criteria for childhood sexual abuse vary by: (1) upper age limit of the child, generally between 12 and 18; (2) severity of abuse, ranging from no physical contact to penetration; (3) minimum age difference between the child and perpetrator of the abuse, from none to 10 years; and (4) whether or not force and/or threat were used. Studies also vary by which of these criteria are defined in their measurement of childhood sexual abuse, and some specify the number of times certain abusive activities must occur in order to meet the criteria. The lack of any uniform operationalization of childhood sexual abuse makes it difficult to compare outcomes across studies. Additionally, no theoretically or empirically based rationale is given for including any particular criteria in respective studies. This may help explain why a consistent definition is lacking. The absence of theory or empiricism to guide our measurement and understanding of childhood sexual abuse leaves the operational definitions vulnerable to researcher assumptions and social or political bias. Further, it is likely that the variability in reported prevalence of childhood sexual abuse is due, in part, to the wide range of operational definitions. A theoretically and empirically based definition is sorely needed if we are to advance the field.

The existing literature on childhood sexual abuse among Latino gay and bisexual men also contends with the difficulties of defining childhood sexual abuse. Nonetheless, the findings show consistent trends in prevalence and type of childhood sexual abuse among Latino gay and bisexual men. Furthermore, preliminary analyses of risky sexual situations and childhood sexual abuse among Latino gay and bisexual men offer empirical support for a more precise operationalization of childhood sexual abuse.

Differentiating Childhood Sexual Abuse from Voluntary Childhood Sexuality Among Boys

A preliminary quantitative analysis of a large representative sample of self-identified Latino gay and bisexual men along a series of sexual risk outcomes found no differences between Latino gay and bisexual men who reported no sex before age 16 and those who reported sex before age 16 with someone 5 or more years older that was **not** against their will (Arreola, 2006). However, comparisons of the combined no-sex and voluntary sex groups to the forced sex group revealed significant differences in risky sexual outcomes. The findings on "risky sexual situations" are further explained in the section by the same title later in this chapter.

Findings from another study of 100 Latino, predominately gay men who had childhood sexual experiences with older partners, found that those who considered their experiences to be sexually abusive ($n = 59$) were younger when the events happened and were more likely to have been physically forced, physically hurt, threatened, and emotionally hurt. Additionally, the men who considered themselves the victims of childhood sexual abuse differed from those who did not in having more alcohol use, unprotected anal sex, and male sex partners as adults (Dolezal & Carballo-Dieguez, 2002).

Together, findings from both studies underscore the importance of understanding the subjective experiences of those whose lives we intend to interpret. It has been assumed that sex in childhood or adolescence with an older individual is necessarily abusive, based on the implied power differential between the younger and older person. Although this pattern may differ for women, these data show that men's interpretations of early sexual experiences as voluntary predict outcomes that are similar to those who do not initiate sex until much later. The finding that those who initiate sex voluntarily before age 16, even if the partner is much older, do not appear to be at greater risk for HIV than those who do not initiate sex until much later indicates that future research must begin to differentiate forced from voluntary sex, at least for boys and particularly during adolescence.

Prevalence of Childhood Sexual Abuse Among Latino Gay and Bisexual Men

Gay/bisexual men of all ethnicities are more likely to have experienced childhood sexual abuse (childhood sexual abuse) than are non-gay/bisexual men. In fact, some research suggests that childhood sexual abuse in boys is underreported to a high degree (Boney-McCoy & Finkelhor, 1995; Feiring, Taska, & Lewis, 1999). When this underreporting is taken into account, childhood sexual abuse levels for gay/bisexual men may approach levels found in girls. Depending on its operationalization and the population sampled, prevalence rates of childhood sexual abuse among gay/bisexual men vary from 17 to 39% (Carballo-Dieguez & Dolezal, 1995; Holmes, 1997; Jinich et al., 1998; Lenderking et al., 1997; Remafedi, Farrow, & Deisher, 1991).

As high as the prevalence of childhood sexual abuse may be among gay/bisexual men, it is consistently higher among Latino gay and bisexual men. In a study of the prevalence of childhood sexual abuse among adult gay and bisexual men across two separate population-based samples of 1,941 gay and bisexual men, 39.4% of Latino gay and bisexual men versus 25% of gay/bisexual men overall reported childhood sexual abuse (Jinich et al., 1998). Childhood sexual abuse was defined as sexual behavior with someone at least 5 years older prior to age 13, or with someone at least 10 years older when between ages 13 and 15.

A more recent study used a random-digit telephone probability survey with self-reported histories of childhood sexual abuse of 2,692 adult MSM aged 18 years or older residing in San Francisco, New York, Los Angeles, and Chicago to specifically examine the prevalence of childhood sexual abuse among Latino gay and bisexual men. The definition of childhood sexual abuse was more precise by including a subjective experience of coercion with someone 5 or more years older. An additional question asked about the respondent's age when abuse first occurred. This study also found a significantly higher proportion of Latino MSM reported sexual abuse before age 13 (22%) than did non-Latino MSM (11%) (Arreola et al., 2005).

Not only is there a greater prevalence of childhood sexual abuse among Latino gay and bisexual men compared with non-Latino gay and bisexual men, but also the abuse has been found to be more severe. Compared with African American boys, Latino boys are more likely to have been sexually abused by an extended family member, such as a cousin, or uncle, experienced more genital fondling, exposed to more sexually abusive behaviors, and experienced more anal abuse (Lindholm & Willey, 1986; Moisan et al., 1997).

Childhood Sexual Abuse, HIV Risk Behavior, and HIV Infection

Probability samples of gay/bisexual men have found that those with a history of childhood sexual abuse were more likely to engage in unprotected anal intercourse with a non-primary partner in the previous 12 months (21%), than those who were not (15%). Furthermore, childhood sexual abuse and higher levels of coercion were associated with an increased risk of HIV infection (Jinich et al., 1998). A telephone probability sample also found that men who reported childhood sexual abuse were more likely than those who did not have histories of childhood sexual abuse to engage in unprotected anal intercourse with a non-primary partner or with a serodiscordant partner, which in turn has been linked to the risk for HIV infection. This pattern holds for Latino gay and bisexual men as well. In a study specifically focused on Latino MSM, a history to sexually abusive abuse was significantly related to an increased likelihood of engaging in receptive anal sex without protection (Carballo-Dieguez & Dolezal, 1995). Research is needed to uncover how and why childhood sexual abuse is related to risk for HIV among Latino gay and bisexual men.

Modeling Childhood Sexual Abuse and HIV Risk Behavior

Rigorous, theory-driven investigations of the link between childhood sexual abuse and HIV risk behavior are scant in the literature. The few proposed theoretical models have been based on findings with women (Koenig, Doll, O'Leary, & Pequegnat, 2003) and have limited empirical data to support their hypotheses. A theoretical model is needed to explain how and why childhood sexual abuse is related to sexual risk behaviors among Latino gay and bisexual men in order to (1) guide further research through testable hypotheses and (2) foster empirically based interventions that reduce the occurrence of childhood sexual abuse as well as interventions to reduce HIV risk specifically among those abused.

However, few studies have focused on uncovering how and why HIV risk patterns are maintained among Latino gay and bisexual men despite their strong intentions to the contrary (Diaz, 1998). One of the limitations in understanding this relationship has been the sole focus on the individual behavioral and demographic correlates of HIV risk. While demographic and individual behavioral characteristics shed light on the correlates of risk, they do not explain how the risk patterns are maintained. Additionally, they fail to account for the contextual, sociocultural, and psychological determinants of HIV risk that compete with Latino gay and bisexual men's behavioral intentions.

Findings from research on the sociocultural, psychological, and contextual predictors of risk, along with implications from the literature on childhood sexual abuse among women, provide indicators of possible factors that mediate and moderate the link between childhood sexual abuse and HIV risk.

Sociocultural Factors

Sexual Silence

The Latino Gay Men's Sexuality Study used in-depth individual qualitative interviews to explore the sexual development and subjective experiences of 30 Latino gay and bisexual men in the San Francisco Bay Area. The study found a very high level of silence about sex generally when growing up, and about gay sex in particular (Arreola, 2006). The men in this study attributed their feelings of uncleanliness and worthlessness when having sex with other men as adults to the silence they experienced in childhood regarding their sexuality. A quote from an interview captures the impact of this sexual silence:

> The idea of keeping it a secret and feelings of guilt and shame around it are still really present when I start having sex as an adult, [resulting in sexuality becoming] separate from ...my individuality. It was like another persona (Arreola, 2006).

This research further concluded that sexual silence resulted in the inability of the family and social environment to facilitate a boy's ability to make sense of and assimilate his developing sense of desire for men with loving and warm feelings. This may lead to a need to keep sexual feelings separate (or silent, even to himself) from the rest of his developing sense of self. In adulthood, this may make it difficult for a man to integrate messages of safe sex into sexual situations and contexts that are already laden with feelings of guilt and disgrace:

> "There was a whole separate secret identity around sex and I knew how to hide that and how to live with that, so it was easy to take living—keeping my sexuality a secret" (Arreola, 2006).

Homophobia

Homophobia has a strong association with HIV risk behavior. In a multivariate model of HIV sexual risk among predominantly English-speaking Latino gay and bisexual men, experiences of homophobia in childhood were found to increase the likelihood of participating in risky sexual situations that mediate the effects of social oppression and psychological distress on sexual risk behavior (Diaz, Ayala, & Bein, 2004). Another study that sought to replicate these findings among predominantly Spanish-speaking MSM found similar results: experiences of discrimination based on homosexual behavior were predictive of HIV risk behaviors (Jarama, Kennamer, Poppen, Hendricks, & Bradford, 2005). Finally, findings from the Latino Gay Men's Sexuality Study suggest that homophobia among Latinos may increase the likelihood that effeminate or gay boys become targets to be sexually abusive by older men who potentially feel threatened by a boy's effeminacy (Arreola et al., 2005).

Homophobia and Psychological Distress

In a quantitative study of 912 Latino gay and bisexual men, the investigators examined the relation between experiences of social discrimination (for example, homophobia) and symptoms of psychological distress (for example, depression and suicidal ideation) (Diaz et al., 2001). Results showed that homophobia (a sociocultural determinant) was a strong predictor of psychological distress (a psychological determinant). The authors concluded that, among Latino gay and bisexual men, a social context of oppression leads to psychological distress that is directly related to mental health (Diaz et al., 2001). Importantly, they also found that psychological distress has been linked to HIV risky behaviors across several studies (Diaz et al., 2004).

Psychological Factors

Psychological Distress

Childhood sexual abuse predicts psychological distress, which predicts risky sexual situations, which predict risky sexual behavior. Consistent with findings among women and men (Weiss, Longhurst, & Mazure, 1999), analyses of the effect of childhood sexual abuse on psychological distress show that among Latino gay and bisexual men, childhood sexual abuse strongly predicts symptoms of depression and anxiety (Arreola, 2005). Given previous findings that psychological distress predicts risky sexual situations among Latino gay and bisexual men (Diaz et al., 2004), it is not surprising to find that multiple logistic regression models found significant effects of childhood sexual abuse on depression/anxiety and risky sexual situations and behaviors, even when all of the factors were included in the model (Arreola, 2005).

One way Latino gay and bisexual men appear to cope with psychological distress is through sex. In the Latino Gay Men's Sexuality Study, one of the men interviewed described reaching adulthood and seducing men as a way of feeling in charge or

> "Successful. I felt like a spider and they were like flies on my (thread) in my trap. I got it. I'm going to get some (sex) tonight. I would feel like I got laid and it was just like an accomplishment like I did it". Afterward, however, he "would feel like a tramp. At the same time I felt like a slut; I felt like a tramp; I felt cheap; I felt sleazy" (Arreola, 2006).

The study suggested that this pattern of using sex as a way to feel better about oneself with the apparent feeling of success during the encounter was often followed by a let down and a need to cope with ensuing self-condemnation. This was not uncommon among the descriptions of casual sex among the Latino gay and bisexual men interviewed. Importantly, these feelings of worthlessness become risky sexual situations to the extent that they create a need to use sex as a way to escape from them, if only for a short time.

Dissociation

Dissociation is a psychological state or condition in which certain thoughts, emotions, sensations, or memories are separated from the rest of the psyche. Pierre Janet coined the term, emphasizing its role as a defensive mechanism in response to psychological trauma (Janet, 1889). While Janet considered dissociation an initially effective defense mechanism that protects the individual psychologically from the impact of overwhelming traumatic events (such as childhood sexual abuse), he believed that continued dissociation after the trauma ended could become maladaptive and psychopathological (Janet, 1889).

Studies with women have found a strong relationship between childhood sexual abuse and dissociation in cases where the childhood sexual abuse was severe (Briggs & Joyce, 1997; Chu, 2000; Johnson, Pike, & Chard, 2001; Mulder, Beautrais, Joyce, & Fergusson, 1998; Neumann, Houskamp, Pollock, & Briere, 1996). As Janet's work suggested, it is likely that the ability to dissociate during childhood sexual abuse is adaptive, especially when there is no control over the situation. However, to the extent that dissociation is generalized to non-threatening situations (such as consensual sexual encounters in adulthood), the ability to make conscious choices about behavior in non-threatening contexts is dramatically limited.

Some research among women attempts to apply the advances made in the treatment of dissociative disorders to broaden our understanding of sexual compulsivity as an unconscious reenactment of early trauma and inescapable stress (Schwartz, Galperin, & Masters, 1995). The extent to which childhood sexual abuse is associated with dissociation among Latino gay and bisexual men is not known. However, given the importance of dissociation in the context of childhood sexual abuse found among women and the high level of severity of childhood sexual abuse among Latino gay and bisexual men, dissociation may be one of the mechanisms that account for the link between childhood sexual abuse and risky sexual behaviors in adulthood. Support for this hypothesis comes from a case study of a 16-year-old boy with a history of childhood sexual abuse who became infected with HIV and who suffered from posttraumatic stress, substance abuse, and depersonalization disorder (a main feature of dissociation) (Allers, White, & Mullis, 1997). The authors concluded that undiagnosed or untreated dissociative disorders do indeed complicate AIDS prevention efforts.

Resiliency Factors

Although resiliency factors that may moderate the impact of childhood sexual abuse among Latino gay and bisexual men have not been examined previously, it is likely that the effect of childhood sexual abuse on psychological factors is moderated by various resiliency factors. Preliminary findings from the Latino Gay Men's Sexuality Study suggest that the extent to which the childhood sexual abuse impacts on psychological factors can be attenuated by the response of close adults to the childhood sexual abuse episode(s), by later therapy directed at addressing those effects, or by a loving and accepting personal relationship in adulthood.

Contextual Factors

Risky Sexual Situations

As noted above in the section on differentiating childhood sexual abuse from voluntary childhood sexuality among boys, preliminary analyses of a large representative sample of self-identified gay and bisexual men suggest that the context of sexual behaviors are different for those with a childhood sexual abuse history compared with those without childhood sexual abuse. When separated into three categories: (1) no history of childhood sexual abuse, (2) childhood sexual abuse without coercion, and (3) childhood sexual abuse with coercion, the data indicate significant differences in sexual contexts depending on childhood sexual abuse history. No differences were found between the first two groups. However, compared with those who had no history of childhood sexual abuse and those who had a history of childhood sexual abuse without coercion, those who reported a history of childhood sexual abuse with coercion were significantly more likely to report sexual contexts involving (1) the use of drugs, (2) an escape from loneliness or depression, and (3) difficulty maintaining an erection (Arreola & Diaz, 2001). Importantly, there was a strong relationship between contexts of sexual risk and actual sexual risk-taking behaviors that predict HIV infection.

Conclusions

Toward a Preliminary Model of Childhood Sexual Abuse and HIV Risk
     Together, the findings from the literature cited above suggest a preliminary model that may help to explain how childhood sexual abuse leads to increased risk for HIV. This preliminary model hypothesizes that childhood sexual abuse leads to dissociation which leads to psychological distress that increases risky sexual situations that result in risky sexual behaviors. Sociocultural determinants, such as sexual silence and homophobia, may moderate the effect of childhood sexual abuse on dissociation. For example, high levels of sexual silence in childhood may increase a child's need to continue to dissociate beyond the period of the trauma because of the implicit shame and lack of support that sexual silence condones. The link between childhood sexual abuse and dissociation may also be attenuated by resiliency factors such as a supportive parental response.
     Dissociation may increase the likelihood of psychological distress to the extent that an adult man, who has been sexually abused in childhood, does not attribute his depression or anxiety to the originally abusive situation (since it is dissociated from consciousness) and so does not find adaptive

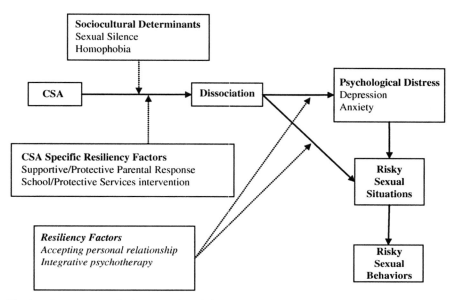

Fig. 2.1 Presents a preliminary model of the mediators and moderators of childhood sexual abuse and HIV risk based on previous studies and preliminary data from both quantitative and qualitative studies presented above (Arreola, 2005)

methods, such as psychotherapy, to cope with his feelings. He may be left to seek alternative coping strategies such as risky sexual encounters. These risky sexual encounters may also be further reinforced by continued dissociation. To the extent that the cues in the adult sexual situations match the original abusive sexual situations, the individual may continue to dissociate as a way to distance himself from the shameful and worthless feelings associated with the abusive event in order to be able to enjoy the encounter. However, as in the findings from the Latino Gay Men's Sexuality Study, this may eventually lead to more feelings of shame and guilt.

An accepting personal relationship or integrative psychotherapy may prove to be important resiliency factors that moderate the effects of dissociation on psychological distress and risky sexual situations. These forms of resiliency may serve the same goal of helping the individual integrate the original experience of childhood sexual abuse. To the extent that he can integrate the abusive event(s), he may be able to attribute shame and guilt feelings to the perpetrator rather than to himself, thereby reducing the need to cope with these feelings through risky sexual behaviors.

The literature on childhood sexual abuse and its sequelae, including HIV risk, among Latino gay men decidedly warrants further development of a research agenda that explains the relationship between the two. The development of a theoretical model that explains how and why these relationships are maintained would steer further research as well as intervention programs to reduce childhood sexual abuse or to treat those who suffer from its effects. Although limited, the literature on determinants of HIV risk provides clues regarding mediating and moderating factors that may maintain the relationship between childhood sexual abuse and HIV risk. The preliminary model presented in this chapter is intended as a heuristic that may guide future work in this research agenda.

The preliminary theoretical model of the relationship between childhood sexual abuse and HIV risk has implications for clinicians working with gay youth, survivors of childhood sexual abuse, or people living with HIV. The model suggests that clinicians must begin to acknowledge the impact of competing sociocultural (such as homophobia) and contextual (such as risky sexual situations, and parental or societal protections, or responses to childhood sexual abuse) factors on individuals' attempts to change their behavior. The extent to which clinicians incorporate an understanding of the sociocultural and contextual environments in their clinical interventions may determine patients' or clients' ability to make changes that are healthier and in accord with their intentions. Another implication of the preliminary model is that clinicians working with Latino gay men who have a history of childhood sexual abuse may need to give attention to the integration of the abuse, specifically, and of sexuality, generally, in order to reduce the likelihood of dissociation during adult sexual encounters.

Finally, the preliminary model has societal and policy implications. As a society, we must begin to take responsibility for the portion of individuals' behavior that is determined by the social norms and policies we espouse that send competing messages of individual responsibility along with those of condemnation or unworthiness. It is of no surprise that these conflicting messages may contribute toward some Latino gay men taking risks that are contrary to their intentions. To the degree that sociocultural, socioeconomic, and political conditions will contribute toward accepting and supportive environments, individuals will be better able to comply with their intentions toward safe, healthy, and loving lives.

References

Allers, C. T., White, J. F., & Mullis, F. (1997). The treatment of dissociation in an HIV-infected, sexually abused adolescent male. *Psychotherapy: Theory, Research, Practice, Training, 34*(2), 201–206.

Anon. (2005). Epidemic is shifting to blacks, Hispanics. Most common transmission is MSM. *AIDS Alert, 20*(8), 89–90.

Arreola, S. (2001). *Aspectos psicosociales y conductas del sexo forzado en ninos y ninas jovenes (Psychosocial aspects and behaviors related to forced sex in young boys and girls)*. Paper presented at the VIII Congresso Mexicano De Psicologia Social & I Congresso Mexicano De Relaciones Personales, Guadalajara, Mexico.

Arreola, S.G. (2005). Sexual risk among Latino gay men: Modeling the link between child-hood sexual abuse and adult sexual risk. Paper presented at the Robert Wood Johnson Medical School, Critical Research Issues in Latino Mental Health 2005 Conference: Biological and Psychosocial Influences on Diagnosis and Treatment, Princeton, New Jersey.

Arreola, S. (2006). Childhood Sexual Abuse and HIV among Latino Gay Men: The price of sexual silence during the AIDS epidemic. In N. Teunis (Ed.), *Sexual Inequalities and social justice*. Berkeley, CA: University of California Press.

Arreola, S., & Diaz, R. M. (2001, October). *Forced sexual abuse and risky sexual situations among Latino gay men*. Paper presented at the Ninth International Conference of the National Organization on Male Sexual Victimization, New York, New York.

Arreola, S. G. (2005). *Sexual Risk among Latino Gay Men: Modeling the link between childhood sexual abuse and adult sexual risk*. Paper presented at the Robert Wood Johnson Medical School, Critical Research Issues in Latino Mental Health 2005 Conference: Biological and Psychosocial Influences on Diagnosis and Treatment, Princeton, New Jersey.

Arreola, S. G., Neilands, T. B., Pollack, L. M., Paul, J. P., & Catania, J. A. (2005). Higher prevalence of childhood sexual abuse among Latino men who have sex with men than non-Latino men who have sex with men: data from the Urban Men's Health Study. *Child Abuse & Neglect, 29*(3), 285–290.

Boney-McCoy, S., & Finkelhor, D. (1995). Psychosocial sequelae of violent victimization in a national youth sample. *Journal of Consulting and Clinical Psychology, 63*(5), 726–736.

Briggs, L., & Joyce, P. R. (1997). What determines post-traumatic stress disorder symptoma-tology for survivors of childhood sexual abuse? *Child Abuse & Neglect, 21*(6), 575–582.

Carballo-Dieguez, A., & Dolezal, C. (1995). Association between history of childhood sexual abuse and adult HIV-risk sexual behavior in Puerto Rican men who have sex with men. *Child Abuse & Neglect, 19*(5), 595–605.

Centers for Disease Control and Prevention. (2001). HIV testing among racial/ethnic mino-rities—United States, 1999 (Vol. 50, pp. 1054–1058): U.S. Department of Health and Human Services.

Centers for Disease Control and Prevention. (2001a). National Center for HIV, STD, and Tuberculosis Prevention (NCHSTP). Last accessed April 6, 2007; Available at: http://www.cdc.gov/hiv/topics/surveillance/basic.htm.

Centers for Disease Control and Prevention. (2001b). NIAID. Last accessed April 6, 2007; Available at: cdc.gov/omh/AMH/factsheets/hiv.htm.

Centers for Disease Control and Prevention. (2002a). Health, United States 2002, Table 33. Last accessed December 10, 2006; Available at: http://www.cdc.gov/nchs/data/hus/tables/2002/02hus033.pdf.

Centers for Disease Control and Prevention. (2002c). NCHS Health United States, Table 54. Last accessed April 6, 2007; Available at: cdc.gov/omh/AMH/factsheets/hiv.htm.

Centers for Disease Control and Prevention. (2004). Health disparities experienced by Hispanics—United States. *MMWR Morbidity & Mortality Weekly Report, 53*(40), 935–937.

Centers for Disease Control and Prevention. (2005). Trends in HIV/AIDS diagnoses—33 states, 2001–2004. *MMWR Morbidity & Mortality Weekly Report, 54*(45), 1149–1153.

Centers for Disease Control and Prevention. (2006a). Epidemiology of HIV/AIDS—United States, 1981–2005. *MMWR Morbidity & Mortality Weekly Report, 55*(21), 589–592.

Centers for Disease Control and Prevention. (2006b). The Global HIV/AIDS pandemic, 2006. *MMWR Morbidity & Mortality Weekly Report, 55*(31), 841–844.

Centers for Disease Control and Prevention. (2006c). Racial/ethnic disparities in diagnoses of HIV/AIDS—33 states, 2001–2004. *MMWR Morbidity & Mortality Weekly Report, 55*(5), 121–125.

Chu, J. A. (2000). Psychological defense styles and childhood sexual abuse. *American Journal of Psychiatry, 157*(10), 1707.

Diaz, R. M. (1997). Latino gay men and psycho-cultural barriers to AIDS prevention. In *In changing times: Gay men and lesbians encounter HIV/AIDS*. (pp. 221–244). Chicago, IL: University of Chicago Press.

Diaz, R. M. (1998). *Latino gay men and HIV: Culture, sexuality, and risk behavior*. New York, NY: Routledge.

Diaz, R. M., & Ayala, G. (1999). Love, passion and rebellion: Ideologies of HIV risk among Latino gay men in the USA. *Culture, Health & Sexuality, 1*(3), 277–293.

Diaz, R. M., Ayala, G., & Bein, E. (2004). Sexual risk as an outcome of social oppression: data from a probability sample of Latino gay men in three U.S. cities. *Cultural Diversity Ethnic Minority Psychoogy, 10*(3), 255–267.

Diaz, R. M., Ayala, G., Bein, E., Henne, J., & Marin, B. V. (2001). The impact of homophobia, poverty, and racism on the mental health of gay and bisexual Latino men: Findings from 3 US cities. *American Journal of Public Health, 91*(6), 927–932.

Diaz, R. M., Ayala, G., & Marin, B. V. (2000). Latino gay men and HIV: Risk behavior as a sign of oppression. *Focus, 15*(7), 1–5.

Dolezal, C., & Carballo-Dieguez, A. (2002). Childhood sexual experiences and the perception of abuse among Latino men who have sex with men. *Journal of Sex Research, 39*(3), 165–173.

Feiring, C., Taska, L., & Lewis, M. (1999). Age and gender differences in children's and adolescents' adaptation to sexual abuse. *Child Abuse & Neglect, 23*(2), 115–128.

Fontes, L. (1995). *Sexual abuse in nine North American Cultures: Treatment and prevention*. Thousand Oaks, CA: Sage Publications.

Guzman, B. (2001). *The Hispanic Population: Census 2000 Brief*: U.S. Census Bureau, Department of Commerce, Economics and Statistics Administration.

Holmes, W. C. (1997). Association between a history of childhood sexual abuse and subsequent, adolescent psychoactive substance use disorder in a sample of HIV seropostive men. *Journal of Adolescent Health, 20*(6), 414–419.

Janet, P. (1889). *L'automatisme psychologique* (Vol. Reprint: Societe Pierre Janet, Paris, 1973). Paris: Felix Alcan.

Jarama, S. L., Kennamer, J. D., Poppen, P. J., Hendricks, M., & Bradford, J. (2005). Psychosocial, behavioral, and cultural predictors of sexual risk for HIV infection among Latino men who have sex with men. *AIDS Behavior, 9(4)*, 513–523.

Jinich, S., Paul, J. P., Stall, R., Acree, M., Kegeles, S. M., & Hoff, C., et al. (1998). Childhood sexual abuse and HIV risk-taking behavior among gay and bisexual men. *AIDS & Behavior, 2*(1), 41–51.

Johnson, D. M., Pike, J. L., & Chard, K. M. (2001). Factors predicting PTSD, depression, and dissociative severity in female treatment-seeking childhood sexual abuse survivors. *Child Abuse & Neglect, 25*(1), 179–198.

Koenig, L. J., Doll, L. S., O'Leary, A., & Pequegnat, W. (Eds.). (2003). *From Child Sexual Abuse to Adult Sexual Risk: Trauma, revictimization, and intervention*. Washington, DC: American Psychological Association Press.

Lenderking, W. R., Wold, C., Mayer, K. H., Goldstein, R., Losina, E., & Seage, G. R., III. (1997). Childhood sexual abuse among homosexual men: Prevalence and association with unsafe sex. *Journal of General Internal Medicine, 12*(4), 250–253.

Lindholm, K. J., & Willey, R. (1986). Ethnic differences in child abuse and sexual abuse. *Hispanic Journal of Behavioral Sciences, 8*(2), 111–125.

Moisan, P. A., Sanders-Phillips, K., & Moisan, P. M. (1997). Ethnic differences in circumstances of abuse and symptoms of depression and anger among sexually abused Black and Latino boys. *Child Abuse & Neglect, 21*(5), 473–488.

Mulder, R. T., Beautrais, A. L., Joyce, P. R., & Fergusson, D. M. (1998). Relationship between dissociation, childhood sexual abuse, childhood physical abuse, and mental illness in a general population sample. *American Journal of Psychiatry, 155*(6), 806–811.

Neumann, D. A., Houskamp, B. M., Pollock, V. E., & Briere, J. (1996). The long-term sequelae of childhood sexual abuse in women: A meta-analytic review. *Child Maltreatment: Journal of the American Professional Society on the Abuse of Children, 1*(1), 6–16.

Paul, J. P., Catania, J., Pollack, L., & Stall, R. (2001). Understanding childhood sexual abuse as a predictor of sexual risk-taking among men who have sex with men: The Urban Men's Health Study. *Child Abuse & Neglect, 25*(4), 557–584.

Remafedi, G., Farrow, J. A., & Deisher, R. W. (1991). Risk factors for attempted suicide in gay and bisexual youth. *Pediatrics, 87*(6), 869–875.

Schwartz, M. F., Galperin, L. D., & Masters, W. H. (1995). Dissociation and treatment of compulsive reenactment of trauma: Sexual compulsivity. In M. Hunter (Ed.), *Adult survivors of to be sexually abusive: Treatment innovations* (pp. 42–55). Thousand Oaks, CA, US: Sage Publications, Inc.

Valleroy, L A., MacKellar, D. A., Karon, J. M., Rosen, D. H., McFarland, W., & Shehan, D. A., et al. (2000). HIV prevalence and associated risks in young men who have sex with men. Young Men's Survey Study Group. *Journal of the American Medical Association, 284*(2), 198–204.

Weiss, E. L., Longhurst, J. G., & Mazure, C. M. (1999). Childhood sexual abuse as a risk factor for depression in women: Psychosocial and neurobiological correlates. *American Journal of Psychiatry, 156*(6), 816–828.

Portrait Four
May and December: Dangerous Intimacies

L. Michael Gipson

Here are some hard to swallow, oft-ignored pills. Adolescent sex with older men contributes to higher HIV infection and substance abuse rates among young men who have sex with men (YMSM). Sex with older men may also be contributing factors to mental health issues that challenge YMSMs far beyond their adolescence. Older men believe that unprotected sex with younger men is safe because these youth, their elders incorrectly deduce, are unlikely to be HIV infected and therefore protection is unnecessary. Younger men looking to their older partners for sexual guidance, including direction regarding appropriate protection measures, adopt unsuitable HIV prevention strategies from elders modeling poor or no prevention methods. In other words, these youth learn not to use condoms and other life-saving barrier methods from their elders, immediately initiating their sex lives behind the eight ball. As if teaching the lessons of unsafe sexual behavior alone were not criminally irresponsible, older men are more likely to have had multiple sexual partners than younger men and are also more likely than their younger counterparts to have experienced injection drug use. These probabilities make older men dangerous to younger men. However, there is enough blame to spread around; new HIV infection rates for younger men demonstrate that the majority of new HIV infections among MSMs are occurring among young adult men of ages 19–25, men most likely infected during their adolescent and college-age years. These statistics demonstrate that older men may need to be just as weary of their young partners, as their younger partners need to be of their elders. But what do all of these statistics mean? Why are young men having sex with older men to begin with? How does it start and what are the implications of such taboo relationship dynamics? Just what is going on between older men and younger men in the gay male community? We'll explore these questions using my own experience and those of young people that I work with through various youth programs serving YMSMs and lesbian, gay, bisexual, and transgender (LGBT) youth in Cleveland.

L. Michael Gipson
LMG Consulting Partnerships, Ltd., Washington, DC

S. Loue (ed.), *Health Issues Confronting Minority Men Who Have Sex with Men.*   57
© Springer 2008

Facts Stranger than Fiction

"I was thirteen years old when they first started pulling their cars up to holla at me." This was a line I spoke as a character named Reverend John T. Sutton in a Cleveland-based HIV prevention play, *Silhouettes of Reality*. John was a heterosexually identified minister, husband, and father who purposely sought out young male victims to infect with HIV. The teenage character John grew up longing for male attention. His longing was met by numerous older men who taught John the value of his body as a sexual commodity, one that he could exchange for semblances of their attention and affection. Some of the men would even dare to say that they loved John as a means to a sexually gratifying end.

Eventually, John became older, less desirable to his elders, and mature enough to determine that he needed his life to be more than just pedophilic sustenance. After his epiphany, John became conflicted and angry because he couldn't clearly determine whether his natural orientation was homosexual or whether he had allowed his adolescent need for male bonding to be corrupted by the sexual proclivities of older men. As John stated in *Silhouettes*, he felt that the men who had taken advantage of his adolescent needs had stolen his choice from him. Not that John's sexual orientation was a choice, but since his identity was not given an opportunity to realize itself unencumbered by pedophilic assaults, it was easy for John to perceive that he had once had a choice in deciding his orientation.

John hated being a man attracted to other men, partially because his identity had been sullied and partially because he only knew homosexuality through the lens of sexual abuse. The men who had used him had taught John that to be gay or bisexual was to be someone dark and carnal, to be used in the backseat of a car in an abandoned parking lot, an enclosed men's room stall, or a secluded bush in a park; to be used and unloved. John had never observed beauty, love, or fulfillment as aspects of a homosexual life.

Years later, when John was grown, he fled to find his desired shelter and solace in a heterosexual marriage and through his religious faith. Disillusioned by the trappings of church and marriage that failed to provide him with relief from his sexual proclivities, John found himself reliving the cycle of abuse he'd been taught with new, young victims who were searching in the dark for love. During John's unsafe sexual activities with young men, who he assumed were HIV negative because of their age, he became HIV infected and subsequently began infecting others.

While John is a fictitious character in imagined circumstances, it is telling that gay teens assisted in creating his character, for his story is all too real and familiar to them and to me. Given the similarities in John and my adolescent stories, John's road was all too easily the road that I could have taken and one that is far from make-believe in the lives of the youth I serve.

My Story

I was 13 when grown men began pulling their cars up to me on the streets of Chicago. I was easy and willing prey. I was dark in a city that reveres lighter complexions; pudgy in a society that depicts the young Black physique as a lean, taut Adonis; and effeminate in a culture that places masculinity on a pedestal. I found little affirmation in the communal places where my peers sought and could more easily find approval. During the difficult years of ages 12–14, home was not a refuge but a suffocation; church was damning; school, a battleground of bullies; and sports, a source of humiliation and ridicule. Ah, but in the arms of grown men who told me that I was beautiful and valuable, I was made to feel special. I was made to feel like I was appreciated and belonged. From age 13, when the first man made sexual advances at me while I was coming home from a pool at Washington Park, I found that men could smell my voracious appetite for attention and affection like sharks to blood.

Initially, I was timid and afraid but also excited by the idea that someone wanted me, desired me. Certainly, nothing of the sort was occurring with the girls in my school and I never dared accost the boys at school for fear of being attacked or "outed" as deviant. By the time I was 14, I found myself seeking men in places where I'd been cruised before and I could tell you exactly where the Chi-town boys were in the late 1980s. At the time I didn't consider myself to be a victim, I naively thought of myself as an equal to my sexual partners. Each and every time that I went for a "walk," I went in search of more anonymous male attention and I told myself that I was experimenting or going through a phase, that I wasn't gay. It was during my 14th summer that I realized that I was not an equal to the men who used my body, but only a child playing an adult game.

You see, it was during my 14th summer when a man old enough to be my grandfather forcibly raped me, a man with whom I told myself, I would only let "things" go so far (only as far as I had let those achieve before him). Only my elder had other plans for me, much more painful and a lot further sexually than my mind had allowed itself to conceive at the time. I foolishly assumed because other strangers had stopped their sexual progression when I requested, that all men would. Repeatedly, I screamed "No!" and "Stop!" while the perpetrator crossed my boundaries, but he didn't listen and I suddenly became tearfully aware that this man was an elder who held power over me and as such I had better cooperate with him. After the incident, I contemplated my options for recourse. I knew that I had cruised my rapist and willingly *began* to participate in sexual acts with him. With those facts in mind, I told myself that no one would believe me when I said that I was raped. Who would believe a fat, ugly 14 year-old boy who cruised men just as heavily as he was being cruised by men? My attacker hadn't used protection and I was terrified of being HIV infected, so 2 months later, I told my mother an elaborate, more palatable tale of how I'd been raped in the park by two strangers at knife point. My distortions were rewarded with the HIV test I eagerly desired and free mental health counseling for my sexual trauma.

For the next 2 years, I rebelled against that fat 14-year old that seemed, to his young mind, anyway, to be a magnet for men. I left Chicago to live in Germany with my army dad. Sure, that my weight accompanied by rather large buttocks were to blame for my appeal, I became bulimic and lost 75 pounds. I began to forcefully pursue girls, and I became more aggressive when people invaded my personal space.

On the outside, I appeared to be a socially active, overachieving youth. However, I was a ball of tormented nerves on the inside. I desperately wanted to be heterosexual and was actively trying to overcome my past with older men. However, I was failing miserably. On military bases and in the German economy, there were even more men interested in a tall, newly slender youth who was just as closeted and conflicted as they were. I would find myself habitually slipping back into my "walks" followed by anguished guilt and relentless prayers to God to remove my desires. Like John in *Silhouettes*, I only knew homosexuality as something sexual and exploitive, something addictive and horribly unchristian, and I didn't want to live my life like that. Miserably, I would attempt bouts of abstinence and try to become emotionally connected to the young women I dated to no avail. Tired and frustrated, I attempted suicide during this period. Having abandoned my attempt prior to completion, I cursed the men who had approached me and wondered whether I would have been heterosexual if it weren't for those men's advances. Had they made me gay?

Neither my nor John's plight and confusion over an authentic sexual identity are unusual among gay and bisexual young men of color. In my HIV prevention and youth development work with young men who have sex with men (YMSMs) and adolescent lesbian, gay, bisexual, and transgender (LGBT) youth, I find mine and John's stories to be fairly common. When I finally did come out as openly gay, I did so with the caveat that my rape had made me that way. There was no pride or self-affirmation in my coming out declaration. So deep was my internalized homophobia, that it would be years after coming out before I readily acknowledged that I had experienced multiple same-sex relations with a peer a full year before that first menacing car honked at me. Even more years passed before I allowed myself to fully remember elementary school crushes on other boys and stereotypical stories of my nonconformist gender expression even as young as age six. Elder men hadn't taken my choice from me as John would say, but they did muddy the waters, provided me with distractions to some real emotional and mental health issues that I needed addressed, and they gave me an out from fully accepting who I am. I am not alone. When I conduct anecdotal surveys of my young men, I find that they disproportionately identify as victims of childhood sexual assault, often by a family member or a close family friend. It is little wonder that so few of them find little pride in their sexual orientation either, so ugly were many of their first same-sex experiences.

I am of the opinion that body image issues in the Black gay male community can find its origins in the anecdotal exploitation tales of my youth and me. By having men place a premium on my sexual attractiveness, I learned at an early, very impressionable age to be overly preoccupied with my physical appearance. This preoccupation assisted me in becoming bulimic in my teens and later in life, muscle dysmorphic. In my body image issues, I find many young compatriots. As a consequence of lessons learned from elder men of color, I work with some young men who base their value solely on their ability to attract. While sex with older men is not exclusively to blame for youth's fixation with their physical appearance—hip-hop, prison, and media culture all collude in idealizing images of lean or muscular men—older men are still a factor. It is important to note that similar body image dynamics can be found among teenage girls who alter themselves once they realize that they are to be dissected and assessed under the critical, and often older, male gaze.

Why Accept Diabetic Sugar Daddies?

One might ask if there are so many negative implications and repercussions for young men, then why do they consistently enter these relationships? In my past and in others, I've seen innumerable variations of and rationales for the May–December theme. Youth who have determined that they are homosexual and actively seek older men, because they youthfully believe that they are "too mature to date guys their age." Openly gay, fatherless youth who fruitlessly search for father figures in their intimate partners, emotional security blankets, to replace the one they never had. Young men looking to profit off older men who will willingly provide these youth with the economic resources (and occasional luxuries) they need to survive in exchange for sex and attention. Older men deemed unsuitable by peers who may require more economic stability and social standing in potential mates, who then prey on younger men to fulfill their need to be seen as valuable, to serve as companions that eases lonely hours, and to be easily manipulated pawns in relationships that inherently favor the elder male in the relationship's power dynamic.

Conversely, there are predatory younger men, who are determined to be perceived by elder men as their equals and are dogged in their zealous pursuit of elders for their sexual, financial, and occasionally emotional partnerships. While the motivations of these youth certainly deserve study and perhaps a strong chiding, the moral ambiguity of men who acquiesce to their young suitors' advances deserves uniform societal condemnation.

What to Do?

I am not a homophobe and having worked daily with YMSM and LGBT youth populations at a youth social service drop-in center has certainly made me sensitive to the nuances and exceptions to the rule among youths' experiences.

However, anecdotal information and a few small studies regarding young men of color consistently demonstrate that there are a substantial number of older men preying on younger men. Practitioners working with LGBT youth are quietly asked by gay rights activists to be silent about the politically untenable issue, since it is a no-win situation for activists already grappling with mainstream and conservative institutions equating gay men with pedophiles. There is little truth to the label since national studies show that 96–98% of child molesters identify as heterosexual.

However, the predators this essay has identified aren't men looking for elementary school-age children. Rather, they are men whose appetites seem to be exclusively reserved for high school and college-age young men. Generally, these men are adhering to the law by limiting their sexual relationships with young men above the age of consent (an age as low as 16 in some states, including Ohio). Despite the fears of gay rights activist, the homosexual or bisexual natures of these men are not the issue either. To the contrary, anyone exploring teen pregnancy and STDs (sexually transmitted diseases) among young women of color can find eerily similar parallels occurring in a heterosexual context. These elder men deserve societal condemnation because their decision making regarding youth is generally self-serving and fails to have these youths best interest at heart. If not our societal condemnation, then at the very least these elder men need strong assistance and encouragement to enroll in psychological counseling to assist them to develop better impulse control and other behavioral changes.

Young men eventually come to learn their elders' dishonorable intentions the hard way once they became older, more mature, less malleable, and consequently less desirable. Young men who relied on their youth and beauty to be "kept" later find themselves with little education, few marketable skills, and a lack of employment history necessary to sustain the lifestyle their "sugar daddies" afforded them. These young men may become bitter about their life station after their waistlines have thickened and minds have sharpened enough to have discovered their voice and boldly articulate their own opinions about their lives. Some allow their bitterness or their sense of hopelessness about their futures evolves into substance abuse and depression.

More frightening than the substance abuse and mental health concerns, is the number of young men who become HIV and STD infected because they never learned how or developed and practiced the necessary skills to protect themselves, whether in a monogamous relationship or not. Their unhealthy relationship cycles may even continue as young men who develop "Peter Pan" complexes or "arrested development" begin looking to younger partners for sexual and emotional validation, modeling more of the behavior they were taught. There are also young men who, like myself, look back in anger and repulsion at the relationship they maintained with their elders, only after having achieved their elder partners' age (or the age the elder partner was during the inappropriate relationship).

So what is to be done? Older men must be willing to bear the weight and responsibility to behave and perform the role of the responsible adult, even when being relentlessly pursued by youth. Someone has to erect boundaries that say "no" to youths' sexual advances and be prepared to say "yes" to feeding youths' emotional hunger for guidance, mentorship, and unconditional love. I assure you having been there and working with kids who are reliving my adolescence before my very eyes, that young men are generally not equipped, interested, or capable of erecting those barriers or enforcing such boundaries. One, the young men initially may only identify the benefits of these relationships and, like all youth, they want desperately to be considered grown and mature by both their peers and elders. May–December relationships seem to provide instant recognition and affirmation by peers, with few detractors among the broader LGBT community. Older men have to be willing to be mentors and not sexual partners, regardless of their attraction. Older men should understand that youth need healthy role models that demonstrate how to practice consistent morals, values, healthy friendships, and intimate relationships with partners of equal standing. Men who continue to exploit youths' socioeconomic challenges and emotional needs keep the gay and bi male community in a state of moral stagnation and assist in its political and social demise by continuing to spread HIV among those representing its future. Gay and bisexual men of color and adult programs should not affirm their peers who consistently behave as "chicken hawks" but hold them to task about behavior that damages the whole community.

Programs working with YMSMs and LGBT youth need not shy away from the moral and legal issues posed by May–December relationships. Practitioners serving youth should consistently enforce zero tolerance policies of May–December relationships within youth programs. Program planners should hold forums, workshops, and seminars that outline the dangers of such May–December relationships for youth and educate youth on the long-term prospects and possibilities of such relationships. Additionally, youth should be assisted developing their own cost-benefit analysis of dating their peers versus dating their elders, so that the youth are able to identify tangible reasons for making healthier choices in partners for themselves. Programs should screen films like *Kevin's Room II,* movies that attempt to depict such relationships in an analytical light, and hold critical discussions about shows like *Queer As Folk*, which idealize such relationships. Once youth and their elders know better, perhaps they will do better. If not, for a Black gay community that is already reeling from the loss of one generation, the cycles and its consequences may be too dire to contemplate or for its young to bear.

III
Mental Illness and Substance Use

Chapter Three
Body Image Disturbance and its Related Disorders

Leslie J. Heinberg and Chris Kraft

Introduction

Body image is a multifaceted, multidimensional concept that embodies the thoughts, feelings, and behaviors that a person has and expresses related to their appearance, weight, and shape. A classic meta-analysis helped demonstrate why body image is so important for psychosocial functioning. This study, a review of the attractiveness literature, demonstrated that the correlation between the objective attractiveness (as determined by expert raters) and an individual's self-rating of attractiveness was only 0.24 for men (and 0.25 for women; Feingold, 1992). This means that only just over 6% of one's body image is explained by actual physical attractiveness to others. Interestingly, however, it is the subjective rating—not the objective one—that is significantly associated with self-esteem (Feingold, 1992). Researchers and clinicians have suggested a continuum model as the best way to conceptualize body image (Thompson, Heinberg, Altabe & Tantleff-Dunn, 1999). This model suggests that body image disturbance can range from none to extreme with most people falling somewhere near the middle and experiencing mild to moderate concern or dissatisfaction (Thompson et al., 1999). However, a number of subgroups and individual differences may place people at greater risk for falling on the extreme end of the continuum (Thompson et al., 1999).

This chapter will address body image, body image disturbance, and its related behaviors in a largely understudied population, minority men who have sex with men (MSM). We will first review the very limited empirical research on men, MSM and minority MSM as well as implications from related populations. It is important to note from the outset that the limited studies that we review focus almost exclusively on self-identified gay men rather than the more encompassing population of MSM. "Men who have sex with men" more

Leslie J. Heinberg
Cleveland Clinic Lerner College of Medicine, Cleveland, OH
Chris Kraft
Johns Hopkins University School of Medicine, Baltimore, MD

S. Loue (ed.), *Health Issues Confronting Minority Men Who Have Sex with Men.*
© Springer 2008

broadly encompasses various groups of men who engage in sexual activities with other men, including those who self-identify as gay, bisexual, transgender, and transsexual and those who self-identify as heterosexual, but have had sexual relations with other men for any of a variety of reasons, including economic gain, assurances of shelter and/or safety, or in exchange for drugs (Cáceres, 2002). This much more broadly defined population has not been given attention within the body image literature. We will next address differing body image ideals (and their related behaviors) that may be applicable to minority MSM followed by brief discussions of different minority groups and two case studies. Finally, we will discuss future directions for research.

Overview of Body Image and Eating Disorders

Body image dissatisfaction (BID) is a concept of great interest to clinicians and researchers because of its strong association with depression, self-esteem, eating-disordered behavior, problematic dieting, and other risky health behaviors (Heinberg & Thompson, 2006). Body image research began in earnest approximately 30 years ago as a result of concerns with, and greater interest in, eating disorders. This led to a large literature investigating BID and eating disorders in females. (The prevalence of eating disorders is approximately nine times greater in women than in men. This may be attributable, at least in part, to detection and diagnostic biases.) This literature, linking body image to dieting and eating disorders, has led to the formation of prevention, early intervention, and treatment programs—again, primarily focusing upon female populations (Stice, 2001).

Eating disorders, particularly bulimia nervosa, have steadily increased over the past 50 years (Currin, Schmidt, Treasure, & Jick, 2005; Eagles, Johnston, Hunter, Lobban, & Millar, 1995) and are associated with significant psychological (e.g., starvation-induced depression, increase in obsessions), social (e.g., social withdrawal, academic, and occupational impairment), and medical (e.g., cognitive impairment, hypokalemia, bradycardia) comorbidities (Joiner, Vohs, & Heatherton, 2000; Lewinsohn, Shankman, Gua, & Klein, 2004; Pomeroy, 2004). Anorexia nervosa has the highest mortality rate of any psychiatric disorder (5% per decade of follow-up) (Sullivan, 1995).

Long considered disorders of Caucasian girls and young women, more recent epidemiological studies demonstrate significant increases in minority and male populations (Hoek & van Hoeken, 2003). Concurrently, there has been an increasing recognition of clinically significant eating and body image dysfunction in boys and men (Andersen, Cohn, & Holbrook, 2000; Pope, Gruber, Mangweth, Bureau, deCol, Jouvent, R., et al., 2000; Pope, Phillips, & Olivardia, 2000). Research has found that men do not differ from women in the pathophysiology, familial aggregation patterns, or biological etiology of eating disorders (Corson & Andersen, 2003). Unfortunately, diagnosis is more difficult in males because of: (1) reluctance to admit having a "women's disorder;" (2) *DSM-IV (Diagnostic and Statistical Manual, Fourth Edition)* criteria that focus on women (e.g., amenorrhea as a criterion for anorexia nervosa); and (3) clinician bias. Other eating disorders such as binge eating disorder and night eating syndrome are actually more common in men (Corson & Andersen, 2003). However, perhaps because of body image's outgrowth from the eating disorders literature, the vast majority of studies examining body image have focused on women. Recently, greater interest in boys and men have indicated that, like women, concerns about appearance, weight, and shape are common and lead to considerable suffering (Corson & Andersen, 2002).

Male Body Image

Survey research demonstrates a significant increase in male BID over the past three decades (Cash, 1997), although it is important to note that such studies do not specify men's sexual orientation or their sexual behaviors. Results demonstrate that 43% of men are dissatisfied with their mid-torso, 52% with their weight, and 43% with their overall appearance. Some researchers suggest that these increases reflect increasing sociocultural pressures regarding one's physique and attractiveness in men. Shifting trends in the thin ideal as well as pressure to achieve that ideal have been well documented through archival research of print media marketed to women (Andersen & DiDomenico, 1992; Garner, Garfinkel, Schwartz, & Thompson, 1980; Wiseman, Gray, Mosimann, & Ahrens, 1992).

Similar trends were demonstrated by examining the two most popular men's magazines, *GQ* and *Esquire* (Petrie, Austin, Crowley, Helmcaup, Johnson, Lester et al., 1996). Article and advertisement content and male models' body sizes were assessed during the period of 1960–1992. Linear trend analyses revealed that, like women's magazines, the number of messages concerning physical activity and health have increased over time. However, in contrast to print media aimed at female audiences, messages concerning weight and physical attractiveness have declined since the late 1970s and measurements of male models' body sizes have not changed significantly since the 1960s (Petrie et al., 1996). Although pressures for thinness were absent for men, the authors hypothesize that the increasing pressure to be involved in fitness activity may lead to unhealthy body-changing practices, such as crash dieting and steroid use (Petrie et al., 1996). Similarly, the influence of media consumption on self-identified heterosexual and gay males' body image (Duggan & McCreary, 2004) has been examined. This study found that consumption of muscle and fitness magazines was positively related to body dissatisfaction (BD) in both gay and heterosexual males but pornography exposure was only related to physique anxiety in gay men.

Unlike women, where there is a relatively universal thin ideal, male body image may be more complex with numerous ideals such as "heroin chic," "metro-sexual," and "body-builder" noted (Warren & Hildebrandt, 2006). Unfortunately, very little work has examined male body image and eating disorder pathology in minority populations. Rather, the extant literature has focused almost exclusively on Caucasian college-aged males (Heinberg & Thompson, 2006), with a small body of work on African American men (Heinberg, Haythornthwaite, Rosofsky, McCarron, & Clarke, 2000; Pulvers, Lee, Kaur, Mayo, Fitzgibbon, Jeffries, et al., 2004) and there are no published studies specifically examining either eating disturbance or body image in Latino men. The lack of data on Latinos has considerable consequences. In a nationwide study of participants in the National Eating Disorders Screening Program, Latino participants were significantly less likely than Whites to receive a recommendation or referral for further evaluation or care, controlling for presenting symptoms (Becker, Franko, Speck, & Herzog, 2003), suggesting that clinician bias may be an important treatment barrier for Latinos. Given that only one-third of individuals with anorexia and 6% of those with bulimia receive mental health care, these lower rates of treatment are significantly alarming.

There has been burgeoning interest in the role of sexual orientation and BD. For instance, studies have evaluated differences in body satisfaction and eating disturbance among homosexual and heterosexual men and women (Morrison, Morrison & Sager, 2004) and boys and girls (Austin, Ziyadeh, Kahn, Camargo, Colditz, & Field, 2004), the "muscular ideal" endorsed by gay men (Yelland & Tiggemann, 2003), and sex-role orientation and risk for body image disturbance (Gettelmann & Thompson, 1993).

Sexual Orientation and Eating Disorders

Sexual orientation has been identified as a potent gender-specific risk factor for eating disorders (ED) and BD in men (Andersen, 1999; Boroughs & Thompson, 2002; Strong, Williamson, Netemeyer, & Geer, 2000). That is, sexual orientation places gay men at greater risk for experiencing ED and BD than heterosexual men. However, homosexuality as a general risk factor for all types of psychopathology has been empirically rejected (Russell & Keel, 2002). Again, it is important to note in presenting these data that the following studies are in self-identified gay males, rather than in a more broadly defined MSM population. Thus, one must be cautious in generalizing results to MSM. In a population-based study, 27.8% of homosexual male adolescents reported BID versus 12% of heterosexual male teens (French, Story, Remafedi, Resnick, & Blum, 1996). Among men with ED, 10–42% self-identify as homosexual or bisexual (Carlat et al., 1997; Russell & Keel, 2002) which is, on average, higher than the base rate of homosexuality in the male population (~6%; Seidman & Rieder, 1994).

Yager and colleagues (1988) found a past prevalence of eating disorders in 2.1% of homosexual men compared with 0.33% of heterosexual men. Similarly, gay men score significantly higher on eating disorder screening measures, suggesting higher subthreshold disorders (Siever, 1994; Williamson & Hartly, 1998). Bingeing and purging symptomatology may be particularly relevant for homosexual males with lifetime prevalence rates 2.5 times higher than heterosexual men (French et al., 1996).

Several theories have been posited to explain why male homosexuality may contribute an inordinate risk for eating disorder. The most commonly-accepted theory is that BID plays a critical role in making homosexual men vulnerable to eating disorders (Hospers & Jansen, 2005). That is, BD which is "fueled by the possibly higher valuation on thinness" (Andersen, 1999: 208) is greater in gay men which, in turn, is largely predictive of the disturbed eating behaviors found in gay men. It is important to note, however, that BID in eating-disordered men may be somewhat different than that in eating-disordered women as the female ideal focuses primarily on thinness, whereas the male homosexual ideal cannot only be focused on being slender, but also on being muscular and may have greater varieties of ideals (Yelland & Tiggemann, 2003). Just as sociocultural pressures that focus on the value of thinness in heterosexual women place them at risk for the development of dieting and disordered eating, the greater sociocultural pressures on gay men (as compared with heterosexual men or lesbian women) to reach an ideal male figure comprises additional risk.

However, other studies suggest that self-reported femininity (i.e., the endorsement of personality traits and behaviors that are stereotypically feminine in nature) is the relevant risk factor for both heterosexual women and homosexual men, whereas masculinity confers a protective effect (Hospers & Jansen, 2005; Meyer et al., 2001). These studies, however, have focused almost exclusively on self-identified gay, Caucasian men.

To date, there has been only one study examining body image and eating-disordered behavior in minority MSM. This preliminary study examined these topics as part of a needs assessment for the AIDS Taskforce of Greater Cleveland, which had noted anecdotal concern about the frequency of eating and body image disturbance among the populations they serve. A total of 18 African American (AA) and Black Hispanic MSM participated (mean age = 20.64; SD = 2.59; mean BMI = 23.49; SD = 3.00). On the Eating Attitudes Test-26 (Garner, Olmstead, Bohr, & Garfinkel, 1982), an eating disorders screening measure, average total scores were not significantly higher than male norms. However, 19% of the sample scored above clinical cut-offs for possible ED. Further, one-quarter of the sample endorsed occasional or more frequent vomiting after meals, with 37.5% reporting an urge to vomit after eating and 31% reporting binge eating "often" or more frequently.

Additional supplemental items were written to query about behaviors that may be more relevant to MSM. On items assessing the frequency of other extreme body-changing behaviors, 25% endorsed regular use of "prohormones" and diet pills, 18.8% used female hormones, 33% had considered using anabolic–androgenic steroids to alter their body shape, and 38% had considered collagen or silicone. Conversely, the minority MSM in this study did not score differently than college-aged male norms on body esteem or situational BD. However, differences were shown on the bodybuilders image grid (BIG; Hildebrandt, Schlundt, Langenbucher, & Chung, 2006), a figure-rating scale that systematically varies body fat and musculature in which participants choose the figures they think best correspond to their ideal and current body. On the BIG, the minority MSM's self-ideal discrepancy for muscularity was almost three times greater than the norms for men working out regularly in a gym and 1.3 times greater than college-aged men. Self-ideal discrepancies for fatness were highly similar to male norms.

Two hypotheses were presented to explain the inconsistent results. First, measures comprising items that are developed and validated on college-aged heterosexual populations may not be appropriate for minority MSM. It was recommended that future work should develop instruments that specifically assess body image in MSM and such measures should be validated in diverse ethnic samples. Second, the diversity of body image ideals within a minority MSM population may lead to excessive variability and loss of possible effects. By collapsing men with diverse ideals into a singular small sample size group, such important differences may be lost. We will discuss the variety of ideals later in this chapter.

Body Image and HIV Risk Behavior

Although a fairly large literature exists examining the body image concerns of individuals living with HIV and AIDS (see Chapman, 2002 for a review), only four studies have examined the influence of body image on HIV risk behavior. In African American adolescent girls, after controlling for depression, self-esteem, and BMI, those who were more dissatisfied with their body image were more likely to fear abandonment as a result of negotiating condom use, more likely to perceive limited control in sexual relationships and more likely to worry about acquiring HIV (Wingood, DiClemente, Harrington, & Davies, 2002). Additionally, there was an association between greater BD and never using condoms during sexual intercourse (Wingood et al., 2002). In a similar population, BD was significantly related to fear of negotiating condom use, whereas greater self-concept predicted refusal of unprotected sex (Salazar, DiClemente, Wingood, Crosby, Harrington, & Davies, 2004). Among college students (sexual orientation was not queried), higher BMIs were associated with increased odds of having a casual sex partner (OR = 2.7) and being intoxicated during last intercourse (OR = 2.1) and using no or unreliable contraception (OR = 1.98; Eisenberg, Neumark-Sztainer, & Lus, 2005).

Conversely, in a gay male population, lower BMI and younger age predicted lower condom usage (Kraft, Robinson, Nordstrom, Bockting, & Simon Rosser, in press). Other studies indicate an increased risk of HIV transmission via intravenous drug use. Compared with females, males with eating disorders are more likely to have substance abuse as a comorbid condition (Andersen, 2002). BID, as expressed by muscle dysmorphia (sometimes referred to as "reverse anorexia"), is associated with very high prevalence of intravenous anabolic–androgenic steroid use (Kanayama, Barry, Hudson, & Pope, 2006; Keane, 2005). Finally, in a male Latino adolescent sample, poor body image— especially for acculturated youth—was a significant risk factor for substance abuse (Nieri, Kulis, Keith, & Hurdle, 2005).

In sum, these findings point to an area of important future research. Eating disturbance and BID are becoming more prevalent among both genders and MSM may be at particularly high risk. Such eating and body image disturbance may result in higher rates of HIV risk behaviors. However, studies have not previously examined ED or BID and their relationship to risk behaviors in a minority MSM population. Future work should explore this link further along with the prevention and clinical implications of body image in HIV risk behaviors.

Body Image and Other Risk Behaviors

Steroid use has been an isolated area of examining male populations in the body image literature. A number of studies have examined steroid use prevalence, its relationship to body image, and desire for weight loss or gain (Blouin & Goldfield, 1995; Drewnowski, Kurth, & Krahn, 1995; Schwerin, Corcoran, Fisher, Patterson, Askew, Olrich, et al., 1996). Investigations suggest that men who abuse steroids may be similar to women with eating disorders (Blouin & Goldfield, 1995). However, studies have failed to examine the differential ethnic influences, sexual orientation, or activity on men's drive for a certain physique, exercise adherence, or steroid use. Further, except for one study previously described (Heinberg et al., under review), studies have not included other drugs—particularly female hormones—that may be used/ abused by MSM populations.

MSM Body Image Ideals

Since very little empirical work has examined body image in MSM, particularly minority MSM, much of the remainder of this chapter is theoretical in nature. This review should be considered heuristic in nature rather than wholly descriptive of the vast experiences likely seen in minority MSM. We will organize the discussion around diverse body image ideals that may be seen in different groups as well as the behavioral implications of these ideals. A brief case report is included to illustrate the diversity of issues experienced by minority MSM with body image concerns.

There are a variety of body types that are valued and respected among men who have sex with men. However, as previously stated in the empirical literature, more is known about men who self-identify as gay versus the more broadly defined MSM population. Before the AIDS epidemic, gay men used to emulate the body image of the strong masculine man that was popular during the late 1970s by the Village People, a widely acclaimed male singing group whose songs contained homoerotic overtones and who were rumored to be gay themselves. This Village People look had a broad range of body types to emulate, ranging from the strong and tough leather man to the lean Indian. These ideals also included ethnic diversity represented through some of the first images of African American homosexual males (Bergling, 2007).

Probably, the most valued and emulated body type, at least among Caucasian self-identified gay men, is the young hairless muscular white male. This body type was strongly influenced by the Calvin Klein underwear ads featuring Mark Wahlberg, a well-known masculine rap artist who became popular in the late 1980s. Mark Wahlberg's body type in the underwear ads was of a muscular, hairless, White male who epitomized the "All-American bad boy." This young, healthy, masculine, and strong body type when achieved by gay males was a clear departure from the stereotypical effeminate male and the disturbing news media images of emaciated gay men in the late 1980s who were said to resemble concentration camp victims due to wasting syndrome from AIDS (Bergling, 2007).

Currently, the body types among gay male Caucasians vary widely from the Mark Wahlberg Calvin Klein underwear ad at one end of the spectrum to the images of the Village People's members. Even though the hairless, muscular, young, bad boy type prevails, there are other body type subgroups that are also valued. One look is the masculine, strong, mature, leather wearing man with plenty of body hair. This subtype was most likely the "masculine" image on which the Village People premised their own images. This subtype of masculinity can be traced back to the days of Tom of Finland, a well-known erotic male artist who was first popular in the 1960s (Bergling, 2007).

The bear look is another Caucasian body type that is valued. This can be a man who is muscular or overweight, has body hair, and can range in age from younger to older. This image of a gay male is strongly linked to the appearance of his body and tends to be a look some gay males grow into as they age, particularly the overweight bear type (Bergling, 2007).

Yet another image consists of the thin, young, boyish body type who can present a gender role from effeminate to androgynous. This look most likely develops in the early 20s when there may be more difficulty for some men to gain body mass from eating or exercise (Bergling, 2007).

One of the most popular body types is the collegiate, Caucasian, masculine, lean-muscled, and hairless body, epitomized in advertising for Abercrombie and Fitch. This type of look may be valued more greatly if the man also has blond hair and blue eyes. Images from gay porn to gay magazines such as the *Advocate* and *Details* abound, depicting the perfect blond hair, blue-eyed, Abercrombie and Fitch ideal (Bergling, 2007).

Minority MSM Body Image Ideals

One gay male body image that has been lacking in the media is men of color. Since the Village People of the 1970s, there have been very few images of African American gay men in the media. Additionally, there have been almost no images of Latino or Asian gay males portrayed. In the general male African American and Latino cultures, there appears to be a strong emphasis on masculinity. Musical artists and sports figures who are African American or Latino are often seen as almost hypermasculine. Strong cultural connections to traditional religions may not only reinforce traditional gender roles, but may also strongly condemn homosexuality. Similar to Caucasian gay males before the 1970s, minority MSM have one primary image of homosexuality presented through the media and that is femininity. What is largely portrayed by the media of Latino or African American gay males are images of campy effemininity or full-on female identity presented through female impersonation. One of the most well-known African American male/female impersonators was Rupaul. She became well known as a glamorous supermodel and performer during the 1990s. Unfortunately, Rupaul was the only image of a gay male of color portrayed in the media (Bergling, 2007).

Gay males of color seeking a role model are left to either take on the effeminate identity or to emulate the Caucasian gay male image. This leaves a strong masculine–feminine dichotomy within the gay male of color cultures. Gay men of color who take on a more effeminate identity may struggle with body image concerns related to weight and body shape and may consequently engage in problematic dieting, diet pill usage, purging, and restricting. Conversely, the body image concerns of minority MSM who internalize a more hypermasculine body image ideal are more likely to relate to muscularity. Amongst these individuals, concerns with steroid usage, exercise addiction, and binge/purge behavior are paramount (Bergling, 2007).

CASE STUDIES

Case Example #1

A is a 21-year-old biological male. His mother is a Latina and his father is an Italian. He grew up in South Florida. A often exhibited more feminine behaviors growing up (e.g., playing with girls' toys, identifying more with girls than boys, discomfort with rough and tumble sports). He was taunted and teased through school because of his atypical gender identity. As he approached middle school, he found himself attracted to males. Around the same time, he developed gynecomastia, a condition where breast tissue develops in males. A was self-conscious of his small breasts and asked his parents if he could have them removed through plastic surgery. After the breast surgery, he tried to take on a more masculine appearance which was strongly encouraged by his parents. After leaving home to attend a prestigious college in the mid-Atlantic East Coast, he reverted back to a more female identity. By his second year of college, he felt his identity was more of a female than a male. He began to perform as a female impersonator and began to get significant validation in his role as female. A entered a number of female impersonator pageants where he was judged on physical appearance. When he was not dressing as female, his identity was that of an effeminate male.

A has a history of body image concerns which revolves around thinness. He began restricting food and at times purging when he first got to college. As a male, he was uncomfortable with his lack of musculature and as a female he disliked his larger boned body and weight that he carried in his waist and stomach. At the same time, he had difficulty finding males interested in dating him, which he attributed to an attraction of gay males to more masculine-looking gay men. He found that the men who were attracted to him as a female were usually bisexual or heterosexual. He feared that they would discover that he was not a biological female and he worried that they were more attracted to him as a "she-male" in a more fetishistic way. He wished to feminize himself even more through the use of female hormones and plastic surgery, in order to assume a female identity on a full-time basis. However, he feared taking on a full-time female identity because of his lack of parental support, the possibility that educational and career opportunities would be limited as a result, and/or the fear of discrimination or abuse. Recently, a close African American male-to-female transsexual friend of his was beaten and burned to death in her apartment by a man she had recently met at a club.

A's body image concerns are influenced by a number of cultural factors. Growing up in the Miami area of South Florida may have created a greater body image focus due to the emphasis on physical attractiveness prevalent within the model and music culture existing in South Florida. Additionally, A's Latina mother and her family placed a strong emphasis on traditional femininity. A's mother is very petite and thin and many of his female relatives have similar body types. A's breast development and the surgical removal of the breast tissue during his adolescence also contributed to his body image concerns. A also spent a significant amount of time with other effeminate and masculine gay males in clubs and bars where the Caucasian gay male culture equated lean muscularity with beauty (Bergling, 2007). A's emphasis on body image increased as she assumed a more female identity, began performing as a female impersonator, and participated and competed in female impersonator beauty pageants, in which he was judged and rated against other contestants. Here, we see various cultural factors that contribute to A's body image concerns: South Florida beauty culture, gynecomastia, Latina femininity standards of thinness, gay male standards of thinness and muscularity, and the standards of female beauty reinforced by beauty pageants.

Case Study #2

P is a 26-year-old Korean American biological male. He initially presented for treatment because of severe body image disparagement related to acne scars and Asian facial features. P was born in Korea but spent most of his childhood and early adulthood being educated in Europe and the USA and had lived in the USA full time since attending college. He self-identifies himself as "straight" but has engaged in numerous sexual encounters with MSM, most of whom he meets anonymously in gay bars.

The patient was preoccupied by disparaging thoughts about his facial scars for most of his waking hours. The scars resulted from cystic acne that occurred during his teen years. Although the acne scars were visible, P largely overestimated their severity, redness, depth, and unattractiveness. That is, rather than recognizing that these were minor imperfections, he thought that they were marked disfigurements that would lead others to be uncomfortable looking at him, would result in staring and teasing, and were the only thing noticeable about his appearance. P spent many hours looking into the mirror, attempting to apply concealer make-up, checking his appearance in any reflective surface, such as a window, and combing his hair in an attempt to camouflage the scars. P was unable to work full-time, which he attributed to his facial appearance making employment an impossibility (i.e., an interviewer would be so repelled by the scarring that he would never be hired). In addition, to concerns about scarring, he voiced frequent complaints about his Asian features, particularly the shape of his eyes and nose. He also was quite concerned about his inability to grow enough facial hair to effectively cover the scars on his cheeks and chin. In the past, he had undergone a number of cosmetic procedures in an attempt to reduce the appearance of his scarring and had considered aesthetic surgery to change his Asian appearance.

Because of the severity of concerns, P was diagnosed with body dysmorphic disorder. Body dysmorphic disorder is a *DSM-IV* diagnosis restricted to cases of extremely severe body image disturbance. Body dysmorphic disorder has the following criteria, which P fully met: (1) a preoccupation with an imagined defect in appearance or if a slight physical anomaly is present, the individual's concern is markedly excessive; (2) the person's preoccupation causes clinically significant distress or impairment in social, occupational, or other important areas of functioning; (3) the preoccupation is not due to another mental disorder (e.g., dissatisfaction with body shape and size in anorexia nervosa) (APA, 1994).

P conceptualized his sexual behavior with men as a direct result of his body image concerns. He noted that his appearance made meeting women difficult but that he could successfully negotiate anonymous sex with men in the dark, bar environment. He asserted that if his skin could improve, he would be a "ladies' man."

Treatment for body dysmorphic disorder largely involves graded exposures and cognitive restructuring. Unfortunately, P was very resistant to the most minimal exposures and left treatment in favor of pursuing additional plastic surgery.

Implications and Future Directions

As this chapter has outlined, there are a variety of body image ideals for men, minority men, self-identified gay men, minority gay men, and MSM. This diversity of ideals makes assessment a challenge. Unlike the almost universal thin ideal that informs the assessment measures frequently utilized in female populations, a "one size fits all" assessment strategy is invalid for minority MSM.

First, body image assessment items that were developed and validated on college-aged heterosexual male populations are inappropriate for minority MSM. For example, the body sites of concerns, situations that cause distress and behavioral consequences (e.g., steroid use) may not tap into the sites, experiences, or behaviors that minority MSM find most distressing. Even instruments that have been normed on self-identified gay men may not be appropriate for use in a more diverse MSM population. Qualitative (e.g., focus groups) and quantitative researches are necessary to better assess the types of body image ideals, degree of disturbance, areas of interference, and behavioral consequences among diverse MSM.

Second, the diversity of body image ideals within a minority MSM population may lead to excessive variability and loss of possible effects. For example, minority MSM who have hypermasculine ideals may be interested in a muscular large physique, be dissatisfied if they do not achieve it, and engage in resultant problematic behaviors related to improving muscle mass. Conversely, minority MSM who favor a leaner look or a more feminine presentation may wish to be thinner and engage in unhealthy dieting or purging behavior in order to try to reach their ideal. By collapsing men with diverse ideals into a singular group and by utilizing a single instrument, such important distinctions will be lost. Future work should develop instruments that specifically assess body image in MSM, include a variety of body image ideals, and such measures should be validated in diverse ethnic samples.

This chapter has also reviewed the diversity of problematic behaviors that may result from body image distress including HIV risk behaviors, excessive dieting, purging, steroid use, and the use of other hormones and substances. Such risk, however, is largely based on studies outside of minority MSM. Although it is hypothesized that results may be generalizable to minority MSM, a clear link has not been established. Further, identification of which minority MSM groups may be at greater risk and which subgroups are at greater risk for specific problematic behaviors and the extent of these behaviors is largely unknown. A better understanding of body image and eating disturbance and their impact on high-risk sexual behaviors among MSM may have an important impact on individual and public health.

Finally, although interventions for body image disturbance have been established and shown to be remarkably efficacious among a variety of populations including body image disturbed women (Butters & Cash, 1987; Grant & Cash, 1995; Dworkin & Kerr, 1987), obese persons (Rosen, Orosan & Reiter, 1995), and individuals with body dysmorphic disorder (Neziroglu & Yaryura-Tobias, 1993; Veale, Gournay, Dryden, Boocock, Shah, Willson, & Walburn, 1996), male populations with body image distress, as a whole, have largely been neglected. The development of culturally competent, multidimensional interventions for body image disturbance in MSM is an immediate need in the field. Once established, such interventions should be tested for efficacy and potentially refined for use among a variety of minority MSM populations and to address a number of male ideals. For example, although basic intervention strategies may be helpful across subgroups, different components may need to be added or refined for those with muscular ideals versus those wishing a more feminine appearance.

References

American Psychiatric Association (1994). *Diagnostic and statistical manual for mental disorders (4th edition)*. Washington: American Psychiatric Association.

Andersen, A. (1999). Eating disorders in gay males. *Psychiatric Annals, 29*, 206–212.

Andersen, A. E., Cohn, L., & Holbrook, T. (2000). *Making weight: Men's concerns with food, weight, shape and appearance*. Carlsbad, CA: Gurze Books.

Austin, S. B., Ziyadeh, N., Kahn, J. A., Camargo, C. A., Coditz, G. A., & Field, A. E. (2004). Sexual orientation, weight concerns, and eating-disordered behaviors in adolescent girls and boys. *Journal of the American Academy of Child and Adolescent Psychiatry, 43*(9), 1115–1123.

Becker, A. E., Franko, D. L., Speck, A., & Herzog, D. B. (2003). Ethnicity and differential access to care for eating disorder symptoms. *International Journal of Eating Disorders, 33*, 205–212.

Bergling, T. (2007). *Chasing Adonis: Gay men and the pursuit of perfection*. Binghamton, NY: Harrington Park Press.

Blouin, A. G., & Goldfield, G. S. (1995). Body image and steroid use in male bodybuilders. *International Journal of Eating Disorders, 18*, 159–165.

Boroughs, M., & Thompson, J. K. (2002). Exercise status and sexual orientation as moderators of body image disturbance and eating disorders in males. *International Journal of Eating Disorders, 31*, 307–311.

Butters, J. W., & Cash, T. F. (1987). Cognitive-behavioral treatment of women's body-image dissatisfaction. *Journal of Consulting and Clinical Psychology, 55*, 889–897.

Cáceres, C. F. (2002). HIV among gay and other men who have sex with men in Latin America and the Caribbean: a hidden epidemic? *AIDS, 16 Suppl* , S23–33.

Carlat, D. J., Camargo, C. A., & Herzog, D. B. (1997). Eating disorders in males: A report on 135 patients. *American Journal of Psychiatry, 154*, 1127–1132.

Cash, T. F. (2002). The Situational Inventory of Body-Image Dysphoria: Psychometric evidence and development of a short form. *International Journal of Eating Disorders, 32*, 362–366.

Cash, T. F., Morrow, J. A., Hrabosky, J. I., & Perry, A. A. (2004). How has body image changed? A cross-sectional investigation of college women and men from 1983 to 2001. *Journal of Consulting and Clinical Psychology, 72*(6), 1081–1089.

Chapman, E. (2002). Body image and the complications of HIV treatment. *Focus, 17*, 1–5.

Corson, P. W., & Andersen, A. E. (2003). Body image issues among boys and men. In T. F. Cash & T. Pruzinsky (Eds.), *Body image: A handbook of theory, research, and clinical practice*. New York: Guilford Press.

Currin, L., Schmidt, U., Treasure, J., & Jick, H. (2005). Time trends in eating disorders incidence. *British Journal of Psychiatry, 186*, 132–135.

Drewnowski, A., Kurth, C. L., & Krahn, D. D. (1995). Effects of body image on dieting, exercise, and anabolic steroid use in adolescent males. *International Journal of Eating Disorders, 17*, 381–386.

Dworkin, S. H., & Kerr, B. A. (1987). Comparison of interventions for women experiencing body image problems. *Journal of Counseling Psychology, 34*, 136–140.

Eagles, J. M., Johnston, M. I., Hunter, D., Lobban, M., & Millar, H. R. (1995). Increasing incidence of anorexia nervosa in the female population of northeast Scotland. *American Journal of Psychiatry, 152*, 1266–1271.

Eisenberg, M. E., Neumark-Sztainer, D., & Lust, K. D. (2005). Weight-related issues and high-risk sexual behaviors among college students. *Journal of American College Health, 54*, 95–101.

Feingold, A. (1992). Good-looking people are not what we think. *Psychological Bulletin, 111*, 304–341.

French, S. A., Story, M., Remafedi, G., Resnick, M. D., & Blum, R. W. (1996). Sexual orientation and prevalence of body dissatisfaction and eating disordered behaviors: A population-based study of adolescents. *International Journal of Eating Disorders, 19*, 119–126.

Garner, D. M., Garfinkel, P. E., Schwartz, D., & Thompson, M. (1980). Cultural expectations of thinness in women. *Psychological Reports, 47*, 483–491.

Garner, D. M., Olmstead, M. P., Bohr, Y., & Garfinkel, P. E. (1982). The Eating Attitudes Test: Psychometric features and clinical correlates. *Psychological Medicine, 12*, 871–878.

Gettelman, T. E., & Thompson, J. K. (1993). Actual differences and stereotypical perceptions in body image and eating disturbance: A comparison of male and female heterosexual and homosexual samples. *Sex Roles, 29*, 545–562.

Grant, J., & Cash, T. F. (1995). Cognitive-behavioral body-image therapy: Comparative efficacy of group and modes-contact treatments. *Behavior Therapy, 26*, 69–84.

Heinberg, L. J., Haythornthwaite, J. A., Rosofsky, W., McCarron, P., & Clarke, A. (2000). Body image and weight loss compliance in elderly African-American hypertensives. *American Journal of Health Behavior, 24*(3), 163–173.

Heinberg, L. J., Pike, E., & Loue, S. (under review). Body image and eating disturbance in minority men who have sex with men: Preliminary observations. *Journal of Homosexuality*.

Heinberg, L. J., & Thompson, J. K. (2006). Body Image. In S. Wonderlich, J. E. Mitchell, M. deZwaan, & H. Steiger, (Eds.) *Annual review of eating disorders: Part 2 – 2006*. Oxford, UK: Radcliffe Publishing Ltd.

Hildebrandt, T., Schlundt, D., Langenbucher, J., & Chung, T. (2006). Presence of muscle dysmorphia symptomatology among male weightlifters. *Comprehensive Psychiatry, 47*, 127–135.

Hoek, H. W., & van Hoeken, D. (2003). Review of the prevalence and incidence of eating disorders. *International Journal of Eating Disorders, 34*, 383–396.

Hospers, H. J., & Jansen, A. (2005). Why homosexuality is a risk factor for eating disorders in males. *Journal of Social and Clinical Psychology, 24*, 1188–1201.

Joiner, T. E. Jr., Vohs, K. D., & Heatherton, T. F. (2000). Three studies on the factorial distinctiveness of binge eating and bulimic symptoms among nonclinical men and women. *International Journal of Eating Disorders, 27*(2), 198–205.

Kanayama, G., Barry, S., Hudson, J. I., & Pope, H. G. (2006). Body image and attitudes toward male roles in anabolic-androgenic steroid users. *American Journal of Psychiatry, 163*, 697–703.

Keane, H. (2005). Diagnosing the male steroid user: drug use, body image and disordered masculinity. *Health (London), 9*(2), 189–208.

Kimmel, S. B., & Mahalik, J. R. (2005). Body image concerns of gay men: The roles of minority stress and conformity to masculine norms. *Journal of Consulting and Clinical Psychology, 73*, 1185–1190.

Kraft, C., Robinson, B. E., Nordstrom, D. L., Bockting, W. O., & Simon Rosser, B. R. (in press). Obesity, body image, and unsafe sex in men who have sex with men. *Archives of Sexual Behavior*.

Lewinsohn, P. M., Shankman, S. A., Gua, J. M., & Klein, D. N. (2004). The prevalence and co-morbidity of subthreshold psychiatric conditions. *Psychological Medicine, 34*, 613–622.

Morrison, M. A., Morrison, T. G., & Sager, C. (2004). Does body dissatisfaction differ between gay men and lesbian women and heterosexual men and women? A meta-analytic review. *Body Image, 1*(2), 127–138.

Neziroglu, F. A., & Yaryura-Tobias, J. A. (1993). Exposure, response prevention and cognitive therapy in the treatment of body dysmorphic disorder. *Behavior Therapy, 24*, 431–438.

Nieri, T., Kulis, S., Keith, V. M., & Hurdle, D. (2005). Body image, acculturation, and substance abuse among boys and girls in the Southwest. *American Journal of Drug and Alcohol Abuse, 31*, 617–639.

Petrie, T. A., Austin, L. J., Crowley, B. J., Helmcaup, A., Johnson, C. E., Lester, R., et al. (1996). Sociocultural expectations of attractiveness for males. *Sex Roles, 35*, 581–601.

Pomeroy, C. (2004). Assessment of medical status and physical factors. In J. K. Thompson (Ed.), *Handbook of eating disorders and obesity* (pp. 81–111). Hoboken, NJ: Wiley Press.

Pope, H. G. Jr, Gruber, A. J., Mangweth, B., Bureau, B., deCol, C., Jouvent, R., et al. (2000). Body image perception among men in three countries. *American Journal of Psychiatry, 157*(8), 1297–1301.

Pope, H. G. Jr, Phillips, K. A., & Olivardia, R. (2000). *The Adonis complex: The secret crisis of male body obsession*. New York: Free Press.

Pulvers, K. M., Lee, R. E., Kaur, H., Mayo, M. S., Fitzgibbon, M. L., Jeffries, S. K., et al., (2004). Development of a culturally relevant body image instrument among urban African Americans. *Obesity Research, 10*, 1641–1651.

Rosen, J. C., Orosan, P., & Reiter, J. (1995). Cognitive behavioral body image therapy for negative body images in obese women. *Behavior Therapy, 26*, 25–42.

Russell, C. J., & Keel, P. K. (2002). Homosexuality as a specific risk factor for eating disorders in men. *International Journal of Eating Disorders, 31*, 300–306.

Salazar, L. F., DiClemente, R. J., Wingood, G. M., Crosby, R. A., Harrington, K., Davies, S. et al. (2004). Self-concept and adolescents' refusal of unprotected sex: A test of mediating mechanisms among African American girls. *Prevention Science, 5*, 137–149.

Schwerin, M. J., Corcoran, K. J., Fisher, L., Patterson, D., Askew, W., Olrich, T., et al. (1996). Social physique anxiety, body esteem, and social anxiety in bodybuilders and self-reported anabolic steroid users. *Addictive Behaviors, 21*, 1–8.

Seidman, S. N., & Rieder, R. O. (1994). A review of sexual behavior in the United States. *American Journal of Psychiatry, 151*, 330–341.

Seiver, M. D. (1994). Sexual orientation and gender as factors in socioculturally acquired vulnerability to body dissatisfaction and eating disorders. *Journal of Consulting and Clinical Psychology, 62*, 252–260.

Strong, S. M., Williamson, D. A., Netemeyer, R. G., & Geer, J. H. (2000). Eating disorder symptoms and concerns about body differ as a function of gender and sexual orientation. *Journal of Social and Clinical Psychology, 19*, 240–255.

Veale, D., Gournay, K., Dryden, W., Boocock, A., Shah, F., Willson, R., et al. (1996). Body dysmorphic disorder: A cognitive behavioural model and pilot randomised controlled trial. *Behaviour Research and Therapy, 34*, 717–729.

Warren, M., & Hildebrand, T. (2006). Proceedings from the Male Special Interest Group. *International Conference for Eating Disorders*, Barcelona, Spain.

Williamson, I., & Hartley, P. (1998). British research into the increased vulnerability of young gay men to eating disturbance and body dissatisfaction. *European Eating Disorders Review, 6*, 160–170.

Wingood, G. M., DiClemente, R. J., Harrington, K., & Davies, S. L. (2002). Body image and African American females' sexual health. *Journal of Women's Health & Gender-Based Medicine, 11*, 433–439.

Wiseman, C. V., Gray, J. J., Mosimann, J. E., & Ahrens, A. H. (1992). Cultural expectations of thinness in women: An update. *International Journal of Eating Disorders, 11*, 85–89.

Yager, J., Kurtzman, F., Landsverk, J., & Wiesmeier, E. (1988). Behaviors and attitudes related to eating disorders in homosexual male college students. *American Journal of Psychiatry, 145*, 495–497.

Yelland, C., & Tiggemann, M. (2003). Muscularity and the gay ideal: Body dissatisfaction and disordered eating in homosexual men. *Eating Behaviors, 4*(2), 107–116.

Portrait Five
Cutting

Anonymous

This is an excerpt from an interview with an African–American gay man in his mid-20s. Jefferson, [a fictive name], is a college student at a private university. He recently came out to his family, although he has known for some time that he is gay. In this part of the interview, he discusses his cutting and purging.

I would describe myself as lonely. I'm sick. Sickening. When I was growing up, my sister looked this way, my brother looked this way. I was like one of a kind. I don't know any darker, dark kid previously, so when I was growing up as a kid in Ohio, it was funny because, like everybody, there's only like four dark people in my whole family so I was a darkie, yeah. I just think I'm sick.

The only reason I cut myself is because I thought it would drain all the bad out of me, to make me feel a different type of way because, I don't know, it was stupid. I'll be sitting there and I was like, I can't take it, but let me try this and I just cut and while I was bleeding, I just feel some, I feel good. Like it's yes, that's how it's supposed to, it was like, I felt better when I was leaking. I didn't like being me. Okay, it was something, escape, it made me not be, or made me feel better about being, right?

Even when I was younger, I was gay. We were only kicking and assing everybody, so it was quite me not to be valued but it was cool. Then, I used to puke because I didn't like the way I looked. That wasn't good either because, um, I always messed with boys, like I don't gain weight at all. Very skinny for my size. I can eat whatever I want to and still be skinny. I got hypoglycemia, like I always keep a snack on me or something. It was stupid. I don't see why I wanted to do it. Back then made me feel like I was feeling good. Like when it came out, it made all the pain inside come out with all the other stuff, so that's why I was into blood and cut myself. It was just I don't know, I don't know how to explain it.

So reading them books, they were talking about people puking and cutting and I'm like, well, I can puke and I can cut. Maybe I feel like cutting me. They were looking fabulous in the magazines. Like, if you can puke and you can cut, you can look like that. Well, I feel like I can puke and cut. Well, see, that was killing me because like I don't know it's stupid.

I know I'm not stupid but doing that, that was somewhat stupid. Because think about it, if I was just not paying no attention, pain and everything it does,

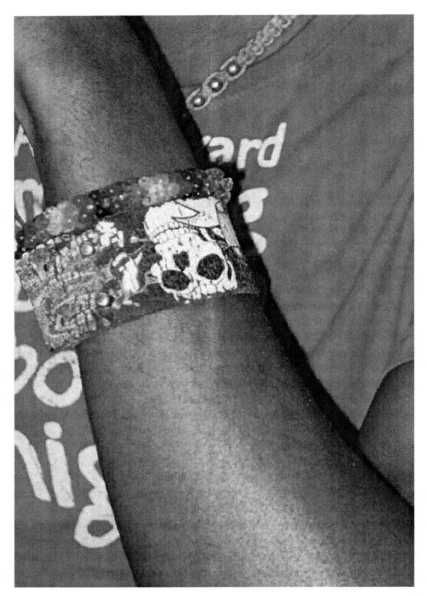

Fig. P5.1

because I was letting everything get, get to me. Like this was pissing me off and I couldn't say nothing because I was so young, so I would do this to my myself or this happened during that day. I can't tell my parents because they weren't paying attention, so I feel the same way about just, it made me feel better about me when I was doing.

So what was bad inside? Being gay for god sakes. Back then, I thought I was
a three. There wasn't nobody that ever told me I was ugly. I was always like,
you're a cute kid and then I heard hot, sexy... I always heard it and I wasn't, for
God sakes look at me, my lips are big, my nose is big, my head is very long, my
body is very skinny.

So what made the change? Getting tired of it. Just was over it, hate it, like
I can't just make me feel every day, I want to do the same thing. You make me
feel like 45 minutes to an hour, all is said and done. I feel this way, that way, but
then after a long while, you start looking at your arms and you start getting
tracks and scrapes and people start asking. I just stopped doing, I just was fed
up. I cut myself with a knife, it hurt, please give me a nice little nick okay.

So, if there was a younger guy cutting or puking [I'd tell him], you don't need
to, because at the end of the day, you're still going to feel that same way you did
5 minutes before you cut yourself. Ain't going to make you feel no type of
difference. Going to give you more of a headache, make you miserable. You
may think, you may seem like every time you do it, you feel just a little bit better
and you can't bear no more but you can. Think about it. Just think about it. In a
situation like what, you said if you don't know what you're doing, if you cut,
you can die or you bleed half out, now you go to the hospital and people looking
at you like you are trying to commit suicide. What you wanting to do? Puking
early could tear-up your esophagus. You'll learn, they'll learn. I've been doing
that. The erosion of the throat, that, please, you don't know what that will do.
The acid that comes up and goes back down. The erosion, I know you don't
need to do it, it's not that serious, never was completely. At the end of the day,
you're still going to be you and if people didn't like you, then they won't like you
now, too, and that's what I think. If they make you feel that bad, stay away
from them, that's what I do, I stay away from them, they make me feel such a
tray full away that I feel like hurting myself or hurting them maybe you can stay
whose company I can do without. That's a clue towards me.

People don't talk to kids, not like real talk to them. Like, basically, well,
yeah, basically a kid wants somebody who can sit there and relate to what they
do, been through, or going through. You can't sit there and try to sugar coat it.

Popping pills is like so ignorant. Trying to kill yourself with the pills... It's
ignorant. Because baby, that never worked. Okay, I'm not going to say it never
worked, but it rarely works. You got to take a whole bottle of pills. Get that two
and a half hour high. They're going to find you stroked in the middle of the
bathroom in a puddle of spit. They're going to make you chew Vaseline, they're
going to make you eat Vaseline. Lube you up with a, like four inch thick pipe,
shove it down your throat and make you spit through her. Your throat is going
to hurt for weeks on end because she has worked your esophagus. For what?
Because you didn't like life that bad? Baby please! I never kill myself, I try to
hurt myself, yes, that was stupid, but I ain't been to the extreme. Pop pills, or
sniff something, or drink, I never did, oh, I started off, okay. I don't want to die,
I want to hurt. Why do you want to hurt? Because I want to make myself feel.
Basically I live to feel so that's why.

Chapter Four
Substance Use among Minority Men who have Sex with Men

Sana Loue and Jaroslaw Richard Romaniuk

Introduction

This chapter addresses substance use among several subgroups of minority men who have sex with men (MSM). This term encompasses several distinct groups of men: those who self-identify as gay, bisexual, or transgender; incarcerated self-identified heterosexual men who, due to their circumstances, engage in voluntary sex with other men; self-identified heterosexual men who engage in sex with other men as a means of survival during incarceration, periods of homelessness, or for economic gain; men who have sex with females and with male-to-female (MTF) transgender persons; and men who self-identify as "same-gender loving" or "sexual freaks" (Goldbaum, Perdue, & Higgins, 1996; Mays, Cochran, & Zamudio, 2004). The chapter focuses specifically on minority men who self-identify as gay (homosexual), bisexual, and/or transgender.

Published literature suggests that the incidence of substance use of all types among gay and lesbian populations is high. The incidence has been estimated to be between 28 and 35% (Kelly, 1991; Lohrenz, Connelly, Coyne, & Spare 1978; Morales & Graves, 1983; Saghir & Robins, 1973; Stall & Wiley, 1988), in comparison with an incidence of 10–12% in the general population (Cabaj, 2000). Although it had previously been postulated that homosexuality itself causes alcoholism (Israelstam & Lambert, 1983), it is now believed that the high incidence of alcohol and other substance use among gay men is attributable to the internal and external psychological effects of heterosexism and homophobia and to genetic and biological factors. Specific risk factors that have been identified include antigay discrimination and harassment (McKirnan & Peterson, 1989; Stall et al., 2001), childhood sex abuse (Paul, Catania, Pollack, & Stall, 2001), low self-esteem (Ghindia & Kola, 1996), a habit of socializing in bar settings (Cabaj, 2000; Paul, Barrett, Crosby, & Stall, 1996; Stall et al., 2001),

Sana Loue
Case Western Reserve University, School of Medicine, Cleveland, OH

S. Loue (ed.), *Health Issues Confronting Minority Men Who Have Sex with Men.*
© Springer 2008

participation in circuit parties (Mansergh, Colfax, Marks, Rader, Guzman, & Buchbinder, 2001), and genetic factors (Cabaj, 2000). Each of these is discussed below in greater detail.

The prevalence of substance use among MTF transgender persons also appears high. A study conducted in San Francisco with 392 transgender persons reported that of the MTF participants, 64% used marijuana, 30% used speed, and 21% used crack cocaine (Clements, 1999). Alcohol and methamphetamine have also been found to be in common use among MTF transgender persons (Rebac & Lombardi, 2001).

Unfortunately, despite the growing recognition of substance use within gay and lesbian populations, relatively little research has focused specifically on the extent of substance use and the prevention and treatment needs of minority MSM. For this reason, we review first the developmental process for the formation of male gender identity within US culture, relying on a framework derived from masculinities studies. We then discuss the psychological and social implications for non-gender conforming male identity development. Since trauma and childhood sexual abuse (CSA) are significant problems among men having sex with men (Paul et al., 2001), we will also describe the effects of trauma and CSA on the mental health and identity formation of MSM. We next review the literature related to substance use within MSM populations generally and then address issues specific to African American, Latino, and Asian and Pacific Islander MSM. We conclude the chapter with specific suggestions for further theoretical and empirical research related to etiology, prevention, and treatment for minority MSM.

Defining Men and Masculinity in the USA

The Development of Masculine Identity

Defining a "man," apart from a biological definition that incorporates hormone levels, chromosomes, and genital organs, is inextricably linked to our definition of "masculinity" (Whitehead & Barrett, 2001). "Masculinities" have been defined as

> those behaviours, languages and practices, existing in specific cultural and organiza-
> tional locations, which are commonly associated with males and thus culturally defined
> as not feminine. So masculinities exist as both a positive, inasmuch as they offer some
> means of identity signification for males, and as a negative, inasmuch as they are not
> the 'Other' (feminine) (Whitehead & Barrett, 2001: 15–16).

The more positive traits that have been associated with masculinity include a willingness to sacrifice self for family; loyalty, dedication, and commitment; the ability to solve problems and the willingness to take risks to do so; and self-reliance, fortitude, persistence, and calm (Levant, 1995). And, although conceptions of masculinity vary across different American subgroups, it has been asserted that

> there is a core which is common to most: courage, endurance and toughness, lack of squeamishness when confronted with shocking or distasteful stimuli, avoidance of display in weakness in general, reticence about emotional or idealistic matters, and sexual competency (Stouffer et al., 1976).

Manhood in the United States, then, has been defined through various restrictive, societally imposed edicts:

1. "No Sissy Stuff." One may never do anything that even remotely suggests femininity. Masculinity is the relentless repudiation of the feminine.
2. "Be a Big Wheel." Masculinity is measured by power, success, health, and status. As the saying goes, "He who has the most toys wins when he dies."
3. "Be a Sturdy Oak." Masculinity depends on remaining calm and reliable in crises, holding emotions in check. In fact, proving you're a man depends on never showing your emotions at all. Boys don't cry.
4. "Give 'em Hell." Exude an aura of manly daring and aggression. Go for it. Take risks (Brannon, 1976).

Similarly, the "masculine mystique" emphasizes restrictive emotionality, health care problems, obsession with achievement and success, restricted sexual and affectionate behavior, and concerns about power, control, competition, and homophobia (O'Neil, 1982). The "elements" of the male role have been said to include "the anti-feminine element," the "success element," the "aggressiveness elements," and the "sexual element" (Doyle, 1989).

It has been argued that, as a consequence, the birthright of every American male is a chronic sense of personal inadequacy (Woolfolk & Richardson, 1978) and that men's true fear "is not fear of women but of being ashamed or humiliated in front of other men, or being dominated by stronger men" (Leverenz, 1986: 451). If this is, indeed, true, then homophobia has little to do with homosexual experience and everything to do with, as one man stated:

> the fear that other men will unmask us, emasculate us, reveal to us and the world that we do not measure up, that we are not real men. We are afraid to let other men see that fear. Fear makes us ashamed, because the recognition of fear in ourselves is proof to ourselves that we are not as manly as we pretend... (Kimmel, 2003: 104).

It has been hypothesized that, as a result, the development of male gender identity involves the construction of positional identities, whereby a sense of the self is solidified through separation from others (Chodorow, 1978). For men who both fear and desire connection with others, organized sports provides a mechanism for interaction, while still focusing on hierarchical position, e.g., being number one (Messner, 2003).

The establishment of positional identity is evident in other domains, as well. One psychiatrist commented:

> Men become depressed because of loss of status and power in the world of men. It is not
> the loss of money, or the material advantages that money could buy, which produces
> the despair that leads to self-destruction. It is the "shame," the "humiliation," the sense
> of personal "failure"... A man despairs when he has ceased being a man among men
> (Gaylin, 1992: 32).

Accordingly, this process of establishing and asserting one's identity is said, then, to explain much of heterosexual male behavior in the United States: men must act in a way that eliminates any possibility that others will get the "wrong idea": withholding any expression of feelings, displaying sexual predation with women, walking and talking in a specified manner (Kimmel, 2003). There are, however, exceptional situations in which men are permitted to behave in ways that, under other circumstances, would negate their masculinity. Depictions of war, for instance, allow men to hold and comfort each other (Easthope, 1986).

It has been argued, though, that the establishment of a male identity has become increasingly difficult for men due to relatively recent profound changes in men's situations: women's increasing exercise of choice in relationships, divorce, and childbearing; the decreasing likelihood that men will enjoy a secure, life-long career or employment situation; the increasing number of dual-income households in lieu of households where the male is the sole breadwinner; and the increasing visibility of groups once relegated to society's margins, such as gay men, women, and persons of color (Whitehead & Barrett, 2001).

Violence, it has been asserted, or the willingness to engage in violence constitutes one mechanism for the establishment of manhood and masculinity or, in other words, positional identity (Kimmel, 2003). This is reflected in the observation that the insults most shaming to men are those that challenge the existence or the extent of their courage or manliness, including their sexual adequacy: "wimp," "coward," "sissy," "fairy" (Gilligan, 2001: 571). One writer observed:

> Little boys learn the connection between violence and manhood very early in life.
> Fathers indulge in mock prize fights and wrestling matches with eight-year-olds.
> Boys play cowboys and Indians with guns and arrows proffered by their elders. They
> are gangsters or soldiers interchangeably-the lack of difference between the two is more
> evident to them than to their parents. They are encouraged to "fight back," and
> bloodied noses and black eyes become trophies of their pint-sized virility (Komisar,
> 1976).

Exclusionary devices offer an additional route for the establishment and maintenance of a positional hierarchy. Through exclusion, those deemed less manly are relegated to lower positions in the hierarchy-women, gay men, men of color, nonnative-born men, men of lower socioeconomic status, etc. Those men deemed to be less "manly" reflect subordinate and marginal masculinities (Whitehead & Barrett, 2001). Through exclusion, "manhood" embodies sexism, racism, and homophobia (Kimmel, 2003).

Stigmatization and Discrimination of Non-Gender Conforming Men

Stigma has been defined as a "mark" that sets an individual apart from others, linking the "marked" individual to an undesirable characteristic or feature, ultimately leading to the individual's rejection and isolation (Jones, Farina, Hastorf, Markus, Miller, & Scott, 1984). Stigma may be associated with behaviors, such as abuse of substances or sexual practices; structural abnormalities or features, such as skin color; functional abnormalities, including mental illness; contagious diseases, epitomized by HIV/AIDS and leprosy; and other sources (Goffman, 1963; Reingold, 2001). The extent to which an individual is isolated may vary as a function of the strength of the individual's association with the undesirable characteristic(s). For some individuals, the extent or intensity of the stigma may be compounded by association with more than one "marking" characteristics, resulting in a "layering" of stigma (Capitanio & Herek, 1999; Herek, 1999; Herek & Capitanio, 1999; McBride, 1998; Reidpath & Chan, 2005). Stigma has been found to be associated with numerous adverse effects (Goffman, 1963), including avoidance of help-seeking (Chesney & Smith, 1999; Dinos et al., 2001), reduced levels of self-esteem (Link, Struening, Neese-Todd, Asmussen, & Phelan, 2001), and persistence of depressive symptoms (Link, Struening, Rahav, Phelan, & Nuttbrock, 1997).

Minority MSM, then, are multiply "marked." They engage in behavior-sexual relations with other men-that by itself may result in stigmatization. Skin color-being non-White-adds yet another level of stigma, which may be further compounded by marking characteristics such as primary language, for instance, Spanish rather than English; place of birth outside of the US mainland, citizenship status; and the portrayal of HIV/AIDS as a "gay disease."

Individuals attempt to manage stigma using a variety of strategies that fall along a reactive—proactive continuum (Siegel, Lune, & Meyer, 1998). Reactive strategies include concealment of the characteristic, selective disclosure of possession of the stigmatizing attribute, and adoption of a personal attribution style, whereby an individual creates distinctions between him- or herself and others with the same condition in order to set him- or herself apart from those who are stigmatized. Proactive strategies include preemptive disclosure, whereby the individuals makes his or her status known, akin to a preemptive strike; participation in public education efforts to dispel public stigma; and social activism, to reframe the issue and public perceptions. Intermediate strategies between these two poles include the gradual disclosure of the condition or characteristic, selective affiliation with those who are nonstigmatizing, the discrediting of one's discreditors, and challenges to the moral attributions associated with particular conditions (e.g., mental illness reflects a character weakness, is moral retribution for past behavior, etc.) (Siegel et al., 1998).

Trauma in the Life of MSM

Stigma and discrimination may affect the lives of MSM not only in the form of social isolation and limited support but in the form of covert and overt abuse and violence that lead to traumatic experiences. Homophobia, also called homonegativism, by itself could be considered trauma for MSM (Herek, 1991; Kort, 2004). However, several characteristics of MSM youth may lead to a specific vulnerability of this minority group (Garofalo & Katz, 2001).

First, individuals may be alienated from their families and peers due to discrimination and the scarcity of role models (Gwadz, Clatts, Leonard, & Goldsamt 2004; Rivers, 2004). In response, many of them run away from home looking for places where they can be accepted and understood and find themselves in very unsafe places (Cochran Stewart, Ginzler & Cauce, 2002). Second, the secrecy surrounding their sexual desires and behaviors may additionally expose gay youth to exploitation and abuse. Some gay youth with more feminine traits and no coping skills in controlling their sexual behavior could attract sexual predators (D'Augellis, Grossman, & Starks, 2006; Doll et al., 1992).

The constellation of these factors may result in increased vulnerability to sexual abuse and exploitation during childhood. In fact, research has also shown that CSA happens more often among men with multiple minority status (Balsam et al., 2004).

CSA has been found to have a devastating effect on youth identity formation (Doll et al., 1992; Sageman, 2003). Research conducted with women (Chu & Dill, 1990; Epstein, Saunders, Kilpatrick, & Resnick 1998; Wyatt, Guthrie, & Notgrass 1992) has shown that CSA often leads to dissociative symptoms, depression, and use of escape-avoidance coping skills including substance abuse. The feeling of loss of control as the result of CSA may lead to symptoms of learned helplessness and feelings of powerlessness and self-destruction (Paul et al., 2001), as well as increased risk of sexual revictimization, problems with sexuality and sex addiction, substance abuse, and HIV infection (Epstein et al., 1998; Heidt, Marx, & Gold, 2005; Kalichman, Gore-Felton, Benotsch, Cage, & Rompa 2004; Kort, 2004; Stewart, 1996). (The relationship between CSA and HIV risk among Latino MSM is addressed in detail by Grant Arreola in this volume.)

The most difficult time in the life of gay men is childhood. This is the time when they begin feeling the incongruity of their own desires and behaviors and those of their male peers. The process of building the self is challenged by the gay child's comparison of his likes and wants and his innocent dreams with the normative reaction of the external social environment, which may include extreme acts of humiliation and violence in response to the child's expression of those dreams and desires (Garofalo & Katz, 2001). Gay youth have limited resources in dealing with school bullying, a phenomenon many face growing up. Without help and support, they often develop the characteristics of a victim. Years after school, one in ten gay men still experience flashbacks related to school bullying (Rivers, 2004). Gay youth with a history of CSA are also a significant group among youth who run away from home (Cochran et al., 2002). Some of them are homeless and use sex for money as a surviving tool. This group of homeless youth has the most negative behavioral and mental health outcomes. Alcohol and drugs help these homeless youth to survive, so they see substance use as an acceptable coping skill. Living on the street is commonly described as a tough life for men, and the men, hardened by their experiences, are seen as threatening and frightening. In reality, detachment from their feelings and struggles with power and control (including delinquency), so often factors in their homelessness, may be the result of poor family support and history of CSA (Ford, Chapman, Mack, & Pearson, 2006).

Another form of powerful victimization is hate crimes. When a gay youth, who already feels alienated from his peers, is the victim of a hate crime, he may come to believe that "he deserves it" (Herek, Gillis, & Cogan 1999). It has been established that hate crimes are underreported to police and authorities. The mental health effects of hate crime are depression, self-condemnation, lack of self-confidence, low self-esteem, and even acute stress disorder (Kaysen, Lostutter, & Goines 2005).

In his discussion of the effects of discrimination on African Americans, Dimsdale (2000) hypothesized that chronic trauma could lead to an elevated autonomic response. The symptoms of somatization as a result of trauma are well established (van der Kolk et al., 1996). Recently, the effects of sexual and physical abuse on gastrointestinal disorders were described (Drossman, Talley, Leserman, Olden, & Barreiro, 1995). Although we can hypothesize that the chronic stress that is a part of the lives of MSM may affect both psychological and physiological health (Cochran & Sullivan, 2003; Herek, Cogan, Gillis, & Glunt 1997), an epidemiological study of sexual minorities is still lacking.

The next section of this chapter focuses on the implications of discrimination and trauma in the lives of MSM and the use of substances as one strategy that may be utilized in an attempt to deal with adverse factors in their lives.

Developmental Issues for Gay-Identified and Non-Gay-Identified Men

Dissociation

The use of substances permits the individual to act on feelings that he may have denied or repressed due to internalized homophobia, trauma, and/or other factors but renders the integration of intimacy and love with sex increasingly difficult. As a result, sex and intimacy among some gay men are often dissociated from each other (Cabaj, 2000). The use of substances in conjunction with sexual activity may persist during the formation of a social and personal identity, resulting in a temporary alleviation, but long-term exacerbation of self-hatred, depression, and lowered self-esteem.

Because of the long history of harassment against sexual minority individuals, it has become a commonplace for members of sexual minority groups to socialize in clubs and bars. Alcohol and drugs may lower inhibitions and relieve feelings of guilt and anxiety related to internalized homophobia, and/or concerns regarding one's body image (Hicks, 2000; McKirnan & Peterson, 1989). It is not surprising, then, that a proportion of gay men abuse or become dependent on alcohol in view of the reliance on bars and clubs as a venue for meeting and socializing with others and, for some, the addition of a genetic predisposition to alcohol dependence.

Methamphetamine and cocaine use have been found to be significant among gay men (Peck, Reback, Yang, Rotheram-Fuller, & Shoptaw 2005; Stall et al., 2001). It has been hypothesized that these drugs may be particularly appealing to gay men because of the highly sexualized subculture within the larger gay community; the elevation in mood and self-confidence, initial increased alertness, and lowering of anxiety and social inhibitions produced by these particular drugs; a reinforcing social environment; and the synergistic effect produced through the ingestion of the drugs simultaneously with sexual activity (Guss, 2000). The use of these drugs temporarily allows the individual to shed his feelings of anxiety, shame, inadequacy, and guilt and experience instead a sensation of omnipotence, desirability, and euphoria. However, continuous use of alcohol, amphetamine, and marijuana can lead to depression and suicidal behavior, including psychotic illnesses reinforcing the vicious circle of negative feelings and substance use (Peck et al., 2005, Rey, Martin, & Krabman, 2004).

Body Image Disorders

Parental expectations, societal demands, and the absence of recognition and validation from both family and their peer group may converge to produce in non-gender conforming boys feelings of shame, inadequacy, hopelessness, rage, isolation, and internalized homophobia. As one scholar has explained, "the trauma and stigma of the invisible body, invisible self, and negated sexuality remains painfully intense. This traumatic injury is felt concretely, in the body, and is experienced as factual and therefore as unhealable" (Guss, 2000: 110).

As a result, individuals may become obsessed with a desire to transform their bodies into one that is perceived to be more desirable, worthy, and exciting. Men who desire a more "masculine" body may pursue their goal through weight training, the use of anabolic steroids, diet, and plastic surgery, while men who wish to appear more feminine, such as MTF transgender individuals who self-identify as men, may utilize estrogen, plastic surgery, and silicone injections to achieve their desired appearance.

Substance Use Among Minority MSM

By all accounts, the level of substance use among African American, Latino, and Asian and Pacific Islander MSM is quite high. Table 4.1 outlines the various published studies that have focused on substance use among minority MSM. The literature suggests that there is a high prevalence of substance use among minority MSM; that substance use may be initiated at an early age; and that polydrug use, including injection drug use, is common among those minority MSM who use substances.

Although these studies provide us with some data about substance use within this population, numerous methodological issues limit the generalizability of their findings and conclusions. These include small sample sizes, variation in the defined target population across studies, and variation in the assessment and measurement of substance use across studies.

Substance Use and HIV Risk

Substance use and abuse have been found to be associated with engaging in unprotected anal sex, a behavior that increases the risk of HIV transmission. Stall, McKusick, Wiley, Coates, & Ostrow (1986) have delineated four mechanisms to explain the connection between substance use and unprotected anal intercourse among gay men:

1. the pharmacological action of the substance may increase sexual desire or the intensity of the sexual experience (direct drug action model);
2. the substance use may decrease the individual's cognitive awareness of the risks associated with the sexual activity and/or the effectiveness of the individual's efforts to use safer sex precautions, such as the use of a condom (cognitive inhibition model);
3. there may exist an underlying vulnerability, such as high sensation seeking, that is associated with the substance use and the sexual risk taking (common underlying vulnerability model); and
4. the substance use may be used strategically by some men to escape the cognitive inhibitions to participating in unprotected anal intercourse in order to experience the increased intimacy associated with unprotected anal sex (escape model, McKirnan, Ostrow, & Hope, 1996; Ostrow & McKirnan, 1997).

The relationship between substance use and HIV risk is further discussed in the work of Leigh & Stalk (1993).

Table 4.1 Selected Studies of Substance Use among Minority MSM

Study	Methodology	Population	Findings
Centers for Disease Control and Prevention, 2005	Data from 33 states with long-term confidential name-based HIV reporting	MSM with diagnosed with HIV/AIDS 2001–2004	Of 5,685 MSM who injected drugs, 42% were White, 39% African American, 17% Latino, 1% Asian and Pacific Islander, 1% American Indian/Alaskan Native
Diaz & Ayala, 2000	Multisite study with Latino MSM	Latino gay men, including large number of Mexican immigrants at Los Angeles site	Among Los Angeles respondents, 45% reported use of at least one nonprescription drug during previous 6 months, including methamphetamine 20% reported use of methamphetamine during previous 6 months
Finlinson, Colón Robles, & Soto, 2006	Multisession qualitative interviews	20 non-gay-identified Puerto Rican MSM, San Juan, Puerto Rico	Early initiation of cigarettes, alcohol, and marijuana ages 10–15 years; period of snorting or smoking cocaine or heroin, ages 15–23 years; transition to IDU ages 17–26 years All participants dependent on heroin and injected it with cocaine
Irwin & Morgenstern, 2005	Randomized clinical trial comparing two behavioral interventions for alcohol use disorders and HIV risk behavior	198 HIV-negative men who had had sexual relations with a man in the previous 90 days, had used alcohol during the previous 30 days, and who had been diagnosed with alcohol abuse or dependence in the preceding 12 months	Severity of alcohol problem similar across ethnic and sexual identities African Americans found to have higher number of drinks per day compared with other subgroups Non-Hispanic Whites, Latinos, and gay-identified men more likely to have used amphetamines or methamphetamine during the previous 6 months

Table 4.1 (continued)

Study	Methodology	Population	Findings
			Non-Hispanic Whites less likely to have used marijuana compared with African American and Latino men
Jimenez, 2003	73-item survey	Convenience sample of 110 self-identified African American and Latino MSM 50 years of age and older	Most respondents reported drug use in conjunction with sexual activity during previous 6 months; 84% reported use of alcohol "just before or during sex," 59% reported marijuana, 23% amyl nitrate ("poppers"), 20% rock cocaine, and/or 20% heroin
			52% self-identified as gay, 29% bisexual, 16% straight or mostly straight
Kral et al., 2005	Data derived from administration of standardized questionnaire utilized in one interview session and HIV testing in conjunction with the Urban Health Study, a serial cross-sectional study	357 MSM 18 years of age and older who injected drugs in San Francisco between 1998 and 2002	HIV-positive MSM-IDU more likely than HIV-negative MSM-IDU to be African American and older and less likely to be homeless
Morales and Graves (1983)	Self-administered questionnaires	266 self-identified gay men, 129 lesbians, 57 bisexual/gay-identified heterosexuals in San Francisco	18% of gay men, 25% of lesbians presented an "at risk" substance use pattern; 21% of minority gay and lesbians evidenced substance abuse problems
			21% of minority gay men and lesbians used alcohol one or more times each day

Table 4.1 (continued)

Study	Methodology	Population	Findings
Thiede et al., 2003	Venue-based cross-sectional survey conducted during 1994–1998 in seven urban areas	Total of 3,492 participants from Baltimore, Dallas, Los Angeles, Miami, New York, San Francisco Bay area, and Seattle	African American and Asian and Pacific Islander MSM less likely than white MSM to report any drug use, use of three or more drugs, use of drugs more than once a week or injection drug use during previous 6 months Latino MSM less likely than White MSM to report any drug use, use of three or more drugs, use of drugs more than once a week during previous 6 months MSM who self-identified as bisexual or heterosexual more likely to report any drug use, use of three or more drugs, use of drugs more than once a week or injection drug use during previous 6 months compared with self-identified gay men
Williams, Wyatt, Resell, Peterson, & Asuan-O'Brien, 2004	Four focus groups	23 non-gay identifying HIV+ African American and Latino MSM	Frequent use of alcohol, crack cocaine, crystal methamphetamine, marijuana, heroin

Treatment Models and Strategies

It is clear that substance use may be integrally related to issues relating to sexuality, sexual orientation, and treatment by others due to one's sexual orientation. These issues may not be addressed at all in most substance use treatment programs and, if they are, it is most often in a heterosexist context (Niesen & Sandall, 1990). For instance, a recent study was conducted of the 11.8% of 911 listed treatment programs in the United States and Puerto Rico that claimed to offer residential, outpatient, and/or partial hospitalization services specifically for lesbian, gay, bisexual, and transgender clients (Cochran, Peavy, & Robohm, 2007). However, a telephone survey of these programs revealed that only 7.4% could identify an offered service that was specifically tailored to the needs of LGBT clients.

Literature suggests that relapse may be more frequent among sexual minority individuals because they are often unable to express themselves openly while they are in treatment because of actual or feared homophobia (Hicks, 2000; Kus & Latcovich, 1995). For instance, some programs have discouraged gay men from discussing their homosexuality or issues related to their relationships out of concern that it would distress others participating in the group treatment process or the belief that the issues were not relevant to recovery (Green & Faltz, 1991; Lewis & Jordan, 1989). Treatment providers may operate from the perspective that all addiction treatment is equal and equally effective for all (Ubell & Sumberg, 1992). Accordingly, there appears to be a general consensus regarding the importance of establishing and maintaining specialized addiction treatment programs for self-identified gay men (Hicks, 2000; Kus & Latcovich, 1995; Skinner & Skinner, 1992).

Specialized programs present a number of advantages in addition to providing a safe forum in which to address issues of sexuality that may be related to one's substance use. First, they offer a setting in which the likelihood of harassment due to sexual orientation is significantly reduced (Ritter & Terndrup, 2002). Second, participation in a treatment program with like-minded individuals who are also trying to address their substance use presents an opportunity to establish a new and healthier support system (Kus & Latcovich, 1995). Third, the treatment program can not only help participants to address issues related to internalized homophobia, but also can assist them to formulate constructive strategies for dealing with societal sexism and heterosexism without relying on substances (Cabaj, 1995). Fourth, gay men may have to address numerous ancillary issues, such as partner violence and parent-child conflicts, whose contexts differ significantly from those experienced by their heterosexual counterparts. Specialized treatment programs permit individuals the opportunity to address such issues without fear of judgment (Cabaj, 1996; Cabaj, 1995).

The interrelationship between the effects of trauma and substance abuse in the lives of MSM deserve special consideration. There are several approaches that deal with the treatment of both trauma and addiction. The most common treatment approach assumes that people should be treated for substance abuse before facing the symptoms of trauma. This approach has been criticized, however, because untreated symptoms of trauma are often powerful triggers for relapse. More recently, an integrated model of treatment that focuses on both trauma and addiction has been recommended (Miller and Guidry, 2001). Cognitive behavioral therapies and living skills trainings are the most commonly used approaches in dealing with the mental effects of discrimination and trauma. In particular, cognitive processing therapy for acute stress disorder has been described as appropriate for gay patients (Kaysen et al., 2005).

Many gay youth and adults have significant resiliency to hostile environments (Garofalo & Katz, 2001). The larger gay community and personal gay friends may serve as significant sources of support and become more important than the not fully accepting family of origin (Green, 2000). Some individuals may have sufficient coping skills to deal with unwanted sexual attention and other forms of abuse. Similarly, as for racial/ethnic minorities, a positive self-identity increases resiliency to the effects of trauma and addiction (Benight et al., 1997, Herek, 1991, Wallace, 1999). This is why therapies for MSM need to include trainings in coping skills and building a positive self-image and self-confidence.

Many gay men may be uncomfortable with treatment programs premised on a belief in God or a higher power as a result of their denunciation and outright rejection by various religious groups (Hicks, 2000; Kus & Latcovich, 1995). It is critical that a treatment program both acknowledges that such sentiments and experience exist and provide an opportunity to explore and addresses aspects of spirituality that may be critical to recovery. It is also believed that the availability of specialized programs that create a safe place for open expression may reduce the likelihood of relapse by allowing individuals enrolled in treatment to address issues of critical importance to their recovery, including relationships and self-esteem (Hicks, 2000).

Kus and Latcovich (1995) have delineated various reasons for the creation of "special interest groups" for gay men wishing to participate in Alcoholics Anonymous (AA) programs:

1. it is easier to trust in a gay group;
2. it is easier to speak with people who have similar experiences;
3. participation in a gay group provides an opportunity to reduce internalized homophobia;
4. participation in a gay group helps a participant to establish a new support system;
5. gay men's groups help individuals to adapt the philosophy of AA to their experience;
6. men who have abandoned their beliefs in God because of the negative attitudes they have experienced from church members and religious leaders can re-establish their faith;

7. attendance in gay men's groups will help the individual develop in service work for other gay men and/or AA;
8. attendance in gay men's groups may encourage participants to become more aware of a responsibility to other gay men and to others in general;
9. participation in gay groups may help individuals to enjoy all aspects of their lives; and
10. participation will help individuals counteract antimasculine and antigay sentiments that they may experience.

Conclusions

The most significant factors affecting the development of MSM identity are discrimination, stigma, and lack of support. Gay youth struggle with understanding their own desires and instincts in confrontation with what they see and hear around them. There is a significant disconnect between a gay man's self-image and the society's image of what a man is supposed to be. To survive, gay men often need to learn how to deny their own feelings and emotions and to adapt to the norms created by heterosexual society. The subgroups of MSM who are also members of other stigmatized and discriminated minority groups (like African American, HIV positive) struggle even more. Different forms of dissociation are common among MSM. Since acculturation to the MSM community often happens in gay bars, one of the forms of dissociation is the use and consequent abuse of mind-altering substances.

Prevention and treatment then needs to be focused on counteracting the demoralizing effects of discrimination and stigmatization of MSM and to take into consideration the specific behaviors and attitudes developed by MSM. One of the most powerful factors in developing a healthy self-identity is involvement in positive relationships with other gay men in gay and gay-friendly communities (Martin & Knox, 1997). Any substance abuse treatment needs to address both the nature of addiction as well as the effects of externalized and internalized homonegativity.

References

Balsam, K. F., Huang, B., Fieland, K. C., Simoni, J. M., & Walters, K. L. (2004). Culture, trauma, and wellness: a comparison of heterosexual and lesbian, gay, bisexual, and two-spirit Native Americans. *Cultural Diversity & Ethnic Minority Psychology*, 10, 287–301.

Benight, C. C., Antoni, M. H., Kilbourn, K., Ironson, G., Kumar, M. A., & Fletcher, M. A. et al. (1997). Coping self-efficacy buffers psychological and physiological disturbances in HIV-infected men following a natural disaster. *Health Psychology*, 16, 248–55.

Brannon, R. (1976). The male sex role-and what it's done for us lately. In R. Brannon & D. David (Eds.). *The forty-nine percent majority: The male sex role* (pp. 1–40). Boston: Addison-Wesley.

Cabaj, R. P. (1995). Sexual orientation and the addictions. *Journal of Gay and Lesbian Psychotherapy, 2,* 97–117.

Cabaj, R. P. (1996). Substance use in gay men, lesbians, and bisexuals. In R. P. Cabaj & T. S. Stein (Eds.), *Textbook of homosexuality and mental health* (pp. 783–799). Washington, DC: American Psychiatric Press.

Cabaj, R. P. (2000). Substance use, internalized homophobia, and gay men and lesbians: Psychodynamic issues and clinical implications. In J. R. Guss & J. Drescher (Eds.), *Addictions in the gay and lesbian community* (pp. 5–24). New York: Haworth Medical Press.

Capitanio, J. P., & Herek, G. M. (1999). AIDS-related stigma and attitudes toward injecting drug users among black and white Americans. *American Behavioral Scientist, 42*(7), 1148–1161.

Centers for Disease Control and Prevention. (2005). Trends in HIV/AIDS diagnoses–33 states, 2001–2004. *Morbidity and Mortality Weekly Report, 54,* 1149–1153.

Chesney, M. A., & Smith, A. W. (1999). Critical delays in HIV testing and care: The potential role of stigma. *American Behavioral Scientist, 42,* 1162–1174.

Chodorow, N. (1978). *The reproduction of mothering.* Berkeley, California: University of California Press.

Chu, J. A., & Dill, D. L. (1990). Dissociative symptoms in relation to childhood physical and sexual abuse. *American Journal of Psychiatry, 147,* 887–892.

Clements, N. K. (1999). *The transgender community health project: Descriptive results.* San Francisco, California: San Francisco Department of Public Health.

Cochran, B. N., Peavy, K. M., & Robohm, J. S. (2007). Do specialized services exist for LGBT individuals seeking treatment for substance misuse? A study of available treatment programs. *Substance Use & Misuse, 42*(1), 161–176.

Cochran, B. N., Stewart, A. J., Ginzler, J. A., & Cauce, A. M. (2002). Challenges faced by homeless sexual minorities: Comparison of gay, lesbian, bisexual, and transgender homeless adolescents with their heterosexual counterparts. *American Journal of Public Health, 92,* 773–777.

Cochran, S. D., & Sullivan, J. G. (2003). Prevalence of mental disorders, psychological distress, and mental health services use among lesbian, gay, and bisexual adults in the United States. *Journal of Consulting and Clinical Psychology, 71,* 53–61.

D'Augellis, A. R., Grossman, A. H., & Starks, M. T. (2006). Childhood gender atypicality, victimization, and PTSD among lesbian, gay, and bisexual youth. *Journal of Interpersonal Violence, 21,* 1462–1482.

Diaz, R. M., & Ayala, G. (2000). *Social discrimination and health: The case of Latino gay men and HIV risk.* Washington, D.C: The Policy Institute of the National Gay and Lesbian Task Force.

Dimsdale, J. E. (2000). Stalked by the past: The influence of ethnicity on health. *Psychosomatic Medicine, 62,* 161–170.

Dinos, S., Stevens, S., Serfaty, M., Weich, S., & King, M. (2001). Stigma: The feelings and experiences of 46 people with mental illness. *British Journal of Psychiatry, 184,* 178–191.

Doll, L. S., Joy, D., Bartholow, B. N., Harrison, J. S., Bolan, G., Douglas, J. M., et al. (1992). Self-reported childhood and adolescent sexual abuse among adult homosexual and bisexual men. *Child Abuse & Neglect, 16,* 855–864.

Doyle, J. A. (1989). *The male experience,* 2nd ed. Dubuque, Iowa: William C. Brown.

Drossman, D. A., Talley, N. J., Leserman, J., Olden, K. W., & Barreiro, M. A. (1995). Sexual and physical abuse and gastrointestinal illness. *Annals of Internal Medicine, 123,* 782–794.

Easthope, A. (1986). What a man's gotta do: *The masculine myth in popular culture.* London: Paladin/Grafton.

Epstein, J. N., Saunders, B. E., Kilpatrick, D. G., & Resnick, H. S. (1998). PTSD as a mediator between childhood rape and alcohol use in adult women. *Child Abuse & Neglect,* 22, 223–234.

Finlinson, H. A., Colón, H. M., Robles, R. R., & Soto, M. (2006). Sexual identity formation and AIDS prevention: An exploratory study of non-gay-identifies Puerto Rican MSM from working class neighborhoods. *AIDS Behavior,* 10, 531–539.

Ford, J. D., Chapman, J., Mack, M., & Pearson, G. (2006). Pathways from traumatic child victimization to delinquency: Implications for juvenile and permanency court proceedings and decisions. *Juvenile and Family Court Journal, Winter.* 13–23.

Garofalo, R., & Katz, E. (2001). Health care issues of gay and lesbian youth. *Current Opinion in Pediatrics, 13(4),* 298–302.

Gaylin, W. (1992). *The male ego.* New York: Viking.

Ghindia, D. J., & Kola, L. A. (1996). Co-factors affecting substance abuse among homosexual men: An investigation within a midwestern gay community. *Drug and Alcohol Dependence,* 41, 167–177.

Gilligan, J. (2001). *Preventing violence.* New York: Thames & Hudson.

Goffman, E. (1963). *Stigma: Notes on the management of spoiled identity.* New York: Touchstone.

Goldbaum, G., Perdue, T., & Higgins, D. (1996). Non-gay-identifying men who have sex with men: Formative research results from Seattle, Washington. *Public Health Reports, 111*(Suppl. 1), 36–40.

Greene, D., & Faltz, B. (1991). Chemical dependency and relapse in gay men with HIV infection: Issues and treatment. *Journal of Chemical Dependency Treatment, 4(2),* 79–90.

Green, R-J. (2000). "Lesbians, gay men, and their parents": A critique of LaSala and the prevailing clinical "wisdom". *Family Process, 39, 257–266.*

Guss, J. R. (2000). Sex like you can't even imagine: "Crystal," crack and gay men. In J. R. Guss & J. Drescher (Eds.), *Addictions in the gay and lesbian community* (pp. 105–121). New York: Haworth Medical Press.

Gwadz, M. V., Clatts, M. C., Leonard, N. R., & Goldsamt, L. (2004). Attachment style, childhood adversity, and behavioral risk among young men who have sex with men. *Journal of Adolescent Health,* 34, 402–413.

Heidt, J. M., Marx, B. P., & Gold, S. D. (2005). Sexual revictimization among sexual minorities: A preliminary study. *Journal of Traumatic Stress,* 18, 533–540.

Herek, G. M. (1999). AIDS and stigma. *American Behavioral Scientist,* 42(7), 1106–1116.

Herek, G. M. (1991). Stigma, prejudice, and violence against lesbians and gay men. In J. C. Gonsiored & J. D. Weinrich (Eds.), *Homosexuality: Research implications for public policy* (pp. 60–80). Newbury Park, CA: Sage.

Herek, G. M., & Capitanio, J. P. (1999). AIDS stigma and sexual prejudice. *American Behavioral Scientist,* 42(7), 1130–1147.

Herek, G. M., Cogan, J. C., Gillis, J. R., & Glunt, E. K. (1997). Correlates of internalized homophobia in a community sample of lesbians and gay men. *Journal of the Gay and Lesbian Medical Association, 2,* 17–25.

Herek, G. M., Gillis, J. R., & Cogan, J. C. (1999). Psychological sequelae of hate-crime victimization among lesbian, gay, and bisexual adults. *Journal of Consulting and Clinical Psychology,* 67, 945–951.

Hicks, D. (2000). The importance of specialized treatment programs for lesbian and gay patients. In J. R. Guss & J. Drescher (Eds.), *Addictions in the gay and lesbian community* (pp. 81–94). New York: Haworth Medical Press.

Irwin, T. W., & Morgenstern, J. (2005). Drug-use patterns among men who have sex with men presenting for alcohol treatment: Differences in ethnic and sexual identity. *Journal of Urban Health,* 82(Suppl. 1), i127-i133.

Israelstam, S., & Lambert, S. (1983). Homosexuality as a cause of alcoholism: A historical review. *International Journal of the Addictions*, 18(8), 1085–1107.

Jimenez, A. D. (2003). Triple jeopardy: Targeting older men of color who have sex with men. *Journal of Acquired Immune Deficiency Syndromes*, 33, S222-S225.

Jones, E. E., Farina, A., Hastorf, A., Markus, H., Millar, D. S., & Scott, R. A. (1984). *Social stigma: The psychology of marked relationships*. New York: W. H. Freeman.

Kalichman, S. C., Gore-Felton, C., Benotsch, E., Cage, M., & Rompa, D. (2004). Trauma symptoms, sexual behaviors, and substance abuse: Correlates of childhood sexual abuse and HIV risks among men who have sex with men. *Journal of Child Sexual Abuse*, 13, 1–15.

Kaysen, D., Lostutter, T. W., & Goines, M. A. (2005). Cognitive processing therapy for acute stress disorder resulting from an anti-gay assault. *Cognitive Behavioral Practice*, 12, 278–289.

Kelly, J. (Ed.). (1991). *San Francisco lesbian, gay and bisexual alcohol and other drugs needs assessment study, vol. 1*. Sacramento, California: EMT Associates.

Kimmel, M. S. (2003). Masculinity as homophobia. In E. Disch (Ed.). *Reconstructing gender: A multicultural anthology*. Boston: McGraw Hill.

Komisar, L. (1976). Violence and the masculine mystique. In D. S. David & R. Brannon (Eds.), *The forty-nine percent majority: The male sex role*. Boston: Addison-Wesley.

Kort, J. (2004). Covert cultural sexual abuse of gay male teenagers contributing to etiology of sexual addiction. *Sexual Addiction & Compulsivity*, 11, 287–300.

Kral, A. H., Lorvick, J., Ciccarone, D., Wenger, L., Gee, L., & Martinez, A., et al. (2005). HIV prevalence and risk behaviors among men who have sex with men and inject drugs in San Francisco. *Journal of Urban Health*, 82(Suppl. 1), i43-i50.

Kus, R. J., & Latcovich, M. A. (1995). Special interest groups in Alcoholics Anonymous: A focus on gay men's groups. In R. J. Kus (Ed.), *Addiction and recovery in gay and lesbian persons* (pp. 67–82). Binghamton, NY: Harrington Park Press.

Leigh, B. C., & Stall, R. (1993). Substance use and risky sexual behavior for exposure to HIV: Issues in methodology, interpretation, and prevention. *American Psychologist*, 48, 1035–1045.

Levant, R. F. (1995). Toward the reconstruction of masculinity. In R. F. Levant & W. S. Pollack (Eds.), *A new psychology of men* (pp. 229–251). New York: Basic Books.

Leverenz, D. (1986). Manhood, humiliation, and public life: Some stories. *Southwest Review*, 71.

Lewis, G. R., & Jordan, S. M. (1989). Treatment of gay or lesbian alcoholics. In G. Lawson & A. Lawson (Eds.), *Alcoholism and substance abuse in special populations*. Rockville, MD: Aspen Publishers.

Link, B. G., Struening, E. L., Neese-Todd, S., Asmussen, S., & Phelan, J. C. (2001). The consequences of stigma for the self-esteem of people with mental illness. *Psychiatric Services*, 52(12), 1621–1626.

Link, B. G., Struening, E. L., Rahav, M., Phelan, J. C., & Nuttbrock, L. (1997). On stigma and its consequences: Evidence from a longitudinal study of men with dual diagnoses of mental illness and substance abuse. *Journal of Health and Social Behavior*, 38, 177–190.

Lohrenz, L., Connelly, J., Coyne, L., & Spare, K. (1978). Alcohol problems in several Midwestern homosexual communities. *Journal of Studies on Alcohol*, 39, 1959–1963.

Mansergh, G., Colfax, G. N., Marks, G., Rader, M., Guzman, R., & Buchbinder, S. (2001). The Circuit Party Men's Health Survey: Findings and implications for gay and bisexual men. *American Journal of Public Health*, 91, 953–958.

Martin, J., & Knox, J. (1997). Self-esteem instability and its implications for HIV prevention among gay men. *Health & Social Work*, 22(4), 264–273.

Mays, V. M., Cochran, S. D., & Zamudio, A. (2004). HIV prevention research: Are we meeting the needs of African American men who have sex with men? *Journal of Black Psychology*, 30, 78–103.

McBride, C. A. (1998). The discounting principle and attitudes towards victims of HIV infection. *Journal of Applied Social Psychology, 28(7)*, 595–608.

McKirnan, D. J., & Peterson, P. L. (1989). Psychosocial and cultural issues in alcohol and drug abuse: An analysis of a homosexual community. *Addiction Behaviors*, 14(5), 555–563.

Messner, M. A. (2003). Boyhood, organized sports, and the construction of masculinities. E. Disch (Ed.), *Reconstructing gender: A multicultural anthology* (pp. 110–126). Boston: McGraw Hill.

Miller, D., & Guidry, L. (2001). *Addictions and trauma recovery: Healing the mind, body, and spirit*. New York: W. W. Norton & Company, Inc.

Morales, E. S., & Graves, M. A. (1983). *Substance abuse: Patterns and barriers to treatment for gay men and lesbians in San Francisco*. San Francisco, California: San Francisco Prevention Resources Center.

Niesen, J., & Sandall, H. (1990). Alcohol and other drug abuse in a gay/lesbian population: Related to victimization? *Journal of Psychology & Human Sexuality*, 3, 151–168.

Ostrow, D. G., & McKirnan, D. J. (1997). Prevention of substance-related high-risk sexual behavior among gay men: Critical review of the literature and proposed harm reduction approach. *Journal of the Gay & Lesbian Medical Association*, 1, 97–110.

O'Neil, J. M. (1982). Gender-role conflict and strain in men's lives. In K. Solomon & N. Levy (Eds.). *Men in transition: Theory and therapy* (pp. 5–44). New York: Plenum.

Paul, J. P., Barrett, D. C., Crosby, G. M., & Stall,, R. D. (1996). Longitudinal changes in alcohol and drug use among men seen at a gay-specific substance abuse treatment agency. *Journal of Studies on Alcohol*, 57, 475–485.

Paul, J. P., Catania, J., Pollack, L., & Stall, R. (2001). Understanding childhood sexual abuse as a predictor of sexual risk-taking among men who have sex with men: The urban men's health study. *Child Abuse & Neglect*, 25, 557–584.

Peck, J. A., Reback, C. J., Yang, X., Rotheram-Fuller, E., & Shoptaw, S. (2005). Sustained reductions in drug use and depression symptoms from treatment for drug abuse in methamphetamine-dependent gay and bisexual men. *Journal of Urban Health: Bulletin of the New York Academy of Medicine*, 82, i100–i108.

Rebac, C., & Lombardi, E. L. (2001). A community-based harm reduction program for male-to-female transgenders at risk for HIV infection. In W. Bocking & S. Kirk (Eds.), *Transgender and HIV* (pp. 59–68). Binghamton, New York: Haworth Press.

Reidpath, D. D., & Chan, K. Y. (2005). A method for the quantitative analysis of the layering of HIV-related stigma. *AIDS Care*, 17(4), 425–432.

Reingold, A. L. (2001). The study of stigmatizing conditions; An epidemiologic perspective. *Stigma and global health: Developing a research agenda*. September 5–7, Maryland.

Rey, J. M., Martin, A., & Krabman, P. (2004). Is the party over? Cannabis and juvenile psychiatric disorder: The past 10 years. *Journal of the American Academy of Child and Adolescent Psychiatry*, 43, 1194–1205.

Ritter, K. Y., & Terndrup, A. I. (2002). *Handbook of affirmative psychotherapy with lesbians and gay men*. New York: Guilford Press.

Rivers, I. (2004). Recollections of bullying at school and their long-term implications for lesbians, gay men, and bisexuals. *Crisis*, 25, 1–7.

Sageman, S. (2003). The rape of boys and the impact of sexually predatory environments: Review and case reports. *Journal of the American Academy of Psychoanalysis & Dynamic Psychiatry*, 31, 563–580.

Saghir, M., & Robins, E. (1973). *Male and female homosexuality*. Baltimore, MD: Williams and Wilkins.

Siegel, K., Lune, H., & Meyer, I. H. (1998). Stigma management among gay/bisexual men with HIV/AIDS. *Qualitative Sociology*, 21(1), 3–24.

Skinner, W., & Skinner, O. (1992). Drug use among lesbian and gay people: Findings, research, design, insights, and policy issues from the trilogy project. In The Research

Symposium on Alcohol and Other Drug Problem Prevention among Lesbians and Gay Men: Proceedings, October.

Stall, R., McKusick, L., Wiley, J., Coates, T. J., & Ostrow, D. G. (1986). Alcohol and drug use during sexual activity and compliance with safe sex guidelines for AIDS: The AIDS behavioral Research Project. *Health Education Quarterly*, 13, 359–372.

Stall, R., Paul, J. P., Greenwood, G., Pollack, L. M., Bein, E., & Crosby, G. M. et al. (2001). Alcohol use, drug use, and alcohol-related problems among men who have sex with men: The Urban Men's Health Study. *Addiction*, 96, 1589–1601.

Stall, R. D., & Wiley, J. (1988). A comparison of alcohol and drug use patterns of homosexual and heterosexual men: The San Francisco Men's Health Study. *Drug and Alcohol Dependence*, 22, 63–73.

Stewart, S. H. (1996). Alcohol abuse in individuals exposed to trauma: a critical review. *Psychological Bulletin*, 120(1), 83–112.

Stouffer, S. A., Lumsdaine, A. A., Lumsdaine, M. H., Williams, R. M. Jr., Smith, M. B., & Janis, I. L., et al. (1976). Masculinity and the role of the combat soldier. In D. S. David & R. Brannon (Eds.), *The forty-nine percent majority: The male sex role*. Boston: Addison-Wesley.

Thiede, H., Valleroy, L. A., Mackellar, D. A., Celentano, D. D., Ford, W. L., & Hagan, H. et al. (2003). Regional patterns and correlates of substance use among young men who have sex with men in 7 US urban areas. *American Journal of Public Health*, 93(11), 1915–1921.

Ubell, V., & Sumberg, D. (1992). Heterosexual therapists treating homosexual addicted clients. *Journal of Chemical Dependency Treatment*, 5(1), 19–33.

van der Kolk, B. A., Pelcovitz, D., Roth, S., Mandel, F. S., McFarlane, A., Herman, J. L. (1996) Dissociation, somatization, and affect dysregulation: the complexity of adaptation to trauma. *American Journal of Psychiatry*, 153(7), 83–93.

Wallace, J. M. (1999). The social ecology of addiction: Race, risk, and resilience. *Pediatrics*, 103, 1122–1127.

Whitehead, S. M., & Barrett, F. J. (2001). The sociology of masculinity. In S. M. Whitehead & F. J. Barrett (Eds.), *The Masculinities Reader* (pp. 1–26). Malden, MA: Blackwell Publishers Inc.

Williams, J. K., Wyatt, G. E., Resell, J., Peterson, J., & Asuan-O'Brien, A. (2004). Psychosocial issues among gay- and non-gay-identifying HIV-seropositive African American and Latino MSM. *Cultural Diversity and Ethnic Minority Psychology*, 10(3), 268–286.

Woolfolk, R. L., & Richardson, F. (1978). *Sanity, Stress, and Survival*. New York: Signet.

Wyatt, G. E., Guthrie, D., & Notgrass, C. M. (1992). Differential effects of women's child sexual abuse and subsequent sexual revictimization. *Journal of Consulting and Clinical Psychology*, 60, 167–173.

Part IV
Homelessness

Chapter Five
Homelessness among Substance-Using Minority Men who have Sex with Men

James M. Holbrook

Who are the Homeless Minority Substance-Using Men who have Sex with Men?

Homeless minority substance-using men who have sex with men (MSU-MSM) constitute one of the most troubled populations living on the streets of the USA today. Our understanding of the homeless MSU-MSM population is incomplete in many ways, as researchers have just begun studying the population over recent years, motivated largely due to the need to better understand the staggering rate of HIV/AIDS that exists within the MSM community, and that appears to be particularly prevalent among minority young men who have sex with men (YMSM) (Seal et al., 2000). This chapter discusses characteristics and behaviors that are commonly a part of the homeless MSU-MSM experience. Because so little is actually known about the circumstances of homeless MSU-MSM, much of the chapter draws from the published literature relating to substance-using men who have sex with men, who may or may not be minority group members (apart from their status as a sexual minority).

In general, this community tends to experience troubling levels of disempowerment due to poverty, non-majority cultural status, stigmatization resulting from the condemnation of non-traditionally heterosexual lifestyles, and threats to personal safety created by public self-identification as non-heterosexual (Elwood, Williams, Bell, & Richard, 1997; Engler et al., 2005). Many members of this group exist on the fringes of the social service systems and, as a result, must sometimes make stark compromises in order to obtain needed help. Too often, it is only through the episodic occurrence of critical issues such as the emergence of sexually transmitted disease symptomatology, acute physical/mental distress resulting from psychopathology and/or substance use, or through involvement with the criminal justice system that the service systems have therapeutic contacts with these individuals. Service providers often fail to

James M. Holbrook
Cleveland, OH

S. Loue (ed.), *Health Issues Confronting Minority Men Who Have Sex with Men.*
© Springer 2008

recognize the needs of many homeless MSU-MSM, many of whom already exist outside of most social and health care systems (Linn, Brown & Kendrick, 2005), due to both the brevity of their contact and their lack of cultural awareness with regard to this population.

Accurate estimation of the number of MSU-MSM who are homeless has proven to be difficult. Estimates of the nightly homeless population in the United States range from 600,000 to 842,000 people (Harvard Mental Health Letter, 2005; National Coalition for the Homeless, 2006). However, there appears to be general consensus among the research community that approximately 20% of homeless and runaway youth are non-heterosexual (Clatts, Goldsamt, Yi, & Gwadz, 2005). YMSM appear to be overrepresented within the homeless youth population as a whole (Clatts et al., 2005). Homeless sexual minorities may tend to congregate in larger cities, as it may be more dangerous for youth to publicly identify themselves as being non-heterosexual in smaller, rural cities (Whitbeck, Chen, Hoyt, Tyler & Johnson, 2004).

Despite the paucity of national statistics available regarding the racial/ethnic makeup of the homeless MSM population, there are some localized studies that may provide the beginnings of a better identification of this group. In a study by Deren and colleagues (2001) that recruited homeless substance-using men who have sex with men (SU-MSM) from street-based hangouts and shelters in five US cities, it was found that 55% of the participants were African American, 31% were White, 9% were Hispanic and 5% were identified as others. Clatts et al.'s (2005) study of YMSM in New York City indicated that of the participants with a past history of homelessness, 49% were Hispanic, 23% were African Americans, 21% were White, and 8% were identified as others. Among YMSM who were currently homeless, 53% were Hispanic, 27% African American, 8% White, and 12% others. This study additionally noted that while Hispanics were more than twice as likely as Whites and African Americans to have a history of past homelessness, they were almost seven times more likely than Whites, and nearly twice as likely as African Americans to be currently homeless. It is unclear whether this information can be generalized to areas outside of New York. However, both of these studies would seem to suggest that minorities may be overrepresented nationally in the homeless MSM population.

The sexual practices and sexual identity of homeless MSU-MSM may not be congruent. Elwood and colleagues (1997) found that among the general MSM population in San Francisco, nearly half of their participants who behaved bisexually actually self-identified as being heterosexual. A Canadian study of the general MSM population by Engler's research team (2005) reported that disparities may exist between one's sexual self-identification (homosexual/gay versus bisexual) and sexual behavior (homosexual versus bisexual).

Clatts and colleagues (2005) found that among their respondents who were currently homeless, 36% self-identified as "Gay," 34.9% as bisexual, 21.7% as heterosexual, 7.2% as other, and 19.3% as transgender. The currently homeless group was found to be substantially more diverse in sexual identities compared with the "never" homeless YMSM group, with over six times more currently homeless subjects indicating being heterosexual, nearly three times more indicating transgender, and almost twice as many indicating bisexual.

Overall, most research that refers to the sexual minority youth population (much less the MSM population) focuses on sexual issues, with substantially less focus on non-sexual issues. However, Cochran, Stewart, Ginzler, and Cauce (2002) reported that sexual minority youth are more likely to report victimization, use drugs, report more sexual partners, and demonstrate generally higher rates of psychopathology than did their heterosexual peers. In addition, Whitbeck and colleagues (2004) reported that homeless sexual minority adolescents are overrepresented among the homeless population in general, suggesting that they are experiencing greater risk factors within their families of origin or pre-runaway social contexts, such as school, peer groups, etc.

The Impact of Homelessness on MSU-MSM

The pathway toward entry into homelessness, particularly for sexual minorities, can have many origins and influences that may be interrelated in complex ways. There is a limited but growing body of research in recent years that better describes precursors to and characteristics of, the homeless MSU-MSM experience. Many studies on homeless youth suggest that an impoverished household, living in a substance-abusing household, and experiencing sexual abuse are all risk factors for future homelessness (Lankenau, Clatts, Welle, Goldsamt, & Gwadz, 2005). Cochran and colleagues (2002) reported that while sexual minority youth tend to leave home for reasons similar to those of their heterosexual peers, such as family conflict, a desire for freedom, and difficulties with a family member, they do so at nearly twice the rate. They also reported that sexual minority youth were more likely to leave due to physical abuse in the home, alcohol use in the home, and conflict with their caregivers over their sexuality. Young gay males have been found to be five times more likely to have left home over conflicts about their sexuality than were their heterosexual peers (Whitbeck et al., 2004). In general, it appears that compared with their heterosexual counterparts, homeless sexual minority youth are at increased risk for leaving their homes due to negative experiences with their caregiver(s).

In addition to the apparent increased presence of early negative experiences among many sexual minority youth, the existing epidemiological literature suggests a high prevalence of drug use and sexual risk among various homeless youth populations (Clatts et al., 2005). Johnson, Whitbeck, and Hoyt (2005) reported that 61% of the homeless and runaway adolescents in their study met criteria for a lifetime substance-abuse disorder and 90% met criteria for another mental disorder. Unfortunately, rates of substance use among sexual minority youth appear to be even higher. Lankenau et al. (2005) found that homeless sexual minority youth used each drug use category (except marijuana) more frequently in the preceding 6-month period than did their heterosexual counterparts.

There is active discussion in the research community regarding the process by which YMSM enter into homelessness, as well as the precursors to and characteristics of the homelessness. Some of the prevalent behaviors that have been identified include: engaging in non-sexual and sexual street survival strategies, using drugs in increasingly dangerous ways, increasing one's exposure to potential victimization and trauma, and increasing the risk of acquiring/ transmitting HIV or other sexually transmitted diseases. There appears to be some disagreement, however, as to when and in what order these behaviors first arise among very young MSM. The previous conventional wisdom in the social services systems seemed to be that homelessness, particularly among youth, often resulted from problematic conduct that was related to drug use (Clatts et al., 2005). Recent studies have indicated differing courses by which many YMSM may enter into street life.

Lankenau and colleagues (2005) described the idea of a "liminal, transitional period" whereby YMSM may initially reside in a relatively stable household while accumulating knowledge ("street capital") and skills ("street competencies") throughout their childhood and adolescence that permits them to engage effectively in a "street career" and survive in the "street economy" after becoming homeless. They defined the street economy as comprising a variety of sexual and non-sexual survival strategies such as trading/survival sex, pornography, panhandling, stealing, selling stolen goods, mugging, dealing drugs, and/or scams or cons.

Lankenau et al. (2005) found that their homeless YMSM study participants tended to have been born into lower socioeconomic status (typically poor or working class households with some based on formal and others based on informal economies, including sex work), and often in marginal neighborhoods. Participants typically experienced great fluidity in their relationships with caretakers (separated/divorced parents, boyfriends, foster parents, step/grandparents passing in/out of their lives), which resulted in disciplinary and developmental challenges. The boys often reported having to move frequently, many times among various parental or foster homes, or leaving to escape abusive caretakers.

These individuals acquired street capital, consisting of latent knowledge related to drug use, sexual activity, criminal behavior, and housing contingencies, through family or household observations and experiences. This knowledge, which facilitated youths' development of survival skills in the street economy, had often been transmitted to the child unconsciously and continuously by family members throughout the youths' childhood and often their adolescence as well (Lankenau et al., 2005). Sexually abused children, for instance, may become aware of a demand for certain sorts of sexual activities, and use this knowledge for economic purposes during times of desperation, such as during periods of homelessness.

Street competencies consist of practical actions and skills that have developed from the accumulation of street capital and that allow an individual to survive in the street economy and to establish a network that will aid him in the fulfillment of his needs. These competencies may include buying or selling drugs, sexual activity, shoplifting, or finding housing. Utilization of these competencies over time results in the development of a "street career," such as homelessness, sex work, or both. That career may evolve, may be disrupted, or may be redirected by a variety of events and experiences (Lankenau et al., 2005).

Importantly, Lankenau's research team (2005) demonstrated that homelessness consistently served as the critical point whereby "street capital" was translated into "street competencies" for YMSMs. Though the early teen years of the subjects marked a period during which they began to develop competencies in the areas of sexual exchanges in drug use and sales, it was typically not until after entering homelessness that these competencies converged to create a "street career". Though incarcerations, hospitalizations, addiction, and injuries may have disrupted the trajectories of these careers at various points, many times these disruptions ultimately served as opportunities to assist the YMSM in their acquisition of more capital that could be utilized on the streets at a later date.

A number of studies indicate the prevalence of early negative life events among homeless youth, many of which are correlated with drug use, particularly among very young MSM (Clatts et al., 2005). In addition, HIV infection rates have remained high among YMSMs, especially for Hispanic and non-Hispanic Black males, despite steady declines among the general MSM population. As YMSM tend to be overrepresented among the homeless population, this would seem to suggest that existing drug and sexual risk interventions are not working among the younger members.

Different temporal patterns of negative life events have been detected among homeless, formerly homeless, and never homeless YMSM groups, in contrast to the prevailing notion that homelessness in youth results primarily from substance use (Clatts et al., 2005). Though variance exists among individual temporal relationships, a specific constellation of negative life events (foster care, running away, entering group home living, making a suicide attempt, and initial police interaction) has been found to precede a YMSM's first incarceration, onset of sex work, and initial drug use. In addition, exposure to this constellation of negative life events tends to occur earlier for those with current or prior homelessness versus those with no history of homelessness. These findings would seem to support a conclusion that drug use (and other severe negative life events) may often follow, rather than precede, homelessness (Clatts et al., 2005).

It has been reported that few YMSM who become homeless had used drugs prior to becoming homeless (Clatts et al., 2005). Of particular interest, Clatts and colleagues reported that the initiation of drug use was often delayed among YMSM with histories of unstable housing and/or homelessness. They concluded that drug use may not be a dominant causal factor of YMSMs' homelessness, and suggested that their findings challenge the often-held assumption that higher rates of participation in the street economy, including sex trading, are causally related to prior or current drug usage.

Key sources of protective influences, such as families, schools, criminal justice system, and mental health systems, were found to be insufficiently effective in intervening in these YMSM life trajectories. Rather, they concluded that sex work and drug use (and therefore subsequent HIV risk) are best understood as "medical consequences to YMSM's adaptation to homelessness, rather than as artifacts of individual pathology" (Clatts et al., 2005).

Use of Sexual/Non-Sexual Street Survival Strategies by MSU-MSM

"Survival sex" or "trading sex" refers to the selling of sex to meet one's needs, most commonly for shelter, food, drugs, or money. The extraordinary risks associated with this behavior make it one of the most dangerous street behaviors. Numerous studies suggest that it is unfortunately an all-too-common experience among homeless youth. Kipke, Unger, O'Connor, Palmer, and LaFrance (1997) reported in a San Francisco-based study that 16–46% of street youth engaged in survival sex. Greene, Ennett, and Ringwalt (1999) relied upon a nationally representative sample in concluding that among the general population of homeless youth, 28% of street youth and 10% of shelter youth have engaged in survival sex as a means of meeting basic needs; they suggested that this is likely a minimum estimate. Tyler and Johnson (2006) reported that 30% of homeless youth in major cities in four Midwestern states had traded sex. Greenblatt & Robertson (1993) reported that one-third of homeless adolescents of age 13–17 in Los Angeles reported trading sex. Lankenau and colleagues (2005) estimated that 25–47% of homeless youth in New York City had traded sex during their homeless careers.

Homeless men, in general, are at risk to engage in survival sex, though there seem to be some differences in relation to sexual identity. For instance, Whitbeck and colleagues (2004) found that gay males are generally overrepresented among street prostitutes, and that gay males were more likely to report survival sex than heterosexual males. Similarly, Greene and colleagues (1999) found survival sex to be more common among gay and bisexual youth than among heterosexual youth in general. Engler and colleagues (2005) also reported that trading sex is more common among bisexual-identified versus gay-identified males, and that the perception of prostitution as "normative" within the gay community may, in fact, make sex work more visible, accessible, and viable for some MSM. Researchers have also found that while gay-identified homeless males are at high risk for trading sex (usually with other men), higher rates of risk for sex trading exist among heterosexual- and bisexual-identified MSM (Lankenau et al., 2005).

Among the general population of homeless youth, survival sex has been found to be an economic survival strategy linked to the circumstances and duration of individuals' homeless episode(s) (Greene et al., 1999). It appears that survival sex is more prevalent among street youth than shelter-based youth, and secondarily among shelter youth with more street experience than those without. In addition, a positive relationship has been noted between engaging in survival sex and duration of time away from home, as well as between survival sex and criminal behaviors for economic gain. Finally, shelter youth with a history of physical abuse by family members are twice as likely to report engaging in survival sex once on the streets (Greene et al., 1999).

Tyler and Johnson (2006) have noted that survival sex is generally a strategy of last resort and is used relatively infrequently by homeless youth in comparison to non-sexual survival strategies such as conning and stealing. In a New York-based study, nine out of ten youth who traded sex were homeless before doing so (Lankenau et al., 2005). Both heterosexual and gay/lesbian/ bisexual (GLB) youth are more likely to use non-sexual survival strategies (i.e., shoplifting, dealing drugs, robbing others, dumpster diving, and panhandling), even when homeless (Whitbeck et al., 2004). Risk factors for engaging in survival sex include having early experiences with physical or sexual abuse, associating with friends who have traded sex, spending more time out on the street as an adolescent than in a supervised living arrangement, being a runaway or in foster care, and having little education or job skills (Tyler & Johnson, 2006).

Elwood and colleagues (1997) concluded that trading sex (in their study, primarily for drugs) is a function of situational forces, usually poverty and homelessness, and is actually an economic behavior related to one's economic and/or social powerlessness. They found no significant differences by gender or ethnicity with respect to trading sex for drugs after controlling for economic forces. Further, they noted the complex interrelationships that exist between deprivation, sex trading, substance use, sexual risk-taking, and HIV transmission, finding that MSM are more likely to trade sex for money, rather than other items such as drugs or food.

Research suggests that very few youth want to trade sex, but most often do so out of desperation and a lack of alternatives (Tyler & Johnson, 2006). The decision to do so may not be entirely voluntary, but may be largely coerced and is therefore a form of victimization. Once homeless, those who trade sex, use drugs, and/or engage in non-sexual survival strategies are at particularly high risk for trauma(s) (Benda, 2006) and may experience numerous negative outcomes directly related to trading sex that include, but are not limited to, sexual victimization, suicide attempts, severe depression episodes, and HIV seropositivity (Tyler & Johnson, 2006). A relationship has been noted, for instance, between street youths' sex trading and a history of attempted suicide (Kidd & Kral, 2002).

Newman, Rhodes and Wiess (2004) reported on important correlates to survival sex among SU-MSM in general (70.3% of the participants were non-White racial/ethnic minorities). Among the SU-MSM in Long Beach, California who traded sex, these factors included co-occurring crack and alcohol use, injection drug use (IDU; no alcohol), current homelessness, non-gay (generally hetero- or bisexual) self-identification, and a history of childhood abuse/maltreatment. They additionally found that drug use (typically methamphetamine, crack cocaine, and marijuana) was the most common reason for males to engage in survival sex. Factors that increased the odds of a SU-MSM engaging in survival sex included: crack use (four times), childhood maltreatment (2.5 times), homelessness (two times), and IDU (two times). It is notable that they found no difference in sex trading by age or ethnicity.

Prevalence and Patterns of Substance Use among MSU-MSM

Johnson et al., (2005) reported that most adolescents are first exposed to alcohol and/or drug use in their high school years. But MSM, particularly those who experience homelessness, unfortunately tend to be exposed to both alcohol and drugs at much higher rates. They may also be exposed to a much wider range of substance use earlier in their lives than many of their peers. Johnson and colleagues (2005) reported that approximately 24–71% of homeless and runaway adolescents of age 16–19 actively abused drugs, and 67.4% of the males met criteria for a substance-abuse disorder. Greene, Ennett, and Ringwalt (1997) stated that for nearly every substance, drug use prevalence was highest among street youth compared with shelter-based and stably housed youth. Gay/lesbian/bisexual/transgender (GLBT) homeless adolescents in Seattle have been found to use more types of drugs and to use them more frequently than their heterosexual peers (Cochran et al., 2002). Drug and alcohol abuse among GLB adolescents has been positively correlated with non-sexual survival strategies (Whitbeck et al., 2004).

Ongoing patterns of use appear to broaden significantly as homeless SU-MSM age out of adolescence and pass into young adulthood. Clatts et al. (2005) reported that among YMSM of age 17–28 in New York City with past and current episodes of homelessness, there exist broad and high levels of exposure to illegal drugs, both presently and during respondents' lifetimes. YMSM with past episodes of homelessness reported lifetime exposure to crack cocaine (22%), powder cocaine (60%), heroin (20%), speed (29%), MDMA (60%), ketamine (34%), and hallucinogens (41%). These rates of exposure and breadth of drug types were substantially larger than for YMSM without histories of homelessness. In addition, YMSM who were currently homeless and actively using substances, including crack-cocaine (18%), powder cocaine (16%), heroin (14%), speed (8%), and MDMA (15%) had higher levels of ongoing use of many substances. A disturbing number of currently homeless SU-MSM (10%) also reported current IDU. Overall, this research group found that currently homeless SU-MSM were more likely to be using crack cocaine and heroin and engaging in IDU than were those SU-MSM who had never been homeless and those with a past history of homelessness.

There appear to be regional differences with respect to the prevalence and use of various drugs used by the homeless SU-MSM population. However, this author was unable to locate any national statistics on the types and prevalence of substances used by MSM based on region. It would appear, based on the existing literature, that most substances are likely available in most major metropolitan areas throughout the USA. However, there may exist differences in prevalence rates based on regional/population preferences, drug availability, and local market forces for various substances.

Regarding these regional/population-based variances, Reback, Kamien, and Amass (2007) reported that alcohol, amphetamines, cocaine, and marijuana are most prevalent among homeless SU-MSM in West Hollywood, California. Semple, Patterson, and Grant (2004) reported that SU-MSM injectors typically prefer cocaine and methamphetamine over heroin, particularly in San Diego, where 28% of SU-MSM injectors preferred methamphetamines. Shoptaw and Reback (2007) reported that, in general, amphetamines tend to be more popular in the western United States, whereas heroin and speedball are desired more in eastern areas. Elwood et al. (1997) reported that crack cocaine has been quite plentiful in many poor, inner-city neighborhoods, particularly those that are predominately African American. Clatts and colleagues (2005) similarly reported that various forms of cocaine appeared to be prevalent in New York City, whereas methamphetamine was less so.

Newman et al. (2004) concluded from their study that the stereotype of the "high [HIV] risk, drug-using MSM as European American methamphetamine user" as the primary target of HIV prevention strategies may no longer be accurate; their study findings suggested that the typical methamphetamine-using MSM is now most likely to be African American. If this population shift among the SU-MSM community exists on a broader scale in the USA, it would have significant implications in regards to the tailoring of future HIV prevention and intervention and substance abuse treatment efforts.

Sexual Risk Behaviors and HIV Seroprevalence among Homeless SU-MSM

MSM are believed to be at the core of the AIDS epidemic, comprising the largest single population segment of persons living with AIDS in the USA since the epidemic was first identified (Newman et al., 2004). Despite an overall decline in AIDS diagnoses within the MSM community over recent years, an increasing proportion of new AIDS diagnoses continues to occur among ethnic minority MSM. In view of the prevalence of sexual and drug behaviors that place an individual at very high risk for contracting and/or transmitting the HIV virus, no group may be more at risk for new HIV seroprevalence than homeless MSU-MSM.

As an example, findings from a San Francisco-based study indicate that MSM participants were 4.6 times more likely to be infected with HIV, and that minority (mostly African American) MSM in San Francisco were 3.4 times more likely to be infected with HIV, in comparison with their White peers (Robertson et al., 2004). Prior syphilis infection, lifetime sex trading, blood transfusion, non-White race/ethnicity, and interaction between lifetime IDU and White race/ethnicity were found to be predictors for HIV seropositivity. Results from a five-city study with primarily African American IDU and crack-using MSM indicate that almost 17% were HIV positive; the prevalence ranged from 11% in St Louis to 21% in Long Beach (Deren et al., 2001).

There appear to be important differences in relation to sexual self-identity and sexual behavior among MSM, which has implications for HIV risk and prevalence within the MSM population. As mentioned previously, there may be differences in a MSM's sexual behavior and sexual self-identification (i.e., being behaviorally bisexual, but self-identify as being heterosexual). In their study of MSM injection drug users in San Francisco, Lewis and Watters (1994) found the highest HIV seroprevalence among gay-identified MSM, the lowest among heterosexual-identified MSM, and intermediate rates among bisexuals.

Of additional importance, many SU-MSM may have both public and private identities which may not be congruent (Deren et al., 2001). Some SU-MSM may publicly hide their sexual orientation and/or their drug use, which may contribute toward the difficulty in identifying this population. In their study, Deren et al. (2001) reported that while 31% of their minority SU-MSM (primarily African American) reported being behaviorally bisexual, only 17% identified themselves as such to others publicly. This finding may present challenges for existing HIV prevention/reduction efforts that focus on services for those MSM who gay identify, as many of those in the SU-MSM population may find these services less appealing due to their public or private non-gay identification.

Sex trading is one of the strongest predictors of future HIV diagnosis (Newman et al., 2004) and survival sex is prevalent among the homeless MSU-MSM community. Of great concern for the MSU-MSM population is that high-risk predictors for HIV include being an MSM male (Reback et al., 2007), being a crack cocaine or injection drug user (Lankenau et al., 2005), living as a homeless and/or drug-using youth (Newman et al., 2004), and engaging in sex trading (Newman et al., 2004; Reback et al., 2007).

Reback and colleagues (2007) reported that methamphetamine IDU has recently become one of the greatest risks for HIV infection and transmission, largely due to the concurrent drug and sexual risk behaviors that are prevalent in the IDU methamphetamine user community. Sexual risk-taking behaviors among MSM that are associated with cocaine or methamphetamine use include unprotected anal/oral/vaginal sex, trading sex for money/drugs, engaging in sex with HIV-positive partner(s), sex with an injection drug user, sex with anonymous partners, and having sex with a partner who has syphilis or gonorrhea (Centers for Disease Control and Prevention, 2007). The presence of hepatitis C may also increase risk (Reback et al., 2007). However, despite the rapid spread of methamphetamine injection across the USA and Western Europe in recent years (Tyler & Johnson, 2006), few studies describe the experiences and behaviors of injecting methamphetamine users in general (Semple et al., 2004), especially among homeless SU-MSM.

Sex was found to drive HIV infection among homeless and marginally housed MSM in one San Francisco-based study and IDU increased this risk

(Robertson et al., 2004). HIV infection was found to be rampant among study participants: 29.6% overall, 34.8% among MSM with lifetime IDU histories, 22.4% among MSM with no history of IDU, and 40.9% among MSM younger than 30 years. Accordingly, while IDU history was found to substantially increase one's risk of infection, it did not independently predict HIV seropositivity among MSM. Of those who were homeless or marginally housed, 32% of those who engaged in IDU tested positive for HIV, compared with 16% of those who did not report IDU (Robertson, et al., 2004). In addition, substantially higher rates of HIV seropositivity occurred among lifetime IDUs and combined crack/stimulant users who were homeless or marginally housed.

It has been asserted that the homeless SU-MSM population, in general, may be acting as a "Bridge Population" through both injection and sexual risk behaviors (Des Jarlais & Friedman, 1998). Semple and colleagues (2004) stated that through injection drug and other IDU behaviors, SU-MSM may be facilitating HIV transmission within the broader drug-injecting community. Through their sexual behavior, they may "bridge" both the IDU and non-IDU populations as well as the larger MSM community.

Prevalence and Patterns of Psychopathology and Trauma

The psychological challenges for the homeless MSM population often begin early in life. Newman and colleagues (2004) reported that the vast majority of homeless MSM experience early trauma and abuse: 82.2% of their study respondents had a history of childhood sexual abuse, parental violence, or both (70.0% parental violence and 53% childhood sexual abuse). Clatts et al. (2005) reported a high prevalence of negative life events among homeless youth, particularly YMSM, beginning from very early in their lives; these events include poverty, poor caregiver experiences, and victimization(s).

Johnson et al. (2005) found that nearly all of their study participants (93%), who included heterosexual and non-heterosexual homeless and runaway adolescents, met criteria for at least one mental disorder and a co-occurring substance-abuse disorder. Of those meeting criteria for substance abuse, 90% additionally met criteria for conduct disorder and 40% for posttraumatic stress disorder. In a study conducted by Kidd and Kral (2002), slightly more than three-quarters of the street youth in their sample had attempted suicide, with associated analyses indicating predominate themes of isolation, rejection/ betrayal, lack of control, and especially low self-worth.

However, it appears that sexual minority youth who are homeless tend to experience even higher degrees of psychopathology compared with their heterosexual peers (Cochran et al., 2002). Sexual minority youth have been found to be more likely to demonstrate higher levels of withdrawn behavior, somatic complaints, social problems, delinquency, aggression, internalizing behaviors, externalizing behaviors, and higher levels of symptomotology in general.

Homeless GLBT youth may also experience more incidents of sexual victimization since first becoming homeless (Cochran et al., 2002).

And, in a sample of 16- to 19-year-old homeless GLB youth, Whitbeck and colleagues (2004) reported finding higher rates of major depression, posttraumatic stress disorder, suicidal ideation, and actual suicide attempts compared with their heterosexual peers. Among the YMSM who were homeless, they found that 42.1% were much more likely to meet diagnostic criteria for major depression than were their heterosexual peers (24.4%). Similar findings resulted from another study of homeless SU-MSM participants: one-half demonstrated clinically significant depression, while 34% reported at least one suicide attempt (Clatts et al., 2005). Of those who had attempted suicide at least once, almost one-half (47%) reported having made multiple attempts. Despite the high rates of distress, clinical depression, and substance use, YMSM demonstrated low levels of help-seeking behaviors in comparison with their peers.

Whitbeck et al. (2004) also detected differences in the prevalence of psychopathology by gender identity. In contrast to the substantially elevated rates of internalized symptom prevalence, homeless YMSM were less likely to meet criteria for conduct disorder and/or alcohol abuse than their heterosexual counterparts. The research team suggested that YMSM are more likely to exhibit symptoms of internalization and less prevalence of externalization symptoms than are homeless heterosexual males.

Homeless SU-MSM have been found to experience an increased prevalence of many psychiatric disorders compared with adult male non-patients and adult male psychiatric inpatients. Using the Brief Symptom Inventory, Reback and colleagues (2007) found elevated levels of distress in multiple areas including somatization, obsessive-compulsive disorder, depression, anxiety, hostility, phobic anxiety, paranoid ideation, and psychoticism. Of the participants who were homeless SU-MSM, 75% met criteria for mood disorder, 43% for antisocial personality disorder, and 33% for major depressive disorder. Their average low GAF scores (48.5±6.3) were associated with symptoms such as suicidal ideation and serious social impairments.

The relationship between trauma and psychopathology within the homeless MSU-MSM population is important. In comparison with their heterosexual peers, GLBT youth have been found to experience higher levels of physical victimization (Cochran et al., 2002) and more experiences of sexual victimization since they first became homeless (Cochran et al., 2002; Whitbeck et al., 2004).

There appears to be a poverty of descriptive research on the role of trauma among the homeless MSU-MSM population. Unfortunately, trauma is an interwoven theme in the daily lives of many of these men. As indicated, victimization often begins early, as evidenced by the disturbing rates of childhood physical abuse, sexual abuse, and neglect that are prevalent among the homeless MSU-MSM community.

Homelessness itself may induce or further exacerbate trauma symptomatology through the loss of routines, important daily social and emotional contacts, and the lack of a safe place (Goodman, Saxe, & Harvey, 1991). Homelessness may be overwhelmingly stressful, often leading to prolonged states of hypervigilance, a sense of vulnerability, severe anxiety, and fear and may lead to the worsening of already-present symptoms as the result of stress or inadequate access to appropriate management plans (Goodman et al., 1991). The traumatic experiences associated with homelessness may have cumulative or additive effects (Benda, 2006).

Interventions and Future Considerations

Homeless MSU-MSM face severe health and safety issues, including homelessness, racial/ethnic and sexual discrimination, sexual and HIV risk behaviors, drug addiction, exploitation/victimization, trauma, psychopathology, and poverty. This population has received increasing attention in recent years as a function of HIV prevention efforts, but has rarely garnered attention otherwise.

Due to the confluence of historical negative life events and ongoing daily struggles that many homeless MSU-MSM must face, a variety of approaches are warranted in order to improve public health outcomes and individuals' quality of life. Though this population may constitute a small proportion of the overall MSM community, it is important to generate more effective HIV prevention/reduction efforts that specifically address the concerns of this population in order to reduce the level of HIV risk in this community (Rietmeijer, Wolitski, Fishbein, Corby, & Cohn, 1998).

HIV counseling and testing have been shown to be effective when used as part of a two-session, client-centered counseling intervention (Rietmeijer et al., 1998). Localized, community-based efforts that tailor services more closely to the experiences of the particular members of this highly diverse community through the use of health communication, prevention marketing, community mobilization and empowerment, and the environmental facilitation of safer behaviors have demonstrated effectiveness (Rietmeijer et al., 1998).

Specialized behavioral interventions using brief, low-intensity intervention programing to address methamphetamine use and its concurrent HIV risk behaviors have been suggested (Shoptaw & Reback, 2007). More intensive drug treatment services may utilize both contingency management and cognitive-behavioral treatments. Greene and colleagues (1999) have recommended the urgent development of intensive long-term services to provide alternatives to trading sex to meet basic survival needs, access to comprehensive counseling and drug treatment services, independent living for those without housing, employment programing, drop-in centers, and outreach services to make contact with those who may be least likely to seek help.

Interventions that are privately accessible and attentive to distinctions in sexual and gender identification, rather than being geared toward public identities, are needed (Deren et al., 2001). A comprehensive treatment approach that incorporates drug, primary care, mental health, and HIV needs should be utilized, particularly with SU-MSM, in order to meet the individual "where he is at" and to assess his readiness to change.

Seal and colleagues (2000) found from their survey of primarily ethnic minority YMSM under age 25 in Milwaukee and Detroit that the young men were interested in having services that were comprehensive and that would address issues related to relationships; sex, sexual identity, and sexuality; substance use; self-esteem and self-worth; and abuse. Desirable programing was characterized as being confidential, fun, and accepting, particularly with regard to sexual identity. The men were specifically interested in resources such as safe spaces for youth, peer educators, mentorship by older MSM mentors, school-based sexuality education, and greater societal and community support (Seal et al., 2000).

Finally, rapid housing intervention efforts to prevent or quickly intervene upon one's entry into homelessness may be of critical importance. Rapidly arranged, behaviorally flexible housing such as the Housing First initiative represents a particularly important complement to any comprehensive care plan.

Additional research is needed in the form of a national representative study if we are to better understand the regional and demographic characteristics of the homeless MSU-MSM population and the health-related needs of this population. Critical research questions include an examination of the differences between the needs and values of youth and adult homeless MSM, the impact of specific substances on behavior, and the efficacy of various interventions to ameliorate the health-related concerns of and improve the quality of life of the homeless MSU-MSM population.

References

Benda, B. (2006). Survival analyses of social support and trauma among homeless male and female veterans who abuse substances. *American Journal of Orthopsychiatry, 76*(1), 70–79.

Clatts, M., Goldsamt, L., Yi, H., & Gwadz, M. (2005). Homelessness and drug abuse among young men who have sex with men in New York City: A preliminary epidemiological trajectory. *Journal of Adolescence, 28,* 201–214.

Cochran, B., Stewart, A., Ginzler, J., & Cauce, A. (2002). Challenges faced by homeless sexual minorities: comparison of gay, lesbian, bisexual, and transgender homeless adolescents with their heterosexual counterparts. *American Journal of Public Health, 92*(5), 773–777.

Deren, S., Stark, M., Rhodes, F., Siegal, H., Cottler, L, & Wood, M. et al. (2001). Drug-using men who have sex with men: sexual behaviours and sexual identities. *Culture, Health & Sexuality, 3*(3), 329–338.

Centers for Disease Control and Prevention (2007). Methamphetamine use and risk for HIV/AIDS. Last accessed June 30, 2007; Available at http://www.cdc.gov/hiv/resources/factsheets/meth.htm

Des Jarlais, D.C., & Friedman, S.R. (1998). Fifteen years of research on preventing HIV infection among injecting drug users: what we have learned, what we have not learned, what we have done, what we have not done. *Public Health Reports, 113*(1) 182–188.

Elwood, W., Williams, M., Bell, D. & Richard, A. (1997). Powerlessness and HIV prevention among people who trade sex for drugs ("strawberries"). *AIDS Care, 9*(3) 273–284.

Engler, K., Otis, J., Alary, M., Masse, B., Remis, R., & Girard, M. et al. (2005). An exploration of sexual behaviour and self-definition in a cohort of men who have sex with men. *The Canadian Journal of Human Sexuality, 14*(3–4) 87–104.

Goodman, L., Saxe, L., & Harvey, M. (1991). Homelessness as psychological trauma. *American Psychologist, 46*, 1219–1225.

Greenblatt, M. & Robertson, M. (1993). Life-styles, adaptive strategies, and sexual behaviors of homeless adolescents. *Hospital & Community Psychiatry, 44*(12) 1177–1180.

Greene, J., Ennett, S., & Ringwalt, C. (1997). Substance use among runaway and homeless youth in three national samples. *American Journal of Public Health, 87*(2) 229–235.

Greene, J., Ennett, S., & Ringwalt, C. (1999). Prevalence and correlates of survival sex among runaway and homeless youth. *American Journal of Public Health, 89*(9) 1406–1409.

Harvard Mental Health Letter (2005). The homeless mentally ill. Last accessed June 6, 2007; Available at www.health.harvard.edu

Johnson, K., Whitbeck, L., & Hoyt, D. (2005). Substance abuse disorders among homeless and runaway adolescents. *Journal of Drug Issues, 4*, 799–816.

Kidd, S. & Kral, M. (2002). Suicide and prostitution among street youth: A qualitative analysis. *Adolescence, 37*(146) 411–431.

Kipke, M., Unger, J., O'Connor, S., Palmer, R. & LaFrance, S. (1997). Street youth, their peer group affiliation, and differences according to residential status, subsistence patterns, and use of services. *Adolescence, 32*, 655–669.

Lankenau, S., Clatts, M., Welle, D., Goldsamt, L., & Gwadz, M. (2005). Street careers: homelessness, drug use, and sex work among young men who have sex with men (YMSM). *International Journal of Drug Policy, 16*, 10–18.

Linn, J., Brown, M., & Kendrick, L. (2005). Injection drug use among homeless adults in the southeast with severe mental illness. *Journal of Health Care for the Poor and Underserved, 16*, 83–90.

Lewis, D., & Watters, J. (1994). Sexual behaviour and sexual identity in male injection drug users. *Journal of Acquired Immune Deficiency Syndromes, 7*, 190–198.

National Coalition for the Homeless (2006). How many people experience homelessness? Last accessed June 30, 2007; Available at www.nationalhomeless.org/publications/ facts/ How_Many.pdf

Newman, P., Rhodes, F., & Wiess, R. (2004). Correlates of sex trading among drug-using men who have sex with men. *American Journal of Public Health, 94*(11) 1998–2003.

Reback, C., Kamien, J., & Amass, L. (2007). Characteristics and HIV risk behaviors of homeless, substance-using men who have sex with men. *Addictive Behaviors, 32*, 647–654.

Rietmeijer, C., Wolitski, R., Fishbein, M., Corby, N., & Cohn, D. (1998). Sex hustling, injection drug use, and non-gay identification by men who have sex with men: associations with high-risk sexual behaviors and condom use. *Sexually Transmitted Diseases, 25*(7) 353–360.

Robertson, M., Clark, R., Charlesbois, E., Tulsky, J., Long, H., Bangsberg, D. et al. (2004). HIV seroprevalence among homeless and marginally housed adults in San Francisco. *American Journal of Public Health, 94*(7) 1207–1217.

Seal, D., Kelly, J., Bloom, F., Stevenson, L., Coley, B., Broyles, A. et al (2000). HIV prevention with young men who have sex with men: what young men themselves say is needed. *AIDS Care, 12*(1) 5–26.

Semple, S., Patterson, T., & Grant, I. (2004). A comparison of injection and non-injection methamphetamine-using HIV positive men who have sex with men. *Drug and Alcohol Dependence, 76*, 203–212.

Shoptaw, S., & Reback, C. (2007). Methamphetamine use and infectious disease-related behaviors in men who have sex with men: implications for interventions. *Addiction*, *102*(1) 130–135.

Tyler, K. & Johnson, K. (2006). Trading sex: Voluntary or coerced? The experiences of homeless youth. *The Journal of Sex Research*, *43*(3) 208–216.

Whitbeck, L., Chen, X., Hoyt, D., Tyler, K., & Johnson, K. (2004). Mental disorder, subsistence strategies, and victimization among gay, lesbian, and bisexual homeless and runaway adolescents. *Journal of Sex Research*, *41*(4) 329–342.

Chapter Six
"My Body and My Spirit Took Care of Me"

Homelessness, Violence, and Resilience Among American Indian Two-Spirit Men

Karina L. Walters, David H. Chae, A. Tyler Perry, Antony Stately, Roy Old Person and Jane M. Simoni

> *It was colonization that introduced structures of homophobia, racism, capitalism, and sexism into most Native nations.*
>
> -Andrea Smith (1998: 190)

Introduction

Public and scientific discourse on health disparities often fails to consider American Indians and Alaska Natives (AIAN or "Natives"), especially those who are gay, lesbian, bisexual, and transgender (hereafter referred to as "two-spirit"). Two-spirit Native men who are living on the streets or in unstable housing are even further marginalized. The invisibility of Native men's health, in general, and two-spirit men's health, in particular, stems from their existence as a people in a colonial nation state that has endured a succession of traumatic assaults on their land, homes, bodies, minds, and spirits. As Warren (1993, cited in Smitha, 1998: 17) noted, "Dysfunctional systems are often maintained through systematic denial, a failure or inability to see the reality of a situation. This denial need not be conscious, intentional, or malicious; it only needs to be pervasive to be effective."

The little research that exists on the health of Native men suggests that they share a disproportionate burden in terms of morbidity and mortality. Specifically, Native men aged 15–19 years are more likely to die by suicide, homicide, motor vehicle accidents, firearm-related incidents, and drowning than any other racial/ethnic group in the United States (U.S.; U.S. Indian Health Service [IHS], 1997). In fact, nearly one-fourth of Native men die by 34 years of age, and nearly one-half die by the age of 54 (United States Indian Health Service [IHS], 2001).

Karina L. Walters
University of Washington School of Social Work, Seattle, WA

S. Loue (ed.), *Health Issues Confronting Minority Men Who Have Sex with Men.*   125
© Springer 2008

Structural inequities such as housing instability as well as episodic and chronic homelessness are thought to play a major role in the health vulnerabilities of Native men. However, the actual extent of homelessness among Natives is unknown. There is inadequate census sampling and tracking and the homelessness of many Natives is hidden. Many Native men reside in temporary treatment centers or hotels/motels; others frequently move around or migrate back and forth from the reservation to the city, staying on sofas and floors of extended family or friends (Lobo & Vaughn, 2003).

Structural, familial, and individual factors contribute to Native's men risk for homelessness and housing instability. Specifically, they are more vulnerable because of their persistent poverty, low levels of social support, substance use disorders (especially alcohol abuse and dependence), lack of affordable or adequate housing, high rates of trauma exposure, and housing instability during childhood or adolescence. Another factor may be discrimination and maltreatment related to sexual orientation. Research indicates that between 13 and 35% of homeless youth identify as a sexual minority (Clatts & Davis, 1999; Lankenau, Clatts, Welle, Goldamt, & Gwadz, 2005).

Although no data specifically on two-spirit homeless men and boys exist to our knowledge, research on homeless gay-identified boys more broadly suggests that 25–47% have engaged in survival sex (Lankenau et al., 2005; Tyler & Cauce, 2002). Moreover, compared with heterosexual homeless youth, sexual minority homeless youth are more likely to report victimization (especially sexual assault); substance abuse; multiple sexual partners; and psychopathology (i.e., depression, suicide, posttraumatic stress disorder or PTSD) than their heterosexual counterparts (Cochran, Stewart, Ginzler, & Cauce, 2002; Whitbeck, Chen, Hoyt, Tyler, & Johnson, 2004; Yoder, Hoyt, & Whitbeck, 1998). One study found that gay, lesbian, and bisexual homeless youth were more likely than other youth to meet criteria for a major depressive episode (41 vs. 29%), PTSD (48 vs. 33%), and suicide attempt (57 vs. 34%; Whitbeck et al., 2004).

Native men who are two-spirit must negotiate their multiple oppressed statuses. Often, they contend with homophobia in Native communities as well as racism in predominantly non-Native gay, lesbian, bisexual, and transgender communities (Fieland, Walters, & Simoni, 2007; Simoni, Walters, Balsam, & Meyers, 2006; Walters, 1997; Walters, Simoni, & Horwath, 2001). Despite considerable heterogeneity between and within the 562 federally recognized tribes in the U.S., shared colonial histories have created common experiences among two-spirits, shaping distinctive conditions of risk and resilience (Fieland, Walters, & Simoni, 2007). Specifically, preliminary evidence suggests that two-spirits experience disproportionately higher rates of anti-gay as well as anti-Native violence, including high rates of sexual and physical assault in childhood and adulthood (Greenfeld & Smith, 1999; Simoni et al., 2006; Walters et al., 2001) and self-reported intergenerational historical trauma (Balsam, Huang, Fieland, Simoni, & Walters, 2004)—experiences that are typically linked to adverse health and psychosocial functioning.

It is important to note that despite their exposure to multiple traumatic stressors, not all two-spirits experience health problems. Researchers have proposed various pathways to explain the association between traumatic stressors and well-being for non-Native populations. In particular, empirical studies have identified cultural factors such as traditionalism (Cuandrado & Lieberman, 1998); Afrocentricity (Belgrave et al., 1997); religiosity and spirituality (Corwyn & Benda, 2000); and identity (Scheier, Botvin, Diaz, & Ifill-Williams, 1997; Townsend & Belgrave, 2000). Emerging research indicates that the very areas of AIAN culture that have been targeted and wounded through colonial processes (i.e., group identity, spirituality, and traditional healing practices) may, in fact, be strongholds of resistance and resiliency (Walters, Simoni, & Evans-Campbell, 2002; Whitbeck, Adams, Hoyt, & Chen, 2004). Although researchers are just beginning to empirically examine many of these factors in Native communities, Natives themselves have long relied on identity, enculturation, spirituality, as well as traditional health and healing practices to sustain their wellness and resistance efforts.

In this chapter, we examined factors that may be associated with housing among two-spirit AIAN men. To help elucidate factors that may both impact as well as be a consequence of housing status, we examine quantitative and qualitative data from the HONOR Project, a cross-sectional study of the health of two-spirit AIAN in seven urban areas of the US: Seattle-Tacoma, San-Francisco-Oakland, Los Angeles, Tulsa-Oklahoma City, Minneapolis-St Paul, Denver, and New York City. The HONOR Project consisted of two distinct components: (1) a quantitative part based on the collection of survey data; and (2) a qualitative portion which consisted of in-depth interviews with community members. In Study 1, we analyzed quantitative data to describe the extent of unstable housing or homelessness, as well as to identify demographic and psychosocial correlates of housing status. In Study 2, we used qualitative data from interviews with two-spirit men who are marginally housed (i.e., living in substance-use treatment facilities, shelters, or abandoned buildings) to elucidate these relationships, focusing on participants' struggles as well as their resilience with regard to housing. Additionally, we identified factors that may precipitate housing instability or result from it, including violence exposure as well as mental and physical health outcomes.

Study 1: Quantitative Survey Component

Procedures and Sample

Participants in the quantitative component of the HONOR Project were recruited as part of a national multisite cross-sectional survey of AIAN

LGBT (Lesbian, Gay, Bisexual, Transgender and/or two-spirit persons). Recruitment included both targeted sampling and modified respondent-driven sampling techniques. In Seattle, the census site, the study was open to the entire Native two-spirit community, and individuals were recruited with posters, booths at relevant events, and word-of-mouth. At the other sites, the site coordinator developed a targeted sampling list of first-wave seeds (approximately 6–8 per site). The seeds consisted of equal numbers of men and women who varied in age and gender expression. Voluntary participants also were solicited via agency newsletters as well as study brochures and posters. All participants provided information about their social networks in order to identify other potential respondents. At the Seattle site, they were then given printed coupons and asked to give one to each social network member they identified who met the study criteria. At the other sites, approximately four eligible "nominees" were randomly selected from the respondent's network lists. For each such "nominee" who contacted the study staff, respondents were compensated $10.00 (they were never informed of which nominees responded). Additionally, each respondent received two additional coupons to distribute to other potential respondents they might later recall or meet (coupons were coded to this effect). Duplicity in this study was limited since each site had one site coordinator.

Eligibility requirements were: (a) self-identifying as American Indian, Alaskan Native, or First Nations AND either being enrolled in a tribal nation OR having at least one-quarter in total American Indian blood quantum (across tribes); (b) self-identifying as gay, lesbian, bisexual, transgender, or two-spirit OR have had sexual relations with someone of the same biological sex during the past 12 months; (c) residing, working, or socializing in the local study site; (d) being 18 years of age or older; and (e) speaking English.

A total of 448 participants were recruited to the HONOR Project. Four participants could not be classified as gay, lesbian, bisexual, two-spirit, or other sexual minority based on self-reported sexual orientation, gender identity, sexual attraction, and sexual behaviors. A total of 444 participants comprised the analytic dataset of the HONOR Project. The current study is restricted to men and transgender participants ($n = 259$).

Eligible individuals who provided written consent were enrolled in the study. Each respondent received $65 for completing a 3–4-hour computer-assisted personal interview in a private location of their choosing or at the study site. All study procedures were approved by the institutional review board of the University of Washington.

Measures

Demographic Characteristics. Demographic characteristics examined in the present study are self-reported degree of Indian blood (<25%, 25–49%,

50–74%, or ≥75%); age; education (less than high school or <12 years; high school or 12 years; some college or 13–15 years; and at least college or 16+ years); employment status (working, not working, retired, and disabled); and annual household income (<$18,000, $18,001–$30,000, $30,001–$60,000, and > $30,000).

Housing Status. Housing status was measured using a single item assessing current living situation. Participants who reported living at a residence they owned or rented or who were living in a dormitory were classified as having stable housing. Those who reported living in someone else's residence where they did not pay rent; in a rooming, boarding, or half-way house; or at a shelter, welfare hotel, group home, or drug or health treatment facility were classified as having unstable housing. Participants who reported living on the streets or in parks, subways, or abandoned buildings were classified as homeless.

Gender Identity. Four categories of gender identity were constructed based on two items assessing biological sex at birth and current gender identification. Participants were classified as men if they reported being biologically male at birth and currently identified as men. Participants who reported being biologically male at birth and currently identified as two-spirit were classified as male/two-spirit. Participants who reported being male at birth and reported currently being a woman or transgender were classified as being transgender M–F. Those who reported being female at birth and currently identified as men or transgender were classified as transgender F–M.

HIV Status. A single item was used to assess HIV status. Participants who reported an HIV-negative result the last time they were tested were classified as HIV-negative; those who reported being HIV-positive were classified as HIV-positive. Participants who reported never being tested for HIV or who reported being tested but never receiving a result were classified as being of unknown HIV status.

Sex Trade. Engagement in sex trade was assessed using a single item. Participants who reported ever exchanging sex for money, drugs, food, or shelter were classified as trading sex.

Suicide Attempt. Attempted suicide was assessed using a single item. Participants who reported ever attempting suicide were classified as ever being suicidal.

Depressive Mood. Depressive mood was measured using the 10-item version of the Centers for Epidemiologic Studies Depression Scale (CESD-10; Radloff, 1977) designed to measure affective, cognitive, and somatic symptoms of depression. Items were measured on a four-point Likert scale (0 = rarely or none of the time; 3 = most or all of the time). Positively valenced items were reverse-coded and all items were summed. Possible scores ranged from 0 to 30, with higher scores reflecting greater depressive symptoms ($\alpha = 0.82$). We also created a dichotomous measure using the cutoff of ≥10 reflecting high risk vs. low risk for clinically significant depression (Radloff, 1977).

Childhood Trauma. Childhood trauma was assessed using the Childhood Trauma Questionnaire (Bernstein et al., 1994), consisting of five subscales:

(1) childhood emotional abuse ($\alpha = 0.86$), e.g., "I thought that my parents wished I had never been born", "People in my family said hurtful or insulting things to me"; (2) childhood physical abuse ($\alpha = 0.87$), e.g., "I got hit so hard by someone in my family that I had to see a doctor or go to the hospital", "People in my family hit me so hard that it left me with bruises or marks"; (3) childhood sexual abuse ($\alpha = 0.93$), e.g., "Someone molested me", "Someone tried to touch me in a sexual way or tried to make me touch them"; (4) childhood emotional neglect ($\alpha = 0.87$), e.g., "I felt loved", "People in my family looked out for each other"; and (5) childhood physical neglect ($\alpha = 0.71$), e.g., "I didn't have enough to eat", "My parents were too drunk or high to take care of the family". Each subscale consisted of five items measures on a six-point Likert scale (0 = never true; 5 = very often true). Positively valenced items were reverse-coded and summed scores for each subscale ranged from 0 to 25. Because items in the original scale were measured on a five-point scale ranging from 1 to 5, we rescaled our summed scores to range from 5 to 25. Using cutoffs defined by the authors, we also constructed the following categories for each subscale: 5–8.9 = none/minimal; 9–12.9 = moderate; 13–15.9 = severe; 16 or more = extreme.

Domestic Violence. Experiences of domestic violence were assessed using two scales: the Experience with Battering Scale (EBS; Coker, Pope, Smith, Sanderson, & Hussey, 2001) and the Index of Partner Physical Abuse (IPA; Coker et al., 2001). The EBS consisted of 10 items assessing whether participants had symptoms of partner battery (e.g., being made to feel unsafe in their home, feeling owned and controlled); the IPA consisted of 14 items assessing incidents of physical abuse by a partner (e.g., being punched, kicked, hit with an object). Participants who reported any symptoms of battery or who reported any specific instances of physical abuse were classified as having experienced domestic violence.

Alcohol Abuse/Dependence. Past year alcohol abuse/dependence was assessed using the Alcohol Abuse and Dependence section of the MINI International Neuropsychiatric Interview (MINI), English Version 5.0.0. (LeCrubier et al., 1997). Participants who reported meeting at least three out of seven criteria for alcohol dependence, such as tolerance and withdrawal, were classified as having alcohol dependence disorder. Participants were only assessed for alcohol abuse, generally considered less severe, if they did not meet criteria for dependence. Participants meeting at least one of four criteria for alcohol abuse, including alcohol-related problems, were classified as having an alcohol abuse disorder. In the current study, participants meeting criteria for alcohol abuse or disorder were combined.

Posttraumatic Stress. Posttraumatic stress was assessed using the Posttrau-matic Stress Diagnostic Scale (PDS; Foa, Cashman, Jaycox, & Perry, 1997). The PDS consists of four sections: (1) a checklist of 11 possible traumas, including imprisonment, assault, and natural disaster, and an additional item assessing "other" traumatic event; (2) a description of the most traumatizing event; (3) assessment of posttraumatic symptoms associated with the most traumatizing event; and (4) the impact of those symptoms on functioning. We used Part 1 to assess the total number traumas endorsed. We used Part 3 to assess total symptom severity, which was calculated as the sum of 17 items assessing symptoms of posttraumatic stress, including emotional, physical, and cognitive symptoms. Symptoms were assessed with respect to the past month, and item values ranged from 0 ("not at all or only one time") to 3 ("five or more times a week/almost all the time"). Responses were summed and possible values ranged from 0 to 51, with higher scores representing greater symptom severity ($\alpha = 0.95$). Because participants who did not report any traumas in Part 1 did not receive subsequent sections of the PDS, they were classified as having no posttraumatic stress symptoms.

Data Analysis

Analyses were aimed at describing the distribution of gender identity, HIV status, sex trading, attempted suicide, depressive mood, childhood traumas, alcohol abuse/dependence, posttraumatic stress, domestic violence, and demographic characteristics by housing status. Mean substitution was used to handle missing data that were part of multiple-item scales with at least 80% complete data. For all other descriptive analyses, only participants with complete data on the variable are presented. Given the small sample size in some cells, we used Fisher's exact tests to examine differences in housing for categorical variables and ANOVAs to examine differences in housing for continuous variables.

Results and Discussion

Socio-demographic characteristics by housing status are presented in Table 6.1. Although a majority of the participants in our sample (63.1%) reported being in stable housing, a substantial percent of respondents (36.9%) were in some form of unstable housing (i.e., either unstable or homeless), with nearly 10% being homeless. Several noteworthy findings emerged when comparing participants in stable housing, unstable housing, and those who were homeless on demographic and psychosocial characteristics. Although we did not find evidence for a statistically significant difference in HIV status by housing, we did find that participants with unknown HIV status were more likely to be either in unstable housing or homeless. This finding has strong implications for HIV prevention policies and the population-level incidence of HIV transmission. Two-spirit AIAN who are not in stable housing may be less likely to get tested for HIV, be less likely to know their HIV status, and subsequently may be more likely to engage in HIV risk behaviors or less likely to engage in safer-sex practices.

In examining mental health outcomes, we also found evidence for serious mental health concerns impacting two-spirit AIAN communities. We found a

Table 6.1 Socio-demographic characteristics of male and transgender sexual minority participants by housing status

	Stable housing (n = 154)	Unstable housing (n = 67)	Homeless (n = 23)
Gender identity, n (%)			
Men	100 (64.9)	39 (58.2)	12 (52.2)
Men, two-spirit	33 (21.4)	20 (29.9)	7 (30.4)
Transgender M-F	15 (9.7)	5 (7.5)	3 (13.0)
Transgender F-M	6 (3.9)	3 (4.5)	1 (4.3)
HIV status, n (%)			
Negative	96 (62.3)	40 (59.7)	14 (60.9)
Positive	50 (32.5)	21 (31.3)	6 (26.1)
Unknown	8 (5.2)	6 (9.0)	3 (13.0)
Trade sex, n (%)			
Never	94 (61.0)	37 (55.2)	16 (76.2)
Ever	60 (39.0)	30 (44.8)	5 (23.8)
Suicide attempt, n (%)			
Never	114 (75.0)	51 (77.3)	17 (73.9)
Ever	38 (25.0)	15 (22.7)	6 (26.1)
Depressive mood, mean (SD)*	10.1 (6.4)	11.7 (7.1)	13.7 (7.2)
Depression, n (%)			
Low risk	72 (46.8)	29 (43.3)	9 (39.1)
High risk	82 (53.2)	38 (56.7)	14 (60.9)
Childhood emotional abuse, mean (SD)	12.3 (6.3)	13.2 (6.2)	11.1 (6.7)
Childhood emotional abuse, n (%)			
None/minimal	59 (38.6)	20 (30.3)	10 (45.5)
Moderate	23 (15.0)	10 (15.2)	4 (18.2)
Severe	20 (13.1)	12 (18.2)	2 (9.1)
Extreme	51 (33.3)	24 (36.4)	6 (27.3)
Childhood physical abuse, mean (SD)	11.2 (6.3)	11.6 (6.3)	9.3 (5.2)
Childhood physical abuse, n (%)			
None/minimal	68 (44.4)	26 (39.4)	13 (61.9)
Moderate	30 (19.6)	13 (19.7)	1 (4.8)
Severe	17 (11.1)	9 (13.6)	4 (19.0)
Extreme	38 (24.8)	18 (27.3)	3 (14.3)
Childhood sexual abuse, mean (SD)	11.3 (7.2)	12.1 (7.3)	11.1 (7.3)
Childhood sexual abuse, n (%)			
None/minimal	83 (54.2)	29 (43.9)	12 (54.5)
Moderate	10 (6.5)	9 (13.6)	1 (4.5)
Severe	15 (9.8)	6 (9.1)	0 (0.0)
Extreme	45 (29.4)	22 (33.3)	9 (40.9)
Childhood emotional neglect, mean (SD)	11.5 (6.3)	10.9 (5.3)	13.8 (6.6)

Table 6.1 (continued)

	Stable housing (n = 154)	Unstable housing (n = 67)	Homeless (n = 23)
Childhood emotional neglect, n (%) **			
None/minimal	59 (38.6)	27 (40.9)	8 (38.1)
Moderate	43 (28.1)	14 (21.2)	1 (4.8)
Severe	16 (10.5)	16 (24.2)	2 (9.5)
Extreme	35 (22.9)	9 (13.6)	10 (47.6)
Childhood physical neglect, mean (SD)	10.1 (4.7)	10.2 (5.2)	10.2 (4.0)
Childhood physical neglect, n (%)			
None/minimal	69 (45.1)	30 (45.5)	8 (36.4)
Moderate	36 (23.5)	14 (21.2)	5 (22.7)
Severe	29 (19.0)	12 (18.2)	8 (36.4)
Extreme	19 (12.4)	10 (15.2)	1 (4.5)
Traumatic events, n (%)			
None	11 (7.1)	6 (9.0)	2 (8.7)
1 or 2 events	34 (22.1)	9 (13.4)	3 (13.0)
3 or more events	109 (70.8)	52 (77.6)	18 (78.3)
Posttraumatic stress, mean (SD) **	7.1 (8.9)	11.9 (12.8)	12.4 (11.4)
Domestic violence, n (%)			
None	77 (50.7)	28 (41.8)	12 (57.1)
Any	75 (49.3)	39 (58.2)	9 (42.9)
Alcohol disorder, n (%)***			
None	103 (67.3)	29 (43.9)	5 (21.7)
Any	50 (32.7)	37 (56.1)	18 (78.3)
Indian blood, n (%)			
<25%	5 (3.3)	6 (9.0)	3 (13.0)
25–49%	38 (24.8)	19 (28.4)	4 (17.4)
50–74%	37 (24.2)	16 (23.9)	6 (26.1)
75% or more	73 (47.7)	26 (38.8)	10 (43.5)
Age, mean (SD)*	40.7 (11.0)	36.9 (10.8)	37.9 (8.1)
Education, n (%)***			
<12 years	16 (10.4)	12 (17.9)	7 (30.4)
12 years	32 (20.8)	29 (43.3)	13 (56.5)
13-15 years	63 (40.9)	18 (26.9)	3 (13.0)
16 + years	43 (27.9)	8 (11.9)	0 (0.0)
Work status, n (%)**			
Working	85 (55.2)	21 (31.3)	4 (17.4)
Not working	37 (24.0)	22 (32.8)	11 (47.8)
Retired	7 (4.5)	4 (6.0)	1 (4.3)
Disabled	25 (16.2)	20 (29.9)	7 (30.4)
Household income, n (%) *			
<$18,000	85 (55.9)	44 (71.0)	22 (95.7)
$18,001–$30,000	26 (17.1)	8 (12.9)	0 (0.0)

Table 6.1 (continued)

	Stable housing (n = 154)	Unstable housing (n = 67)	Homeless (n = 23)
$30,001–$60,000	25 (16.4)	7 (11.3)	1 (4.3)
= $60,000	16 (10.5)	3 (4.8)	0 (0.0)

*p < 0.05
**p < 0.01
***p < 0.001

very high prevalence of depression in our sample, with more than half of participants overall meeting the more conservative CESD-10 cutoff of ≥10 for high risk of depression (54.9%). We also found significant differences in levels of depression by housing status, with homeless participants having the highest mean score (mean = 13.7), followed by those who were in unstable housing (mean = 11.7); and with those in stable housing have the lowest levels of depression (mean = 10.1). We also found that homeless participants had the highest levels of posttraumatic stress symptoms (mean = 12.4), followed by those in unstable housing (mean = 11.9) and stable housing (mean = 7.1). Our results indicated a very high prevalence of alcohol abuse/dependence in our sample overall (43.4%), as well as evidence for significant differences by housing status. Participants in unstable housing or who were homeless were more likely to have an alcohol disorder (56.1 and 78.3%) compared with those in stable housing (32.7%). These results suggest that negative mental health and substance use outcomes may occur in tandem with poorer housing outcomes among two-spirit AIAN, and that primary and secondary prevention and treatment strategies should address not only more structural-level inequalities in housing, but also issues of individual-level psychological well-being and substance use that may occur in tandem with housing outcomes, particularly depression, posttraumatic stress, and alcohol disorders.

Although we did not find evidence for significant differences in childhood abuse variables in our sample (physical, emotional, sexual) and no evidence for differences in physical neglect, we did find significant differences in childhood emotional neglect by housing status. Our results suggest that participants who experienced extreme childhood emotional neglect may be more likely to be homeless. Experiences of adversity during childhood, specifically childhood neglect, may have long-standing negative housing consequences in this population.

Our analyses also revealed interesting patterns in our demographic variables by housing status. We found that participants in stable housing were older. In addition, as expected, participants in stable housing had higher levels of education, were working, and had higher levels of household income, whereas participants who were in unstable housing or were homeless had lower levels of education, were more likely to be not working or disabled, and were less affluent. In accordance with what we had predicted, pathological socioeconomic conditions may be correlated with adverse housing outcomes among two-spirit AIAN.

Together, these results indicate that poor housing outcomes are a serious concern among two-spirit AIAN men and transgender people. In addition, we identified a number of demographic and psychosocial factors that may be risk factors for unstable housing or homelessness; or may be consequences thereof. Our findings suggest that mitigating negative housing outcomes in this population should entail a multifaceted approach that addresses not only socioeconomic circumstances that may underlie housing instability or homelessness, but also mental, behavioral, and early childhood factors. An important caveat to our results is the inability to determine the causal direction of our associations, given the cross-sectional nature of our data. For example, it is uncertain whether poorer mental health outcomes associated with housing instability or homelessness were risk factors for poor housing outcomes; or whether housing instability was a risk factor for negative indicators of psychological well-being. Similarly, it is difficult to conclude whether disorders related to alcohol consumption occurred prior to housing instability or homelessness, versus whether alcohol abuse/dependence was a means of coping with stressors associated with poor housing outcomes.

In order to better understand the meaning of the associations that we had found as well as elucidate both consequences of and mechanisms leading to housing instability and homelessness among two-spirit AIAN, we examined transcripts from in-depth interviews in the qualitative component of the HONOR project.

Study 2: Qualitative Component

Sample

Working in concert with local and regional two-spirit communities and Native agencies, local site coordinators identified key two-spirit activists and leaders for participation. Over 60 of the two-spirit leaders identified by site coordinators participated in an approximately 3-hour interview, covering topics ranging from terminology and identity to health concerns and community strengths. In this study, we used theoretical sampling, entailing a review of transcripts, to select five respondents with histories of unstable housing or periods of homelessness in their life span.

Selected participants were in their late 40s to late 50s and represented tribal diversity—from the Great Lakes, northern plains, northwest, and northeast. All had spent a considerable part of their childhood on the "rez" or in tribal communities and all currently lived in urban/suburban or rural locales. To respect confidentiality in reports of the findings, we use pseudonyms, omit tribal affiliations, and exclude any details that would link the participants to a particular community.

Interview Procedures

Utilizing narrative and indigenist research methods, Native interviewers provided the opportunity for two-spirit leaders to give their *testimonios*, a type of oral history and life story (Bishop, 2005; McMahan & Rogers, 1994; Smith, 2005). We acknowledge that the research process has been and is simultaneously linked to liberation as well as histories of oppression and racism. *Testimonios* provided two-spirit men the opportunity to reclaim and tell their stories in their own ways and to give voice to their collective histories (Smith, 2005). Therefore, the focus of the interview was not to recall "accurate" historical events; rather, the focus was on the meanings that familial, spiritual, communal, and historical events have had in shaping turning points or key life experiences for two-spirit and collective identities as well as mental health processes.

We recognize that these narratives function in various ways. They are explicitly political in that they describe and resist oppressive forces. They serve to create, in part, a collective memory and a sense of collective identity in the development of two-spirit movement unity and solidarity (Gongaware, 2003). And, embedded in these narratives are the indigenist ways of knowing, worldviews, "deep metaphors", and ways to theorize lived lives and connect with past histories but also with ancestral ties in relation to future generations (Marker, 2003; Smith, 2005a). We have chosen to use the two-spirit men's own words, as much as possible, to illustrate similarities and differences in how Native two-spirit men "talk" about or give testimony to their lived experiences around homelessness, violence, and resilience.

Data Analysis

We used a modified form of a feminist interpretive method of narrative analysis called the Listening Guide, originated by Brown, Tappan, Gilligan, Miller, and Argyris (1989). Each narrative was "listened to" by having multiple readers (including two two-spirit men) read the transcripts multiple times with the intention of "listening" to different aspects of a particular topic (e.g., housing instability) and then rereading the transcripts to listen or focus on a different aspect of the topic of interest each time. Sections of the transcripts were color-coded, creating a visual map of the narratives' layers in which identifiable, coherent "voices" could be heard. One of the two-spirit authors "listened" by recording her thoughts simultaneous to color-coding the transcripts and thus worked reflexively in interpreting the transcripts, cutting and pasting, and finally coding the voices generating "themes" that emerged across the transcripts.

Results and Discussion

All five of the two-spirit leaders and activists we interviewed reported experiencing childhood risks for homelessness (i.e., caregiver fluidity, consecutive or unstable housing; Lankenau et al., 2005). Three experienced actual homelessness (i.e., time on the streets ranging from less than 2 months to more than 10 years) in three major cities throughout the United States. In this section, we will highlight some of the key themes that arose for the men who survived living on the streets and will then turn to key themes across all five men regarding trauma, discrimination, mental health, and resilience.

Qualitative researchers have noted that sexual minority youth who are homeless have street capital and a repertoire of street competencies that assist in them in surviving the streets (Granovetter, 1985; Lankenau et al., 2005). By "street capital," we mean knowledge gained in childhood through observations and experiences related to drug use, sexual activity, housing contingencies, and criminal behavior within the family or community that translated into knowledge for survival on the streets as young adults (Lankenau et al., 2005). "Street competencies" refer to pragmatic skill sets that derived from living on the streets, which then abetted survival in the local street trade (e.g., survival sex). Both street capital and competencies create social embeddedness within street networks and crews (Granovetter, 1985; Lankenau et al., 2005).

"I still have wanderlust in my blood": Early exposure to consecutive housing and caregiver fluidity. All of the men experienced significant fluidity in their relationships with familial and institutional caregivers throughout their childhood. All frequently experienced new and multiple guardians for extended periods of time throughout their childhood and youth. In particular, grandparents played a significant role in child-rearing for the majority of men, and four out of the five attended residential boarding school for at least a few years of their childhood and a few had experienced foster care placement with nonrelatives.

> We went [to boarding school] because our parents split up and so, um, they thought that was the best place for us until they figured out what they wanted to do... then I was in foster care, and transitional housing and ... went through a lot of the teenage stuff getting into trouble and running away, stayed at relatives in the summertime.
> —Chance

> I've lived in a lot of different places, so I won't go into every single place I lived, because it would be a long story, but I've moved around a lot.
> —Dennis

It is important, however, to distinguish traditional indigenous fluid caregiving practices from unhealthful or disruptive fluid practices that are borne out of colonial trauma (e.g., placement with a relative due to desired exposure to other familial influences versus abuse at home). Specifically, nearly all of the men, despite the problems associated with caregiver fluidity that are reported in the literature, contextualized fluidity within indigenist traditions.

> I was raised in ... a small Indian community... where a lot of elders lived and they all raised their grandkids while the parents were out...that's what they tell you, that's how I was raised...I mean my brothers and sisters weren't the only ones raised by my grandparents, my other first cousins [were too]...and so it was just tradition, we would go and stay with them.
>
> —Gerry

Additionally, participants who did not experience homelessness but did experience caregiver and housing fluidity sometimes considered out-of-home placements as beneficial, improving familial conditions.

> When my grandparents passed away... we ended up staying in an [Indian] children's home...so we stayed there and visited with our mom on weekends while she went to school... after she graduated... I chose to stay at the Indian school...I enjoyed it...it was really nice.
>
> —Gerry

"I decided to go over the edge, because I wanted to come out the other side": **Pathways to homelessness.** Frequent housing transitions combined with inconsistent, poor caregiving were related to increased vulnerability for homelessness for some participants.

> We [siblings] all ran away from the state [foster care], we all just went out on our own.... I pretty much grew up on the streets of [city] from that point on [age 14].
>
> —Chance
>
> A lot of my memories of when I was young... being in the projects, then going back to the reservation, then to boarding school... then running away from boarding school... staying with relatives... then when [in early teens].... I came to [city] and the next thing, oh! had no food, no money...stayed mostly on the street.
>
> —Del
>
> We grew up in an alcoholic home and all of us kids started using drugs and alcohol when we were young...um, so I had a really chaotic household... you don't ask for support from another because you maybe tried it and it's not, it's not really going to be offered.
>
> —Dennis

Some of the men reported that parental alcohol or drug use significantly increased their vulnerability to homelessness.

> We all went to the city, took off to look for my mother... that's when I came to the city, with no place to stay... my mother was pretty much homeless... an alcoholic and addict... so we went downtown looking for her... during that time we didn't have enough food... about a month later we found her... we were pretty much all homeless.
>
> —Chance

After witnessing parental drug use, three out of five of the men began challenging rules, authority, and laws relatively early, dropping out of school, running away, and stealing property. Street capital then later proved valuable in street survival when they were homeless.

> When I was about 14, I ran away from [reservation] and went to [city] and lived there with some [teen] Natives...seems like I got kicked out of almost everywhere I was at-boarding school, group homes, foster homes, relatives' homes."
>
> —Chance
>
> I'm like get some food for us, so I'm like sitting there because we had no food, had no money, ah—we were stealing food stamps from some poor mother.
>
> —Del
>
> Somebody left their purse and I picked money out of it... at this point we were homeless and with [stolen money] I would buy hotel rooms and stuff like that.
>
> —Del

Additionally, parental drug use and childhood housing instability frequently placed older siblings in the role of caregiver, ultimately forcing many of them to turn to survival sex to provide for their younger siblings.

> Even when I had my own family [as a teen parent], I pretty much took care of my younger [siblings]... I was pretty much their parent, you know, in a lot of ways, emotionally, and you know physically...all the way up to parent roles in teachers's meetings.
>
> —Chance

"If you're not living on the edge, you're taking up too much space": Transforming street capital into street competencies. Much of the street capital gained via housing instability and caregiver fluidity in childhood translated into valuable street survival skills or street competencies. Typically, all of the men who engaged in survival sex did so after experiencing a period of homelessness which was typically precipitated by some life crisis, such as escalating drug use or long periods of no shelter or housing or access to food.

> I'm waiting down on the corner where everybody is like you know, goin' around tryin' to pick people up and this guy stops, and I'm like, 'oh my God, should I?' we did our thing and... drop me off at this [place] where a lot of the Native street kids hung out... my [relative] knew cause I pulled out money and I'm like ... you want anything to eat?
>
> —Del

Ultimately, street capital and street competencies led to street careers that not only made sense but formed the basis for a pragmatic way of surviving on the streets (Lankenau, 2005). Survival sex emerged as a normative practice for survival, obtaining food, or money for shelter for self and relatives on the street.

> I was just walking down the street in that area because it was really close to where the Natives hung out, and this guy pulled over and offered me some money to do stuff with him and the amount of money he offered me, I was like, wow, we could eat... so from that point on is when I started prostituting.
>
> —Chance
>
> We didn't have enough food... I would like just disappear you know and come back and they were, you know, happy cause they got to eat, got a place to stay...I tried to do straight jobs and just couldn't make the money you could on the streets.
>
> —Chance

Many of the respondents noted that going into survival sex work may be different for two-spirit men than their heterosexual peers who were on the street. In fact, one respondent noted that psychological coping included rationalizing the work as being consistent with sexual expression and liberation.

I thought, wow! I get to do what I fantasize about and get paid for it. I mean, how could you beat that and then on top of that I didn't have to go to school and be in a homophobic environment... when I look back on it, it was a way for me to protect myself psychologically.

—Del

Another respondent noted that one street competency was being able to tell the difference between sex trade and sexual expression.

Know the difference between somebody you wanted to be with and then somebody you were with for money... I could separate that.

—Chance

Nevertheless, there were identified psychological and emotional costs to sex work.

When you work the streets, there's a whole disconnection, you know, I mean to cut off all the natural feelings that you have in a relationship... you have to cut all those off and at first I didn't think it would really affect me...um later, down the road [it did].

—Chance

Street capital related to alcohol translated into street competencies for surviving sex trade work.

I drank in order to [trade sex] but after [awhile] there was just too many things you had to be aware of that... I knew I had to have a clear head you know because I could be in to dangerous situations and not only with a trick, but um you know with other people on the streets and...undercover cops ... I never partied until I was finished with working the streets, and then, getting buzzed after that...that's basically how I handled myself.

—Chance

Street competencies included the ability to become embedded in the social network of the crews on the streets, among other homeless individuals, and, in particular, other homeless Natives.

There were a lot of people at the place where I hung out... mainly the younger males hung out and the reason why was because we were under age. We couldn't get into bars... so what was interesting about that was I was now in an atmosphere of ah, being with other people [who] accepted me.

—Del

These street crews formed circles of support that for some became a place where a true sense of belonging and acceptance were first experienced.

It felt to me like it was a pretty accepting [of my gayness] community, so accepting that I didn't want to ever, I didn't ever want to leave it... it was a sense of belonging and acceptance.

—Del

Street crews also formed important protective functions for its members, imparting important survival skills.

I've always been really friendly, so while I was down there people would be like you know, you're too friendly, these people are gonna beat you up... 'cuz they think you're sniffing out people... I just thought I was being friendly...after that, I was like, I'm not gonna keep to myself, but you know, I [won't] ask any questions."

—Del

I understood [on the street] that gay was not the best thing to be and so one of the guys on the street... he was a good guy... a good friend. He always watched out for us. He told me, he said, 'anybody ever messes with you, you tell me, I'll take care of it.

—Del

Other street competencies included stigma management, attitude and affect management, and cognitive flexibility—all street competencies that translated well into life competencies off of the streets.

At one point [another homeless man] he says to me, 'are you gay, are you bi?', I didn't want to tell anybody I was gay, so I said I was bi... less stigma to it.

—Del

If you're down there for even a couple of years, you pick a little attitude, the hardness... that's just the life and if you don't have the attitude, you don't survive.

—Chance

Living as a street person it's just you realize that all of this out here is um, parameters – are all internal parameters that you can just break. That you don't have to open a bank account, you don't have to subscribe to this...it [was my] exploration of what boundaries were and all of that.

—Ray

"It was all about finding the human in me": Translating street competencies into life competencies. Among the men who experienced homelessness, eventually all had disruptions in their street careers by their early 20s. For most of them, leaving street life came at a point when they migrated back home to their reservations and had access to family or friends who were accepting of their two-spirit identity combined with their own developmental readiness to initiate a new developmental stage in their life, including obtaining their GED, entering the military, entering college, entering the arts community, entering a monastery, or a drug treatment program.

When I was 18, I left the streets and went back to the reservation and I stayed with these friends of mine... they were accepting."

—Del

Several respondents noted that other family members had lived on the streets at one point, but later got off of the streets and "gave back" to their communities and were sources of pride and inspiration for the disruption in their own street careers.

My favorite uncle lived on the streets...well over a decade... it took him a while but he got sober, went to school, to graduate school, and eventually ended up becoming [an administrator] who specifically works with American Indian men. So it was just phenomenal and I wanted to somehow give something back, in honor of him.

—Ray

Most of the street survivor narratives described translating street competencies into life competencies across a host of settings. Particularly effective to stem off discrimination, many of the two-spirit men would not shy away from potential perceived threat to body, mind, or spirit and would invoke cool poses or initiate encounters to demonstrate dominance, strength, and non-victim attitudes learned on the streets.

> I learned [on the streets] you need to find your power place and nobody will mess with you and so when I got down there [to college campus], I would be like, and I did this with skin heads before... I wouldn't get off the sidewalk, I wouldn't walk around, I'd walk right through the middle of 'em...look 'em right in they eye and they'd get out of the way.
>
> —Del

> "There I was, walking around like I was really butch, and you know... having been out on the street, you would walk down the street and look people in the eye and you'd be like, 'hey, how's it goin', what's up?' and people would be like, 'what's up, man?' and they'd just [keep] walkin' by."
>
> —Del

Another street competency included not caring about what others think—the streets allowed some of the respondents to let go of social norms and this helped some of them to psychologically buffer against prejudicial or discriminatory attitudes in non-street worlds.

> I got to understand that a life like that [on the street] was too much difficult and it just wasn't for me. But I got to experience it, and I'm so glad I did, I mean it, it really humanized me in a way, I mean I think that is what it was all about—finding the human in me.
>
> —Ray

> If I do run into a person..., I'm like ah, you know, I just don't care what people think. I don't. It's their issue.
>
> —Ray

> I grew up my whole life and you know, people have called me faggot... I says it doesn't bother me... people don't intimidate me because I can handle myself physically... I can take care of myself.
>
> —Del

Surviving on the streets and the "get down to business" tactics of street survival also translated into life competencies in college for many of the men.

> I realized ... I'm down here for school and this [drinking and partying] is messing it up and so I can't do this anymore and so I quit... I said, 'ok, this is what I'm gonna do... I'm down here for business. I got to get down to business so I just really got into school.
>
> —Del

Finally, compassion and empathy gained on the streets translated into teaching others and leadership positions for all of the men who were formerly homeless.

> What helped [me be a trainer] was my previous time on the street...cause our main emphasis was to stop violence against anybody in any form based on race, creed, color, religion, ability, you know, everything.
>
> —Del

"I know people who were beat with tire irons": Violence and trauma experienced by two-spirit men. All of the men identified high levels of violence exposure in childhood and adulthood, either through witnessing violence or directly experiencing a physical assault or rape. One respondent reflected on the high levels of violence experienced in tribal communities, targeting two-spirit people.

> We also have a lot of violence, we have a lot of hatred, hate crimes, a lot of self-hatred, [Indian] people are like oppressing one another and so you get this very high level of tolerance [of violence], it's like, ok, we've got these gay people, these gay people in our communities and. . . I know people who have been beat with tire irons, I know people who have been killed, I know people who, who's homes have been burned down. . .um, things like that.
>
> —Dennis

Some respondents talked about being physically attacked for being two-spirit.

> We were attacked—I had people come to my house and say, 'let's blow this fag's house up! You know, stuff like that. These are Indian people, Indian people. And it was very, very heartbreaking to see them do that.
>
> —Gerry

Being attacked by Natives was identified as particularly stressful and all of the violence narratives focused on making sense of being attacked by other Natives, whereas discrimination narratives focused on making sense of verbal assaults or racist affronts with non-Natives.

> [Violence and discrimination] made me think about being gay and traditions of Native Americans. . . we [two spirits] were very accepted in our traditions, you know, in our culture—not often spoke about it, it was just accepted as you were, you know. . . you were just who you were and you were part of that tribe. . .but today, with Christian influences, it's made a lot of Native Americans know that you can discriminate and they don't accept everybody anymore. . .it's totally thrown our Indian ideology into a turn, a twist.
>
> —Gerry
>
> A Caucasian person will say, 'oh my God, you know, I feel for you.' And usually I'll just say 'thank you', you know? But deep down I [laughs] say, okay, so now you don't hold yourself accountable. . . it's like a fundraiser. . .people put a penny in and go, 'oh see, I've helped them. . .I feel sorry for you' in their minds. . .'wasn't that good.' And then, they don't work to change.
>
> —Ray

Some of the men contrasted urban and reservation violence and lamented that urban settings were violent for them as well.

> I learned hatred here [names city] and I learned about it here. I never knew that back in Oklahoma, but I learned it here. I learned discrimination here, even though we have it back there, it's a little different, but I learned personal discrimination here. I had people come up and attack me at pow wows here—shove me, try to hit me and stuff, call me faggot and queer, you know? [that] never happened to me back home.
>
> —Gerry

Many of the men deeply contextualized their acceptance of various survival strategies that other two-spirit men employ to survive in homophobic or dangerous environments.

> I would hear through the grapevine, through friends of mine who were gay saying did you hear about so and so....they beat him up down at the 49 [after hours pow wow social], and I'd be like really? And I started thinking to myself, who am I to tell them to come out when it would harm them...I can't be around protecting all these people. I protected myself, I could say I'm willing to be out, but I can't subject anybody to that.
>
> —Del

> Nobody does that to me anymore [discriminates against], I won't sit there and take it anymore. Back then I stood there and put my tail between my legs and I would cry about it, but I'm older now, I've got teenagers looking to me, for being respectful.. for advice. Never will that happen to me ever... No, I'm just going to live my life and if [discrimination] comes to me, I will confront it now... I had to learn you have to be responsible for yourself and your life.
>
> —Gerry

A few of the men talked about childhood violence that they had experienced.

> I experienced something pretty horrendous for a number of years that really retarded my, um... it really put a dark cloud over that part of who I was and am. So it took a while to kind of get it back...the [childhood rape and abuse] actions were so horrific that I couldn't get over it and the only way I could was denial, [well], it wasn't even denial. My body and spirit took care of me, they just kind of put it way down so I couldn't think about it...[being] raped consistently and beaten [by relatives] and it was pretty severe.
>
> —Ray

Some of the men identified coping strategies in dealing with the violence aftermath.

> I blocked it out for the longest time and threw myself into everything...as a student I sort of excelled, I read voraciously, I was always doing something. So I was medicating myself by filling up that hole with things... it didn't really come back to me until I was an adult...I couldn't trust relationships for a long time.
>
> —Ray

One interviewer wondered aloud to a respondent if searching for his sexual identity and coming to terms with it was the reason for his homelessness, but the respondent was clear that his street life was connected, in part, to his struggle to reconcile the childhood violence he had experienced.

> Interviewer: I'm wondering was homelessness an attempt to integrate some of this stuff around your sexuality?

> Respondent: No, it wasn't sexuality, it was who I was. Sexuality was just part of it. It was [violence] a lot of stuff from childhood, I was trying to, and I couldn't put it together.

"The reason I'm sober today is because I choose to live honestly": Alcohol and two-spirit men. All of the men talked about their relationship to the spirit of alcohol in their lives. Most of the narratives reflected use of alcohol as a means to self-medicate from pain, whether pain from living on the streets to pain of negotiating and integrating a two-spirit identity.

> I went into black and white thinking that I could just drink and start having sex, and so that's what I started doing, it was, you know, being able to inhibit your feelings [of isolation] by medicating them with drink...I was probably quelling a lot of [feelings] with drugs and alcohol.
>
> —Del

> I was drinking alcoholically from the time I was 13...by the time I started doing my sexuality, I was pretty well into partying and stuff, then I dropped out of school for a couple of years and moved to [city].
>
> —Dennis

> People who are having sex with people of the same gender...often are doing it when they're drunk, on the sly... or they're married...they're doing it not in a self-honest way and I think that damages the spirit.
>
> —Gerry

Nearly all of the men identified a major turning point in their relationship to alcohol having to do with identity integration and self-acceptance.

> There I was sitting... not really knowing who I was because I wasn't really sharing who I was with them [family]. And so I decided to change that...part of it began when I was getting sober...it was really like, not just the coming out part, cause I was always pretty much told everybody, but there's another acceptance that you have to reach, like self-acceptance. I said, 'okay, this is who I am' , you know? Owning it I guess is what it really is.
>
> —Ray

> I think being a gay person, two-spirited person, a strength is acceptance, that we learn to accept ourselves and then accept everybody else, you know. I think that's something important, cause today, we aren't told to accept ourselves.
>
> —Gerry

> The whole process of dealing with my sexual identity... at its core is really about being a human being and a child of the Creator, that's my core.
>
> —Dennis

> Basically, I look within ourselves for support, you have to be your own support...if you have no family, no distant relatives or Native American community available for support, you have to look within yourself and that's where you become a backbone.
>
> —Gerry

Others also expressed compassion and understanding for other two spirits who are still struggling in their journey and called on the sober two-spirit community to be more understanding and accepting.

> Some of them do have issues with drugs and alcohol...ongoing issues with mental health based on that. And to me they're the ones that are most important you know and the struggle that I have with the Native community in general is they leave them out. Because of their two spiritedness for one part and because they're having struggles with drugs and alcohol—so they're kind of doubly [oppressed] there.
>
> —Del

If I'm gonna be involved in a two spirit organization, it's gonna be open to anybody, whether they drink, they used, or do whatever, because if we're gonna support people, we're gonna support them wherever they're at.

—Del

Respondents who had experienced homelessness talked about the difficulty in getting housing while drinking and living on the streets. Many identified homophobia of service providers as exacerbating difficulty in finding shelter or housing.

I think it's the homophobia because they provide services to people who are having issues with drugs and alcohol... you can even have mental health issues, and they feel comfortable with them [homeless, alcoholic, and mentally ill], but if you're two spirit then it becomes a whole different ball of wax because then they're like saying, 'okay, can we house these people... what will other people think?'

—Del

"I just wanted to die": Depression, PTSD, and Suicidality. All of the men reflected on struggles and resilience in their spiritual and mental health. Many identified social stressors that triggered their depressive and suicidal episodes, in particular, social isolation, extreme job stress, or traditional health practices disconnection.

I stopped a lot of practices that gave me an outlet. I stopped praying in the morning...smudging myself. Things like that... I just lived under a lot of stress.. my job was too much for me, I couldn't handle it...I literally broke apart. I fell apart and just had a nervous breakdown and engaged in unsafe sex like crazy. I mean it was suicide. It was pretty deliberate [to become HIV+].

—Ray

I know mental health—being gay, you go through a lot of stages of or forms of depression...you have moments of depression where you think, 'oh God, I'm never going to find nobody or relationships are bad ...that's a big impact because it'll cause a lot of drinking and stuff.

—Gerry

Many talked about mild depression rooted in struggles with church, family, and a sense of belonging. For some, depression escalated into suicidal ideation and for others, depression was manifest in "trying out heterosexuality" to gain acceptance or psychological peace.

I even contemplated dating a woman [while in college]. I got to the point where I was so distraught and going through such depression that I just wanted to die, and I couldn't kill myself because of our religious beliefs. So, I would be like, I just wish that semi [truck] would just turn off and kill me.

—Del

I think a lot of people live with PTSD, I think because of the whole, whole process of coming out. I think a lot of [two spirit] people live with depression because of who we are as [Indian] people and living with generational shame and dealing with ethno-stress – you know, that is daily.

—Ray

All of the respondents identified spirituality, spiritual traditions, and traditional health practices (e.g., smudging) as key elements in healing, developing, and growing into health and wellness.

> Depression is something that is a really big issue. I think the key once again is creating a really strong sense of self-identity through spiritual connection, building a spiritual foundation.
>
> —Ray
>
> I always knew that prayer was really powerful, so you can live like in any situation and you know, I always knew that I was protected.
>
> —Chance

Others translated this growth into growth of the community and assisting other Natives.

> I've found my power place... to live and my heart is working with two-spirit people and is to help, not just two-spirit people, but Native people.
>
> —Del

"Our People, we're known as praying people, I think most tribes are": Spirituality and navigating life journeys. All of the men invoked the power of prayer and spirituality throughout their narratives, especially in assisting them through life on the streets and other stressors they encountered.

> We always were taught to pray and when we were growing up, we would always pray, for everything, morning, evening, meals, everything.
>
> —Gerry
>
> I'm kind of back in a really good space where I'm saying, 'okay, I'm here universe. Because I know that if I have faith in life, life has faith in me. And it's very strange, I just jump because I know I'm going to land on my feet.
>
> —Ray
>
> I think a lot of the traditional medicines are important, you know. We use a lot, still do... a lot of parts can help you heal, a lot of mediation, a lot of singing—I use my dancing and singing to help me with my stressors.
>
> —Gerry

"Maybe who I am is not about my bedroom, maybe who I am is about me walking the world just like you are walking the world": Two-Spirit Resilience and Resistance. All of the men invoked journey metaphors in their narratives, reframing their stressors and coping as part of life journeys that made them strong.

> Because we had to go through a journey, we've had to explore who we are, I mean it's given us the capacity to look beyond the box...we're very fortunate that we've gone through hell and the we have [laughs] and we've lived with the oppression...because oppression can be liberating, spiritually, I mean.
>
> —Ray
>
> We've been marginalized, oppressed, repressed, suppressed, and those of us that turn around, and I think we have, learned to embrace who I am and really find strength in that self-knowledge and I think it's well worth that we've had to do that. So, I think the ruling class is really missing out [laughs] on a lot of things because they're getting their own way.
>
> —Ray

I can't say that I have a strong heart because I'm a gay person. I have a strong heart because I've gone through all this stuff you know…The journey is not really about coming out. The journey is living honestly, dealing with the crap in your life and moving beyond it, not repeating it anymore, it's you taking care of others, living in a traditional manner in the sense you're living out the culture, you know, the good, the good way that we were given to live. I think that's what we all, if we all did that, we'd be doing pretty good.

—Dennis

Resistance to colonization and internalized oppression was evident throughout the journey metaphors.

When you do accept who you are…you don't apologize anymore for who you are, you don't apologize to people, you don't say you know, well, I wish I weren't this way or um pretend I'm somebody I'm not… accept me or don't, I don't really care… maybe I really think it comes down to how my heart has been strengthened by having to go, to take this journey that I had to take. How my belief in my Creator, my relationship to my Creator has been strengthened because I had to take this journey and how I think even more my relationship to my culture has been strengthened because of this journey of growing up in an alcoholic family, the journey of being male… of being poor… or whatever.

—Dennis

Summary

This chapter has provided an exploratory analysis of Native two-spirit men and their housing experiences, tending to aspects of struggle and resiliency. In our analysis, we found a high proportion of two-spirit men experiencing some form of unstable housing and homelessness at some point in their life span. Although we cannot conclude directionality from the survey data, the qualitative findings illuminated some of the potential precipitating factors leading to temporary and, in some cases, prolonged homelessness and housing instability.

Specifically, the association between extreme childhood neglect and homelessness for the survey sample was consistent with the qualitative sample narratives that reflected parental emotional and physical neglect and, in some cases, outright abandonment of the whole household. This resulted in placing some of the men in highly developmentally and culturally inappropriate roles including ones as primary caregiver, emotional caretaker, and breadwinner for the entire household at very young ages. Future research will need to discern the relationship between dysfunctional caregiver fluidity (also referred to here as colonial trauma response caregiver fluidity) and extreme childhood emotional neglect. Future research will need, in particular, to disentangle the colonial trauma response aftermath in parental caregiving trends (Evans-Campbell & Walters 2006; See Evans-Campbell, Lindhorst, Huang, & Walters, 2006 and Evans-Campbell, Fredriksen-Goldsen, Stately, & Walters, in press, for a more detailed description on historical trauma and violence and parenting among Natives) from culturally based traditional approaches to caregiving with the positive value of multiple caregivers. Specifically, men's narratives that reflected multiple caregivers who were emotionally supportive and consistent in their support for the respondents were quite different than narratives related to multiple caregivers who were not able (for a variety of reasons from their own addictions, homelessness, or age/disabilities) to provide consistency in emotional caregiving or boundary setting (e.g., not bothering to look for the youth when they ran away).

Overall, the survey data revealed incredibly high rates of trauma exposure, elevated PTSD, and depressive symptomatology among the sample as a whole. Moreover, taken together, the qualitative and survey data reveal the potential triangle of risk (Simoni et al., 2004)—trauma, alcohol and drug use and poor health outcomes—including sexual risk behaviors (from the narratives), poor mental health (PTSD and depression), and housing instability and homelessness. Future research will need to examine the triangle of risk, in particular, the mediating effects of alcohol and drug use on housing stability and mental health outcomes. It is important to note that not all two-spirits who experience traumatic stressors and violence have poor health outcomes and housing instability. As some of the narratives indicate and as per the Indigenist Stress-Coping Model (Walters & Simoni, 2002), there are many other protective factors, such as social support, self-acceptance, identity integration, and spirituality, that may buffer the effects of childhood abuse and dysfunctional caregiver fluidity on housing stability and mental health.

Moreover, buffering much of the deleterious effects of housing instability involved access to education, gainful and productive work, and financial resources. Parallel to this, participants spoke to the importance of the internal and collective experience of and access to traditional ways, Native cosmologies, as well as an "Indianness" or indigeneity in order to cope and survive periods of homelessness, housing instability and destabilization in family networks.

It is especially important to note that even among the two-spirit men who were homeless in the qualitative sample, they all had managed to move off the streets and into stable housing, and lead successful and healthful lives as well-respected indigenous two-spirit leaders across the nation. All of the qualitative narratives reflect themes of resilience, strength, generosity, and the indigenous value of "giving back" to their communities and to Native communities as a whole (Walters, Evans-Campbell, Simoni, Ronquillo, & Bhuyan, 2006).

The interpretation of these data becomes problematic if analyzed outside of the larger context of the streets on which the participants lived, in addition to the confines of practitioners, and researchers' offices. A typical byproduct of the colonial process that continues today is the lack of contextualization of health and mental health data—from a fourth world perspective (Walters & Simoni, 2002). Endemic to this process is the positioning of such data especially related to Native populations as normal and even expected. Poor health outcomes, health disparities, and structural and bodily destruction are deemed *understandable* and *natural* to "the Native experience" in US society.

As evidenced in the HONOR Project, much of these destructive processes are anything but normal and natural. Rather, taken in context of fourth world conditions, they become processes experienced intergenerationally which also persist pervasively across social and health structures. The fourth world perspective takes into account the very real *structural* conditions under which generally Native—and especially two-spirit men—live. Thus, contemporary conditions such as unstable housing, for example, are not simple byproducts of individual circumstances, but conditions borne from a complex historical web of colonial structures (e.g., genocidal and ethnocidal policies) set in place over generations. In turn, these structures directly connect to the systematic destruction of Native families (e.g., boarding schools) and lifeways that bear directly on two-spirit health and wellness from the communal level down to the individual level. Health disparities for two-spirit men must therefore be understood and contextualized within socio-political systems that are rooted in colonialism, racism, and gendered violence against AIAN (Smith, 2005a). These foundational differentials play out at state and interpersonal levels, which systematically serve to perpetuate and exacerbate conditions (e.g., lack of adequate housing) facilitating the growth of health disparities (e.g., escalating rates of HIV), structural inequalities (e.g., homelessness); and health risk behaviors (e.g., survival sex).

Considering a more contextualized view of this data, a number of practice implications emerge. Policies and programs serving Native populations generally ought to effectively plan and promote services responding to local health and mental health needs, while bearing in mind the enduring prevalence of health disparities. Most obviously, stable and supportive housing should be a high priority for social service providers. In 1996, the US federal government passed the Native American Housing Assistance and Self-Determination Act (*cf.* Prucha, 2000). Several of the provisions indicate the need to develop, maintain, and operate affordable housing in safe and healthy environments on Indian reservations and in other Indian areas for peoples with low income. However, this Act does not include provisions to adequately address the needs of urban Indians, who represent a higher proportion of Native residency in the US versus reservation and rural areas. There is a need, then, to better implement housing programs in accordance with these federal policies.

Moreover, attention to housing cannot exist only at the policy level; effective response must also include attention to the psychosocial needs of two-spirit men in any geographic location. Given the data presented in this chapter, housing services should necessarily provide case management or other interventions related to the broader and contingent health and mental health disparities of these men. Some of these disparities, as evidenced here, include trauma, depression, isolation, neglect, and alcohol and other drug abuse. In a more contextualized perspective, these disparities illustrate, the lack of access to Native traditions, supports, and community structures that foster nurturing and positive identities and networks. The services responding to these disparities can be seen, then, as interventions around lifeways and skills that are ultimately preventive measures against unstable housing and homelessness, immediately and in the future.

Even more pressing, though, is the need for attention to the multiple oppressions occurring daily and systemically. Attention to "their needs" is not just about providing access to indigenous ways, but also tending to the heterosexism, gendered violence, and racism that is experienced contemporarily in Native and non-Native communities where two-spirit men are living. Likewise, medical centers, non-governmental organizations, and other social and health service agencies would benefit from critically examining the operations of colonialism, racism, and ethnocentrism within their structures. Implicit in this critical awareness must be the attention to the class differentials that not only affect Native communities, but also are part and parcel in the relationships among professionals and community groups. Ultimately, "best practices" around the housing needs of Native two-spirit men not only involves accessing structures to shelter the men, but moreover to access the structures that infringe upon and contribute to continued negative health effects in the lived experiences of these men. This at once supports an attention to the multiple oppressions working against these men, as well as directing providers to see reflexivity as a critical practice within themselves and the systems in which they work.

References

Balsam, K. F., Huang, B., Fieland, K. C., Simoni, J. M., & Walters, K. L. (2004). Culture, trauma and wellness: A comparison of heterosexual and lesbian gay, bisexual and two-spirit Native Americans. *Cultural Diversity and Ethnic Minority Psychology, 10*, 287–301.

Belgrave, F.Z.; Townsend, T.G., Cherry, V.R, Cunningham, D. M. (1997). The influence of an Africentric worldview and demographic variables on drug knowledge, attitudes, and use among African American youth. *Journal of Community Psychology.* Vol 25(5), 421-433.

Bernstein, D. P., Fink, L., Handelsman, L., Foote, J., Lovejoy, M., & Wenzel, K. et al. (1994). Initial reliability and validity of a new retrospective measure of child abuse and neglect. *American Journal of Psychiatry, 151*(8), 1132–1136.

Bishop, R. (2005). Freeing ourselves from neocolonial domination in research. In N. K. Denzin & Y. S. Lincoln (Eds.), *The SAGE handbook of qualitative research,* 3rd ed. (pp. 109–138). Thousand Oaks, CA: Sage Publications, Ltd.

Brown, L. M., Tappan, M. B., Gilligan, C., Miller, B. A., & Argyris, D. E. (1989). Reading for self and moral voice: A method for interpreting narratives of real-life moral conflict and choice. In M. J. Packer & R. B. Addison (Eds.), *Entering the circle: Hermeneutic investigation in psychology* (pp. 141–164). Albany, NY: State University of New York Press.

Clatts, M. C., & Davis, W. R. (1999). A demographic and behavorial profile of homeless youth in New York City: Implications for AIDS outreach and prevention. *Medical Anthropological Quarterly, 13*(3), 365–374.

Cochran, B. N., Stewart, A. J., Ginzler, J. A., & Cauce, A. M. (2002). Challenges faced by homeless sexual minorities: Comparison of gay, lesbian, bisexual, and transgender homeless adolescents with their heterosexual counterparts. *American Journal of Public Health, 92*(5), 773–777.

Coker, A. L., Pope, B. O., Smith, P. H., Sanderson, M., & Hussey, A. J. (2001). Assessment of clinical partner violence screening tools. *Journal of the American Medical Women's Association, 56,* 19–23.

Benda, B.B; Corwyn, R. F.(2000). A theoretical model of religiosity and drug use with reciprocal relationships: A test using structural equation modeling. *Journal of Social Service Research. Vol. 26(4)*, 43-67.

Cuandrado, M., & Lieberman, L. (1998). Traditionalism in the prevention of substance misuse among Puerto Ricans. *Substance Use and Misuse, 33(14)*, 2737–2755.

Evans-Campbell, T., Fredriksen-Goldsen, K., Stately, A., & Walters, K. L. (In Press). Caregiving experiences among American Indian Two-Spirit men and women: Contemporary and historical roles. *Journal of Gay and Lesbian Social Services.*

Evans-Campbell, T., Lindhorst, T., Huang, B., & Walters, K. L. (2006). Interpersonal violence in the lives of urban American Indian and Alaska Native women: Implications for health, mental health, and help-seeking. *American Journal of Public Health, 96(8)*, 1416–1422.

Evans-Campbell, T., & Walters, K. L. (2006). Catching our breath: A decolonization framework for healing indigenous families. In Rowena Fong, Ruth McRoy, & Carmen Ortiz Hendricks (Eds.) *Intersecting Child Welfare, Substance Abuse, and Family Violence: Culturally Competent Approaches*. Alexandria, VA, CSWE Publications.

Fieland, K. C., Walters, K. L., & Simoni, J. M. (2007). Determinants of health among Two-Spirit American Indians and Alaska Natives. In I. H. Meyer & M. E. Northridge (Eds.), *The health of sexual minorities: Public health perspectives on lesbian, gay, bisexual and transgender populations* (pp. 268–300). New York: Springer.

Foa, E. B., Cashman, L., Jaycox, L., & Perry, K. (1997). The validation of a self-report measure of posttraumatic stress disorder: The Posttraumatic Diagnostic Scale. *Psychological Assessment, 9(4)*, 445–451.

Gongaware, T. B. (2003). Collective memories and collective identities. *Journal of Contemporary Ethnography, 32*(5), 483–520.

Granovetter M. (1985). Economic action and social structure: The problem of embeddedness. *American Journal of Sociology, 91*, 481–510.

Greenfeld, L. A., & Smith, S. K. (1999). *American Indians and crime* (BJS Publication No. NCJ 173386). Washington, D.C.: U.S. Department of Justice.

Lankenau, S. E., Clatts, M. C., Welle, D., Goldamt, L. A., & Gwadz, M. V. (2005). Street Careers: Homelessness, drug use, and sex work among young men who have sex with men (YMSM). *International Journal of Drug Policy, 16(1)*, 10–18.

LeCrubier, Y., Sheehan, D., Weiller, E., Amorim, P., Bonora, I., & Sheehan, K. et al. (1997). The MINI International Neuropsychiatric Interview (M.I.N.I.) A Short Diagnostic Structured Interview: Reliability and Validity According to the CIDI. *European Psychiatry, 12*, 224–231.

Lobo, S., & Vaughn, M. M. (2003). Substance dependency among homeless American Indians. *Journal of Psychoactive Drugs, 35(1)*, 63–70.

Marker, M. (2003). 'Indigenous voice, community & epistemic violence: The ethnographer's "interests" and what "interests" the ethnographer'. *Qualitative Studies in Education, 16(3)*, 361–375.

McMahan, E. M., & Rogers, K. L. (1994). *Interactive oral history interviewing*. New York: Routledge.

Prucha, F. P. (2000). Documents of the United States Indian Policy. (3rd edition). Lincoln, NB: University of Nebraska Press.

Radloff, L. S. (1977). CES-D scale: A self-report depression scale for research in the general population. *Applied Psychological Measurement, 1*, 385–401.

Scheier, L. M., Botvin, G. J., Diaz, T., & Ifill-Williams, M. (1997). Ethnic identity as a moderator of psychosocial risk and adolescent alcohol and marijuana use: Concurrent and longitudinal analysis. *Journal of Child Adolescent Substance Abuse, 6(1)*, 21–47.

Simoni, J. M., Sehgal, S., & Walters, K.L. (2004). Triangle of Risk: Urban American Indian women's sexual trauma, injection drug use, and HIV sexual risk behaviors. *AIDS and Behavior*, 8 (1), 33-45.

Simoni, J. M., Walters, K. L., Balsam, K. F., & Meyers, S. B. (2006). Victimization, substance use, and HIV risk behaviors among gay/bisexual/two-spirit and heterosexual American Indian men in New York City. *American Journal of Public Health, 96(121),* 2240–2245.

Smith, A. (1998). Walking in balance: The spirituality-liberation praxis of Native women. In J. Weaver (Ed.), *Native American religious identity: Unforgotten gods* (pp. 178–198). Maryknoll, NY: Orbis Books.

Smith, A. (2005). *Conquest: Sexual violence and American Indian genocide.* Cambridge, MA: South End Press.

Townsend, T. G., & Belgrave, F. Z. (2000). The impact of personal identity and racial identity on drug attitudes and use among African American children. *Journal of Black Psychology, 26(4),* 421–33.

Tuhiwai Smith, L. (2005a). On tricky ground: Researching the Native in the age of uncertainty. In N. Denzin & Y. S. Lincoln (Eds.), *The SAGE handbook of qualitative research,* 3rd ed. (pp. 85–107). Thousand Oaks, CA: Sage Publications, Ltd.

Tuhiwai Smith, L. (2005b). *Decolonizing methodologies.* London: Zed books.

Tyler, K., & Cauce A. M. (2002). Perpetrators of early physical and sexual abuse among homeless and runaway adolescents. *Child Abuse and Neglect, 26,* 1261–1274.

United States Indian Health Service. (1997). *Trends in Indian health 1997.* Last retrieved on 6-28-07; Available at http://www.ihs.gov/publicinfo/publications/ trends97/trends97.asp

United States Indian Health Service. (2001). *Trends in Indian health 2000–2001.* Last retrieved on 6-28-07; Available at: http://www.ihs.gov/NonMedicalPrograms/IHS_Stats/Trends00.asp

Walters, K. L. (1997). Urban lesbian and gay American Indian identity: Implications for mental health social service delivery. *Journal of Gay and Lesbian Social Services, 6,(2) Winter,* 43–65.

Walters, K. L., Simoni, J. M., & Evans-Campbell, T. (2002). Substance use among American Indians and Alaska Natives: Incorporating culture in an "Indigenist" stress-coping paradigm. *Public Health Reports, 117*(Suppl. 1), S104–S117.

Walters, K. L., & Simoni, J. M. (2002). Reconceptualizing Native women's health: An "indigenist" stress-coping model. *American Journal of Public Health, 92(4),* 520–524.

Walters, K. L., Simoni, J. M., & Horwath, P. F. (2001). Sexual orientation bias experiences and service needs of gay, lesbian, bisexual, transgendered, and Two-spirited American Indians. *Journal of Gay & Lesbian Social Service, 13*(1/2), 133–149.

Walters, K. L., Evans-Campbell, T., Simoni, J., Ronquillo, T., & Bhuyan, R. (2006). "My Spirit in my heart": Identity experiences and challenges among American Indian Two-Spirit women. *Journal of Lesbian Studies, 10*(1/2), 125–149.

Warren, K. (1993). A feminist philosophical perspective on ecofeminist spiritualities. In C. Adams (Ed.), *Ecofeminism and the sacred.* New York: Continuum.

Whitbeck, L. B., Adams, G. W., Hoyt, D. R., & Chen, X. (2004). Conceptualizing and measuring historical trauma among American Indian people. *American Journal of Community Psychology, 33*(3–4), 119–130.

Whitbeck, L. B., Chen, X., Hoyt, D. R., Tyler, K. A., & Johnson, K. D. (2004). Mental disorder, subsistence strategies, and victimization among gay, lesbian and bisexual homeless. *The Journal of Sex Research, 41(4),* 329–342.

Yoder, K. A., Hoyt, D. R., & Whitbeck, L. B. (1998). Suicidal behavior among homeless and runaway adolescents. *Journal of Youth and Adolescence, 27*(6), 1573–6601.

Part V
HIV/AIDS

Chapter Seven
National Trends in HIV Transmission Among Minority Men who have Sex with Men

Daniel J. O'Shea

This chapter focuses on the history and recent trends in the course of the HIV/ AIDS epidemic in the USA in relation to its impact on men who have sex with men (MSM) of color. A review of HIV/AIDS surveillance is followed by a discussion of related sexual and substance use risk behaviors; and other barriers to prevention and care, including MSM identity and stigma, and cultural/ socioeconomic issues. Finally, examples of successful strategies for both prevention and access to care are provided.

Surveillance

The first cases of HIV/AIDS epidemic were recognized and reported in June 1981. Between 1981 and 2005, approximately 1.7 million individuals were infected with HIV in the USA; 32% (more than 550,000) of these have died. From a peak of more than 150,000 HIV infections during the mid-1980s, the annual number of new US HIV infections has declined and stabilized since the late 1990s to approximately 40,000. An estimated 1.1 million individuals were living with HIV/AIDS in the USA in 2005, including 425,910 diagnosed with AIDS. Approximately 25% of individuals with HIV are not aware that they are infected (Centers for Disease Control and Prevention, 2006a; Glynn & Rhodes, 2005; Henry Kaiser Family Foundation, 2006a; Centers for Disease Control and Prevention, 2006f).

MSM were dramatically and disproportionately impacted by the HIV/AIDS epidemic since cases were first reported and tracked, and continue to represent the highest HIV incidence of any risk group. Although the numbers and proportion of HIV diagnoses among MSM decreased as the epidemic progressed through the 1990s, recent surveillance data show increases in HIV diagnoses for MSM (Centers for Disease Control and Prevention, 2006f).

Daniel J. O'Shea
County of San Diego Health and Human Services Agency, San Diego, CA

S. Loue (ed.), *Health Issues Confronting Minority Men Who Have Sex with Men.*
© Springer 2008

Among men of color, the leading cause of HIV infection is sexual contact with other men. For AIDS cases reported among US males in 2005, MSM or MSM with injection drug use (IDU) was the HIV exposure category in 58% of cases among Asian/Pacific Islanders (A/PIs), 48% of Latinos/Hispanics, 63% of Native Americans (American Indians/Alaska Natives) and 40% of African Americans/Blacks (Health Resources and Services Administration, 2003).

In 1989, men of color comprised 31% of new AIDS cases among MSM in the USA; less than a decade later in 1998, they accounted for over 50% of new MSM AIDS cases (Health Resources and Services Administration, 2003). Of 30,956 men diagnosed with AIDS in the USA in 2005, 54% were MSM, and 54% of these were men of color (Centers for Disease Control and Prevention, 2006a).

The Impact on MSM

At the end of 2005, of the estimated 342,148 *male* adults and adolescents *living* with HIV/AIDS in the 33 states with confidential name-based HIV infection reporting since 2001, 68% were MSM; 50% of these were MSM of color (Centers for Disease Control and Prevention , 2006a). The disproportionate impact on MSM is evidenced in that only about 5–7% of male adults and adolescents in the USA identify themselves as MSM. African American and Latino MSM also belong to racial/ethnic groups disproportionately affected compared to their share of the population. African Americans represented 47% of estimated living AIDS cases in 2005 and Latinos 17%, compared with 12% and 13%, respectively, of the US population according to the 2000 census (Centers for Disease Control and Prevention, 2006a; Grieco & Cassidy, 2001). Even so, evidence suggests that AIDS surveillance data significantly underrepresent the rate of HIV/AIDS among men of color (Health Resources and Services Administration, 2006a).

The Centers for Disease Control and Prevention's (CDC) Young Men's Survey conducted between 1994 and 2000, targeting young men frequenting bars, dance clubs, and other venues where MSM congregate in seven cities, found high HIV infection rates, especially among men of color. HIV prevalence for survey participants aged 23–29 was 32% among African Americans and 14% among Latinos, compared with 7% for Caucasians (Health Resources and Services Administration, 2003).

HIV-positive MSM of color frequently become infected at an earlier age than their Caucasian counterparts, but are also often diagnosed with HIV/AIDS later in the course of the disease (Health Resources and Services Administration, 2003). A higher proportion of people of color, in general, already have AIDS at initial diagnosis (Health Resources and Services Administration, 2006b). CDC analysis of surveillance data collected from 1996 to 1998 in 25 states with HIV-reporting systems revealed that the proportion of men who were aged 13–14 at initial diagnosis was 16% among African American men, 15% among A/PI men, 15% among Native American men and 9% among Caucasian men, with a greater proportion of the men of color diagnosed with AIDS at the same time (Health Resources and Services Administration, 2003).

Special Issues for Native Americans

Surveillance data for HIV and AIDS among Native Americans are limited or incomplete. States with large Native American populations, including California, New York, and Washington, only recently began conducting HIV surveillance, or have only done so for a few years. The relatively low number of HIV and AIDS cases among Native Americans may be due to racial misclassification and underreporting. Misclassification of Native Americans with HIV/AIDS as another race has been shown to vary widely, from 3% in Alaska to 56% in Los Angeles (Centers for Disease Control and Prevention, 2006d).

Unknown HIV Status

Many MSM of color may be unaware of their HIV status for a variety of reasons, including denial, lack of access to services, and other, more pressing basic need priorities. This is of particular concern since research has shown that many HIV-positive individuals who are aware of their status change behaviors to reduce their risk of transmitting the virus. Increasing the proportion of people who know their HIV status can therefore help decrease overall HIV transmission (Centers for Disease Control and Prevention, 2006f).

Not knowing one's HIV serostatus is risky for MSM of color, particularly African American men and their partners. A survey conducted through the CDC's National HIV Behavioral Surveillance System of MSM over the age of 18 who frequented specific venues in five cities found that 25% were HIV positive (46% of African Americans; 21% of Caucasians, and 17% of Latinos). Almost half (48%) of those who were positive were unaware of their status; 64% of the "unaware" MSM were African American, 18% Latino, 11% Caucasian/White, and 6% multiracial. Within each racial/ethnic group, 67% of participating African American MSM, 48% of participating Latino MSM, 50% of participating multiracial/other MSM, and 18% of participating Caucasian MSM who tested positive were unaware of their infection (Centers for Disease Control and Prevention, 2005). In another recent study summarized by the CDC (2006f), 77% of young MSM testing HIV-positive did not believe that they were infected; 74% had previously tested negative and 59% believed that they were at low or very low risk. Approximately 90% of young African American MSM who tested positive were unaware of their infection, compared with 60% of young Caucasian MSM. A third study of 150 HIV-infected African American MSM who tested positive while participating in the Young Men's Study revealed that 93% (139) were not aware of their status. Of these, 71% believed it unlikely or that there was "no chance" they were infected (Health Resources and Services Administration, 2003).

Sexual Risk Factors

Sexual risk factors for MSM of color include unprotected sex and sexually transmitted diseases (STDs). Lack of condom use during anal insertive sex with someone other than a primary partner of known HIV serostatus continues to be a significant threat to the health of MSM, putting sexual partners at greatest risk for HIV and STD transmission. Improved HIV treatment, substance use, complex sexual decision making, seeking sex partners on the Internet, and failure to practice safer sex have contributed to an evident increase in unprotected anal intercourse (Centers for Disease Control and Prevention, 2006f).

A/PIs, while approximately only 1% of USA AIDS cases, include subgroups in some metropolitan areas at higher risk for HIV infection. A study of 503 A/PI MSM aged 18–29 years in San Francisco revealed high rates of STDs, with 48% reporting unprotected anal sex in the past 6 months and overall HIV prevalence at nearly 3%. For this group, factors associated with HIV infection were Thai ethnicity, US birth, older age, or prior attendance at a circuit party or special MSM social event (Centers for Disease Control and Prevention, 2006c).

The presence of *STDs,* an important health issue for MSM, is indicative of high risk sexual behavior that facilitates HIV transmission. Genital lesions caused by STDs can serve as an entry point for HIV into the body, and the presence of some STDs increases the probability of contracting HIV by three to five times. An HIV-positive individual with certain STDs is also more likely to transmit HIV to sexual partners (Centers for Disease Control and Prevention, 2006b). Prevalence of STDs among MSM, including MSM of color, has increased significantly in recent years. The Gonococcal Isolate Surveillance Project noted that the proportion of positive gonorrhea test results among MSM increased from 4% in 1988 to 19.6% in 2003. Rates of syphilis among MSM have increased recently in several large urban areas, including San Francisco, Chicago, New York, and Seattle. Rates of STDs and HIV infection were reported highest among African American MSM in the MSM Prevalence Monitoring Project encompassing nine US cities (Centers for Disease Control and Prevention, 2006f).

People of color, in general, experience high STD prevalence. Among all racial/ethnic groups, the CDC (2006b) reports the highest rates of STDs for African Americans, with African Americans 19 times more likely than non-Hispanic Whites to have gonorrhea and about six times more likely to have syphilis. Latinos are twice as likely to have gonorrhea or syphilis as non-Hispanic Whites, and three times more likely to have chlamydia (Centers for Disease Control and Prevention, 2006e). The CDC reports that high rates of chlamydia, gonorrhea, and syphilis also occur among Native Americans, who have the second highest rates of all racial/ethnic groups for gonorrhea, chlamydia, and syphilis (their rate for syphilis is tied with Latinos) (Centers for Disease Control and Prevention, 2006d).

The Internet has provided new opportunities in the past decade for MSM to anonymously find and meet sex partners with similar interests without leaving home or risking face-to-face rejection for suggesting unsafe sexual behaviors. Certain risky behaviors have been normalized among Internet users by creating broader awareness of these activities and/or new connections between those who engage in them. At the same time and through the same venues, the potential for using the Internet as a mechanism to reach a large and more targeted audience for HIV prevention interventions has also been enhanced (Centers for Disease Control and Prevention, 2006f). In a recent study of the use of gay-related Internet chat rooms by young MSM of color (YMSMC) who have sex with other men of color, Fields et al. (2006) supported development of Internet outreach protocols for online HIV prevention interventions with at-risk YMSMC.

Lack of sexual partner communication and risk assessment skills among MSM is another significant challenge for HIV prevention. Open and honest communication before engaging in sexual activity is critical. Assumptions by HIV-positive MSM that a partner must be infected or he would insist on using a condom, or by HIV-negative MSM that a partner also is not infected or he would use a condom can have unintended, disastrous consequences. Even disclosure of HIV status may be insufficient since some MSM, particularly younger MSM and MSM of color, may not be aware that they are infected with HIV (Centers for Disease Control and Prevention, 2006f).

Psychosocial problems experienced by some MSM, including MSM of color, increase the likelihood of risky sexual behaviors. These include depression, childhood sexual abuse, substance use, and/or domestic violence. Co-occurrence of more than one of these issues may have an additive impact greater than that of each individual problem, thereby creating additional risk factors for HIV infection (Centers for Disease Control and Prevention, 2006f).

Complacency about risk and burnout among MSM has surfaced in the last decade since the introduction and success of antiretroviral therapy (ART). Data indicate that some MSM are challenged to sustain safer sex practices and underestimate their risk for HIV. The success of ART has minimized negative aspects of HIV disease by significantly reducing morbidity and mortality, thereby creating a misconception of the true impact of living with HIV, with the unintended consequence of increasing risky sexual behaviors among some MSM. Some mistakenly assume that taking medications or having a low or undetectable viral load means that they or their partners are no longer infectious (Centers for Disease Control and Prevention, 2006f). Other research among MSM correlates optimism about HIV treatments with a greater willingness to have unprotected anal intercourse.

Younger MSM without the experience of seeing firsthand the devastation caused by AIDS before the era of ART may also have less motivation to practice safer sex, as evidenced by higher infection rates than older MSM. Twenty-five years into the epidemic, however, even some older HIV-positive and HIV-negative MSM are challenged to sustain long-standing efforts to practice safer sex. A study of HIV-positive MSM in four cities showed that fatigue and burnout from long-term, continuous exposure to prevention messages and engagement in safer sex behavior may contribute to a decision to have unprotected anal intercourse (Centers for Disease Control and Prevention, 2006f).

In their study of barebacking identity among 1,168 HIV-positive gay and bisexual men from New York City and San Francisco, Halkitis et al. (2005) found that men of color were less likely to identify themselves as barebackers. Those who did self-identify as barebackers were more likely to be slightly younger, to report use of injection and noninjection drugs, to be more sexually compulsive, to evidence lower levels of personal responsibility for safer sex, to report higher rates of unprotected insertive and receptive anal sex and insertive oral sex with partners, regardless of their HIV serostatus, and to have missed a dose of medication.

Antiretroviral Therapy: The success of ART in enabling many MSM to live longer and healthier lives with HIV also means more HIV-positive MSM can be and are sexually active with the potential to transmit HIV to their sex partners. Many MSM reduce their risk behaviors after being diagnosed with HIV, taking personal responsibility for protecting others from HIV; some, however, continue to engage in risky behaviors. This underscores the importance of and need for HIV prevention efforts focused on HIV-positive MSM. Some prevention initiatives focusing on HIV seropositive individuals ("prevention with positives") have been found to be effective in reducing or stopping risky behaviors (Centers for Disease Control and Prevention, 2006f).

Both clinical- and community-based settings may be appropriate for prevention with positives for MSM of color. A study of sexual behaviors and condom use by 179 sexually active HIV-positive adults of color attending a primary care clinic by Absalon, Della-Latta, Wu, & El-Sadr, (2005) identified high-risk sexual behaviors among HIV-positive African Americans and Latinos and suggested the clinic as an ideal place for prevention with positives' interventions.

Substance Use

As a blood-borne infection, HIV can be directly transmitted through sharing syringes and other equipment for drug injection. Indirectly, IDU has contributed to the spread of HIV far beyond the circle of those who inject and share. Sexual partners of injection drug users are also at risk for acquiring HIV, and children born to mothers who contracted HIV through sharing needles or having sex with an IDU may become infected as well. In 2005, 1,742 MSM diagnosed and reported with AIDS also had the dual risk of IDU (4% of all AIDS cases, 8% of adult/adolescent male AIDS cases, and 11% of all MSM AIDS cases). At the end of 2005, an estimated 24,012 MSM with a dual risk of IDU were reported *living* with *HIV/AIDS* in the 33 states with confidential name-based HIV infection reporting since 2001 (5% of all estimated persons living with HIV/AIDS in the 33 states; 7% of estimated adult/adolescent males living with HIV/AIDS, and 10% of all estimated MSM living with HIV/AIDS) (Centers for Disease Control and Prevention, 2006a).

Use of alcohol and illegal drugs, both injected and noninjected, is a prevalent contributing risk factor for acquiring HIV and other STDs among MSM, including MSM of color, through the tendency toward risky sexual behaviors while under the influence. Drug use can also affect treatment success by altering the ability to take antiretroviral medicines exactly as prescribed. According to the 2004 National Survey on Drug Use and Health, the rate of current illicit drug use was twice as high for Native Americans and multiracial individuals than other races or ethnicities (Centers for Disease Control and Prevention, 2006d).

In their analysis of data from 253 alcohol-abusing HIV-positive MSM, 79% of whom were men of color, Parsons, Kutnick, Halkitis, Punzalan, & Carbonari, (2005) reported significant relationships between the use of several substances and high-risk sexual behaviors for HIV transmission. Over 80% reported engaging in sexual behaviors with casual partners; of these, almost half (47%) reported unprotected anal insertive intercourse with casual partners of unknown status, 19% with HIV-negative casual partners, and 41% with HIV-positive casual partners. Researchers also found a positive relationship between the quantity of daily alcohol ingestion and viral load, a finding that has significant implications for HIV disease progression and treatment. Of special concern is the growing epidemic of methamphetamine ("meth" crystal) use among MSM and MSM of color. A stimulant drug, meth is associated with both high-risk sexual behaviors and the sharing of injection equipment when the drug is injected. As with alcohol and other "party" drugs, such as methylenedioxymethamphetamine (MDMA or "ecstasy"), ketamine ("Special K"), gamma hydroxybutyrate, and nitrate inhalants ("poppers"), meth is used by some MSM to decrease social inhibitions and/or to enhance sexual experiences. This is sometimes done in dangerous combinations with prescription drugs for sexual performance, such as viagra, and HIV medications to enhance the effect of the drugs or alcohol (Centers for Disease Control and Prevention, 2006f).

A study of Filipino Americans using meth in the San Francisco Bay area suggested a strong association between meth and behavioral risk factors for HIV, including infrequent condom use, commercial sex activity, and low rates of HIV testing. Over half of the young A/PI MSM in another study reported using "party drugs," hallucinogens, crack, and amphetamines. The researchers reported a correlation of drugs or alcohol use among these MSM with unprotected anal intercourse (Centers for Disease Control and Prevention, 2006c).

Other Barriers to HIV Prevention And Care

Barriers to testing, prevention, and care for minority MSM include stigma, historically poor access to care, and negative perceptions of the health care system. Through the concerted efforts of HIV providers, the gap has diminished for some MSM of color, but a significant proportion remain out of care or other services, many unaware of their status (Health Resources and Services Administration, 2003). Health Resources and Service Administration (HRSA) (2003: 2) notes that:

> The AIDS epidemic is, in many ways, one in which the 'easy-to-reach' populations have been reached and the people remaining out of care face barriers that may seem insurmountable to them, especially among certain communities of minority MSM. An extraordinary proportion of MSM of color are at heightened risk of contracting the virus, or they are already infected with HIV—but many do not know it. And for reasons ranging from stigma to being overwhelmed with challenges in meeting basic human needs, such as food and shelter, some people do not want to know it.

Reflective of the racial and ethnic minorities to which they belong, many MSM of color have poor access to health care due to poverty and lack of health insurance. MSM of color struggle not only with stigma associated with being a person of color, but also as a sexual minority (MSM), and, if infected, as a person with dreaded HIV disease. MSM of color sometimes face or fear condemnation from their family, friends and/or other network of support, church, community, and service providers (Health Resources and Services Administration, 2006b). (For a discussion of stigma, HIV disclosure, and sexual orientation, see the chapters by Kang and Rapkin and by Zea that follow.)

MSM Identity and Stigma

Many MSM of color, including significant numbers of African American and Latino MSM, self-identify as heterosexual, rather than gay or bisexual, with stigma associated with homosexuality often a contributing factor (Centers for Disease Control and Prevention, 2006b, 2006e). In the African American community, this behavior is exemplified in the "down low" phenomenon in which African American men who have both male and female sexual partners don't identify themselves as gay or bisexual. The CDC (2006b) noted that in a study of HIV-infected persons, only 6% of African American women reported having had sex with a bisexual man, but 34% of African American MSM reported having had sex with women.

This experience is not unique to African American men; another review noted that 18–35% of heterosexual-identified Latino men reported having had anal or oral sex with another man (Centers for Disease Control and Prevention, 2006f). For Latino MSM, several unique cultural factors discourage openness about homosexuality and, therefore, any discussion of associated risk behaviors. These include: "*machismo*, the high value placed on masculinity; *simpatia*, the importance of smooth, nonconfrontational relationships; and *familismo*, the importance of a close relationship with one's family" (Centers for Disease Control and Prevention, 2006f: 4). The director of Betances Health Center in New York City, which serves primarily Latino populations, reported that although most HIV-positive males report heterosexual contact as their HIV risk factor at intake, subsequent treatment and counseling reveals the patient to be an MSM. "If they're in denial of their own sexual orientation, they're much more likely to deny their HIV risk, too" (Health Resources and Services Administration, 2003: 3).

A 2000 report on MSM of color commissioned by the federal Health Resources and Services Administration (HRSA) highlighted the role that stigma plays in keeping people out of care. Key informants in the roundtable discussions for the study discussed the condemnation that MSM face from their families, communities, and service providers and also the general perception of same-partner sex as unacceptable (Health Resources and Services Administration, 2003). Participants verified that MSM of color are less likely to identify as gay or bisexual than Caucasian MSM. In a CDC-sponsored study of 7,871 HIV-positive MSM (excluding those with dual IDU risk), Blair, Fleming, and Karon (2002) noted that 21% of African American MSM, 13% of Latino MSM, and 12% of A/PI MSM identified themselves as heterosexual, compared with 5% of Native American and 5% of Caucasian MSM. Accordingly, HRSA (2006b: 1) concluded that

> prevention and health outreach targeting sexual minorities may not be effective among this group—and MSM may be especially reluctant to seek services at organizations perceived to be gay oriented. Many minority MSM identify with their racial identity more than their sexual identity; thus, messages aimed at the gay community often do not reach them.

Additionally, MSM of color are less likely to live in gay-identified neighborhoods and, as a consequence, missed by prevention programs and outreach activities focused in those neighborhoods (Centers for Disease Control and Prevention, 2006f).

These studies highlight the need to develop outreach and prevention messages targeted to MSM who do not identify as gay or bisexual, and ensure access to providers and interventions that are not perceived as gay (Health Resources and Services Administration, 2003). Although 75% of Washington, DC's Whitman-Walker Clinic HIV-positive clients are African Americans, the clinic has struggled with the misperception among many people of color that the clinic only serves gay Caucasian men. To counter this notion, Whitman-Walker opened a satellite men's clinic in a predominantly African American neighborhood and deliberately did not call it a gay men's clinic to encourage African American MSM, particularly those who do not identify as gay, to use these services (Health Resources and Services Administration, 2003).

Cultural and Socioeconomic Issues, Discrimination, and Poor Access to Health Care

Stigma is not the only factor preventing MSM of color from receiving HIV care, outreach, or prevention information. Social and economic circumstances, racism, poverty, and lack of access to health care are also significant barriers to accessing services or getting needed information. Lack of awareness of HIV status by MSM of color, a significant issue for young African American MSM in particular, is also a barrier to getting care (Health Resources and Services Administration, 2003). The fact that African American and Latino men are more likely than Caucasian men to be diagnosed with HIV in later stages of infection, frequently with a concurrent AIDS diagnosis, implies a cultural bias to not accessing testing or health care while healthy, but only after symptoms develop (Centers for Disease Control and Prevention, 2006f). Additionally, as noted in HRSA-sponsored roundtable discussions and interviews with MSM in 2000, many MSM of color perceive medical services as unwelcoming to them. This may be underscored by affected MSM of color for whom English is a second language, and for Native American and A/PI MSM who belong to many diverse cultures with a variety of associated languages. Few educational and informational materials have been translated into A/PI and Native American languages (Health Resources and Services Administration, 2003). Following are some cultural and socioeconomic issues specific to racial/ethnic and other affected groups to which MSM of color belong.

African Americans

In 1999, nearly one-quarter of African Americans were living in poverty. Higher AIDS incidence has been found to be associated with lower income. This may be due, at least in part, to the socioeconomic problems that are associated with poverty, such as limited access to high-quality health care and HIV prevention education (Centers for Disease Control and Prevention, 2006b). Data from the HIV Cost and Services Utilization Study (HCSUS) indicate that 22% of HIV-positive African Americans were uninsured and more likely to delay medical care due to a lack of transportation, severity of illness, and/or other competing needs (Henry Kaiser Family Foundation, 2006b).

Latinos

There is no single Latino culture or identity in the USA. Large numbers of Latino Americans or their parents emigrated from many different countries and cultures. For recent immigrants, lack of knowledge about HIV/AIDS and social isolation may increase their risk of exposure to HIV. HIV risk factors vary among Latinos by country of birth; for example, Puerto Rican-born Latinos are more likely to contract HIV as a result of IDU, while the primary risk factor for Mexican-born is MSM (Centers for Disease Control and Prevention, 2006e).

Almost 23% of US Latinos live in poverty. According to a multisite study of HIV-positive Latinos, 47% of Mexican-born MSM and 59% of Puerto Rican-born MSM reported annual incomes of less than $10,000 (Centers for Disease Control and Prevention, 2006e). HCSUS data found 24% of all HIV-positive Latinos were uninsured (Henry Kaiser Family Foundation, 2006c).

Asians and Pacific Islanders

The term "Asian/Pacific Islander" describes approximately 40 cultures and many nationalities—Chinese, Filipinos, Koreans, Hawaiians, Indians, Japanese, Samoans, Vietnamese, and others—and more than 100 languages and dialects. Each group varies in language, customs, and history. Many foreign-born A/PIs, in particular, may experience cultural and language barriers to services and information. Although overall socioeconomically diverse, more than a million A/PIs live at or below the federal poverty level. Given this staggering cultural, linguistic, and socioeconomic diversity, the tailoring of prevention and outreach messages to A/PIs remains daunting. Many A/PIs tend to underutilize health care and prevention services. One study of 653 HIV-positive A/PIs found that few used HIV case management services, housing assistance, substance use treatment, or health education services (Centers for Disease Control and Prevention, 2006c).

Native Americans

Native Americans comprise less than 1% of the US population, but reflect considerable diversity. The classification of "Native American" encompasses 562 federally recognized tribes and at least 50 state-recognized tribes. Each tribe is characterized by its own culture, beliefs, and practices and may be further distinguished by language groups. Almost one-quarter (24.3%) of Native Americans in the USA live in poverty, twice the national average, with associated lower levels of education and poorer access to health care. Native Americans experience a decreased life expectancy in comparison with all other racial/ethnic groups; an increased incidence of many diseases, such as diabetes, tuberculosis, and alcoholism; and decreased levels of access to care.

All of these factors enhance susceptibility to other health issues, including HIV (Centers for Disease Control and Prevention , 2006d).

Although Native Americans with AIDS are more likely to have been diagnosed while residing in a rural area, many who are at high risk in rural areas have limited access to testing. In addition, due to the close-knit nature of the Native American communities, confidentiality and privacy are of particular concern. Individuals may be reluctant to seek HIV testing due to concerns about confidentiality, such as might arise if an individual were to encounter a friend or other known individual at a health care facility. One-half of Native Americans responding to a Behavioral Risk Factor Surveillance System survey in 1997–2000 had never been tested for HIV; in the southwestern USA it was even higher, at 58% (Centers for Disease Control and Prevention, 2006d).

Ex-inmates

HIV-positive men of color leaving correctional facilities face unique challenges, with many unaware of HIV status, out of care for HIV, or both. If socio-economic and health care needs are not addressed expeditiously, many relapse into the same behaviors that led to incarceration and/or HIV infection in the first place. HRSA (2003) noted that among participants in a joint HRSA–CDC Corrections Initiative, many ex-offenders returning to their communities are as unprepared for employment as they were at the time of their incarceration and, with criminal records, may be unable to find employers who are willing to hire them. Ex-inmates are also often estranged from their families or other networks of support. Although some programs provide appropriate transition to the community by assessing need, establishing linkages to health care, and provid-ing assistance to obtain needed services and benefits, most ex-inmates are not aware of or do not have access to such programs (Health Resources and Services Administration, 2003).

Young Men

Specific barriers to care for adolescent and YMSMC include a lack of trans-portation to clinics, a lack of resources to pay for services, an unresponsive health care system, stigma, homelessness, and mental health issues. Clinic staff may be uncomfortable with the youth's presentation and both clinic staff and the youth themselves may be unprepared to address the multitude of legal issues that young men bring, including status as minors, undocumented status, and/or homelessness. Gay or HIV-positive youth may have been disenfranchised by their families following their disclosure of their sexual orientation. In such situations, a stable living situation may be more of a priority to them than health care. Many may also have mental health disorders, which can complicate treatment. Mental health assessment of a sample of youth served by the Adolescent Medicine Program at the CORE Center (AMaC) in Chicago revealed that 83% had symptoms for depression, 73% for posttraumatic stress disorder, 65% for anxiety disorders, and 32% for psychotic disorders (Health Resources and Services Administration, 2003).

Prevention Efforts

The Centers for Disease Control and Prevention issued a new initiative in 2003, Advancing HIV Prevention, comprised four strategies: making HIV testing a routine part of medical care, implementing new models for diagnosing HIV infections outside of medical settings, preventing new infections by working with HIV-infected persons and their partners, and further decreasing perinatal HIV transmission. To be effective, the CDC acknowledges that the interventions for MSM must be tailored to specific target audiences, such as African American or Latino MSM (Centers for Disease Control and Prevention, 2006f). In their study of race/ethnicity, HIV prevalence and related risk behaviors among young MSM in seven urban centers in the United States, Harawa and colleagues (2004: 526) concluded that

> Understanding racial/ethnic disparities in HIV risk requires information beyond the traditional risk behavior and partnership type distinctions. Prevention programs should address risks in steady partnerships, target young men before sexual initiation with male partners, and tailor interventions to men of color and of lower socioeconomic status.

Culturally specific prevention efforts with basic information about HIV and promotion of testing also need to be targeted to older MSM of color, some of whom may not self-identify as gay or bisexual. In a study of 110 older (50+) African American and Latino MSM, Jimenez (2003) noted that almost three-quarters believed that they were at minimal risk for HIV. These older MSM of color were, by contrast, found to be sexually active, frequently engaging in sex with multiple partners, and using drugs during sex. The study also suggested that race and age with associated perceptions of gay or HIV-related stigma may be important factors in forming sexual identity or disclosing same-sex behavior among older MSM of color and need to be considered in developing appropriate interventions.

HIV prevention efforts have shown some success in reducing sexual risk behaviors. One review published in 2002 noted an average decrease of 26% in unprotected sex among men receiving an intervention. Examples of some successful programs targeting MSM cited by the CDC are: "Many Men, Many Voices," an STD/HIV prevention group intervention for gay men of color and MSM who do not identify themselves as gay or bisexual; "Mpowerment," a community-building format for young MSM that utilizes HIV prevention, safer sex, and risk-reduction messages; "Popular Opinion Leader," which identifies, enlists, and trains key opinion leaders to encourage safer sex as the norm in the social networks of MSM; "Healthy Relationships," which develops the self-efficacy skills of HIV-positive people; and "Peers Reaching Out and Modeling Intervention Strategies (PROMISE)," which uses peer advocates (including men who do not identify themselves as gay) to help people adopt practices to reduce or eliminate risk factors for HIV infection (Centers for Disease Control and Prevention, 2006f).

Reaching MSM of Color and Bringing Them into Care

Successful outreach to MSM of color requires the utilization of aggressive case finding; the provision of high quality and nonjudgmental services; emphasis on the relationship between substance use, sexual activity and HIV risk, and support in addressing this interrelationship; cultural competence; and support and encouragement to recognize HIV risk, obtain testing, and access and remain in care. Reliance on peers is often a critical component to the successful achievement of these goals. To accomplish this, many providers have enhanced existing clinic programs instead of creating an entirely new program. Five RWCA providers interviewed by HRSA used a combination of community-based and peer outreach initiatives to reach MSM of color. Once in care, comprehensive care and support services successfully kept them engaged in services (Health Resources and Services Administration, 2003). These and some other program successes are briefly described below.

The **Boriquen Family Health Center in Miami, Florida** serves a large clientele of HIV-positive Latino MSM; 60% of men enrolled in HIV care are from Cuba and Puerto Rico, speaking mostly Spanish and 30% from Haiti, speaking primarily Creole. Histories of substance abuse and trading sex for drugs are common. Stigma due to HIV status, homosexuality and substance abuse, and a lack of trust of "mainstream" medical providers present significant barriers to accessing HIV-positive and at-risk MSM of color. In response, the HIV clinic seeks to make all clients feel comfortable to receive the care they need, regardless of their status, background, or orientation. The clinic developed a five-step process designed to foster a nonjudgmental environment and support clients in accessing and remaining in care: (1) develop trust; (2) educate; (3) provide HIV counseling and testing; (4) use peers to lead outreach efforts, build relationships with potential clients, and provide support to men who come in for counseling and testing; and (5) follow up with clients (Health Resources and Services Administration, 2003).

To reach MSM of color, the clinic conducts outreach through linkages with religious organizations that serve people of color and in areas frequented by MSM. In addition, outreach is conducted at "high risk sites," such as shooting galleries and areas frequented by homeless individuals. With a focus on developing trust, the first interaction is solely about building a relationship. Subsequent encounters stress that clients are not being judged and that outreach workers care about them. Education about HIV and other STDs, which includes one-on-one counseling and discussion, is often accepted only after trust has been carefully fostered. MSM coming to the center are welcomed by Latino and Haitian MSM peer educators who have been trained to be sensitive to their culture, beliefs, and values and to make the prospective clients feel welcome and accepted. Services offered at the center include voluntary HIV counseling and testing, primary medical care, dental care, psychotherapy, and nutrition services. Anonymity and confidentiality are emphasized. For instance, neither "HIV" nor "AIDS" appear on public signage. Rather, the HIV clinic is called the Phoenix Program. Success in high rates of return for test results is attributed to the focus on developing a trusting, caring relationship between potential clients and peers and follow-up by the same peer with individuals who do not return for test results (Health Resources and Services Administration, 2003).

Staff at **Betances Health Center in New York City** is also culturally and linguistically diverse and competent, reflective of the surrounding communities served and languages spoken, and fosters a nonjudgmental environment with strict confidentiality. The comprehensive array of HIV/AIDS services provided on-site includes noninvasive testing, counseling, primary medical care, case management, support groups, nutritional counseling, adherence support, and harm reduction, with access to alternative treatments. At the time of the interview with HRSA (2003), 56% of the clinic's 380 HIV-positive clients were men, and of those, 40% (85) were MSM, although few acknowledged their MSM risk factor at intake. The clinic reported using a comprehensive outreach strategy of peer-based, one-on-one interventions, and community-wide HIV counseling and testing activities to bring MSM of color into care, including men leaving corrections and living in transitional housing. Word-of-mouth from friends, in tandem with the center's long-standing positive community reputation and reputation for the maintenance of confidential relationships with sexual minority men, resulted in increasing success in attracting MSM of color to the clinic. Once connected in care, case management, and ancillary services, including counseling to address HIV, addiction and/or harm reduction, and a peer-based adherence program, have proven critical to keeping clients in care over time (Health Resources and Services Administration, 2003).

Strategies to reach MSM of color by the **Whitman-Walker Clinic in Washington, DC,** which has been challenged to dispel the misperception that it serves only gay White men, include hiring culturally competent staff and opening a separate men's clinic in a largely African American neighborhood. This clinic provides a one-stop array of services including primary medical care, dental care, HIV/AIDS support services, mental health, substance abuse treatment, legal services, and voluntary HIV counseling and testing. In addition, its Men's Wellness Clinic offers confidential STD testing, hepatitis A and B vaccination, and risk-reduction counseling. Prevention initiatives at Whitman-Walker targeting HIV-negative MSM of color include the Black Men's Health Network, which provides street outreach and group interventions, and collaborates with faith and community-based organizations; and

Acuarela, a similar program targeting Latino men. "Proud and Positive," a prevention with positives initiative, also targets MSM of color (Health Resources and Services Administration, 2003).

The statewide **California Bridge Project** reported identifying 325 HIV-positive individuals who had never received HIV medical care, with average time of one-and-a-half years from HIV diagnosis to contact with project staff (Molitor et al., 2006). Nearly three-fourths were people of color and almost half MSM. Project staff effectively linked 29% of these individuals to medical care through intensive outreach, averaging over 15 contacts per client from first contact to linkage. Following an assessment of clients' risk behaviors, mental and physical health status, and actual and perceived barriers to care, project staff focused their efforts on linking clients to medical care. Their success, which was attributed in part to the racial and ethnic similarity between themselves and their prospective clients, is reflected in the fact that Latinos were more than twice as likely and African Americans more than three times as likely as non-Hispanic Whites to be linked to medical care.

Ninety percent of clients at the **Comprehensive HIV Center at St Vincent's Hospital and Medical Center in Greenwich Village, New York City**, are people of color; 42% are Latino, 40% African American, and one-half are MSM. The center has built a reputation for compassionate care and endeavors to make clients feel comfortable in accessing and receiving services, purposely avoiding any categorizing of its clients. The center uses numerous strategies to reach MSM of color including the employment of culturally and linguistically competent staff members who reflect the client populations and the languages they speak; outreach to churches, community organizations, social service agencies, and schools; outreach efforts to the African American community coordinated by an African American staff physician; follow-up by a staff nurse to find patients who have stopped returning for services, particularly useful for patients with substance abuse issues; incentives for current clients who bring in people they know for testing, with those testing positive referred to staff physicians; rapid HIV testing with those testing positive also immediately linked to care; and the "Talk Safe" program, specifically targeted to HIV negative or untested MSM of color. "Talk Safe" provides up to ten free counseling sessions on harm reduction and HIV preventive behaviors, as well as information on how to access HIV care (Health Resources and Services Administration, 2003).

Winiarski, Beckett and Salcedo (2005) reported on the effectiveness of an inner city HIV mental health program integrated with primary care and emphasizing cultural responsiveness. Primary care clients used mental health care at a higher rate than did comparison subjects. Utilization of these services was associated with a reduction in reported mental health problems, HIV-related physical symptoms, use of alcohol and powdered cocaine, and improvement in social functioning.

The CORE Center in Chicago, IL offers comprehensive outpatient care to individuals and families affected by HIV/AIDS, including primary medical care and social services. Most of the HIV-positive youth receiving care in the

Chicago area receive services through the AMaC. Center priorities include physical comfort, language, privacy, diversity, and respect for the clients. To find HIV-infected youth, including YMSMC, many of whom are not receiving needed care, AMaC uses four approaches:

> First, the program focuses on communities identified as epicenters for HIV and associated comorbidities (such as STIs and TB). Second, AMaC works within sub-populations and subcultures, especially youth from communities of color, adolescent women, and adolescent MSM, groups that traditional outreach and education programs often have difficulty reaching. Third, the program reaches out to youth who fit youth profiles developed from data collected in the case-finding program and from primary care services (e.g., youth with high variability in sex partners, a history of drug use, gang affiliations, or a history of STDs). Last, the program identifies and works with networks of youth (defined as an HIV-positive youth and his or her friends and sexual partners), who are often characterized by similar risky behaviors and comorbid factors (Health Resources and Services Administration, 2003: 6).

HIV-positive peer health educators have proven extremely effective in reaching and engaging youth at risk for HIV, people of color, and other populations disproportionately affected by the epidemic. Peers, including "youth buddies" described below, form the cornerstone for AMaC's services (Health Resources and Services Administration, 2003).

Services for adolescents and youth must consider mental health and social needs and psychosocial development in addition to medical needs. Once youth are connected to care, AMaC uses a multifaceted team approach to keep them engaged in care and to address their multiple needs. Teams include medical providers, case managers, peer "youth buddies," peer health educators, and social support groups. In contrast to other programs, CORE Center staff highlights the importance of gathering information up-front about the sexual history of clients, including the sexual behavior of men with men. This approach allows men to discuss their sexual activities with other nonjudgmental adults and may bring feelings of relief in being able to do so. Participation in social support groups provides not only lunch, but also opportunities to discuss critical issues, including family relationships, the adoption of prevention behaviors, and adherence to ART. "Youth buddies," HIV-positive young people, provide one-to-one counseling and engage clients in discussions about obligations and medication side effects. These discussions are more believable to the youth clients because they occur with "buddies" of a similar age, rather than with adult providers (Health Resources and Services Administration, 2003).

Conclusion

MSM of color are dramatically and disproportionately impacted by the HIV/ AIDS epidemic and continue to have the highest HIV incidence of any risk group, facilitated by continuing or reemerging unsafe sexual and drug-using behaviors. Many MSM of color have adopted HIV prevention behaviors, and many who are HIV-positive are in care and benefiting from treatment. However, a significant number of others continue to engage in high-risk behaviors, remain out of care and/or are unaware of their HIV status. Interventions for MSM must be tailored to specific target audiences by sexual orientation, race/ethnicity, age, and geographic location and/or culture. Cultural competency, awareness of stigma, and aggressive case finding have proven effective in reaching MSM of color and engaging them in HIV prevention and care.

References

Absalon, J., Della-Latta, P., Wu, F., & El-Sadr, W. M. (2005). Sexual behaviors and condom use of HIV-infected men and women of color attending a treatment and care clinic. *Journal of the National Medical Association, 97*(Suppl. 7), S25–S31.

Blair, J. M., Fleming, P. L., & Karon, J. M. (2002). Trends in AIDS incidence and survival among racial/ethnic minority men who have sex with men, United States, 1990–1999. *Journal of Acquired Immune Deficiency Syndromes, 31*(3), 339–347.

Centers for Disease Control and Prevention. (2005). HIV prevalence, unrecognized infection, and HIV testing among men who have sex with men—five U.S. cities, June 2004–April 2005. *Morbidity and Mortality Weekly Report, 54*(24), 597–601. Atlanta, Georgia: U.S. Department of Health and Human Services, Centers for Disease Control and Prevention. Last accessed October 27, 2006; Available at http://www.cdc.gov/MMWR/preview/mmwrhtml/mm5424a2.htm

Centers for Disease Control and Prevention. (2006a). *HIV/AIDS surveillance report: Cases of HIV infection and AIDS in the United States and dependent areas, 2005, 17*, 1–46. Atlanta, Georgia: U.S. Department of Health and Human Services, Centers for Disease Control and Prevention. Last accessed December 12, 2006; Available at http://www.cdc.gov/hiv/topics/surveillance/resources/reports/2005report/pdf/2005SurveillanceReport.pdf

Centers for Disease Control and Prevention. (2006b). CDC HIV/AIDS fact sheet: HIV/AIDS among African Americans. Atlanta, Georgia: U.S. Department of Health and Human Services, Centers for Disease Control and Prevention (February 2006). Last accessed October 27, 2006; Available at http://www.cdc.gov/hiv/topics/aa/resources/factsheets/aa.htm

Centers for Disease Control and Prevention. (2006c). CDC HIV/AIDS fact sheet: HIV/AIDS among Asians and Pacific Islanders. Atlanta, Georgia: U.S. Department of Health and Human Services, Centers for Disease Control and Prevention (April 2006). Last accessed October 27, 2006; Available at http://www.cdc.gov/hiv/resources/factsheets/API.htm

Centers for Disease Control and Prevention. (2006d). CDC HIV/AIDS fact sheet: HIV/AIDS among American Indians and Alaska Natives. Atlanta, Georgia: U.S. Department of Health and Human Services, Centers for Disease Control and Prevention (April 2006). Last accessed October 27, 2006; Available at http://www.cdc.gov/hiv/resources/factsheets/aian.htm

Centers for Disease Control and Prevention. (2006e). CDC HIV/AIDS fact sheet: HIV/AIDS among Hispanics. Atlanta, Georgia: U.S. Department of Health and Human Services, Centers for Disease Control and Prevention (June 2006). Last accessed October 27, 2006; Available at http://www.cdc.gov/hiv/resources/factsheets/hispanic.htm

Centers for Disease Control and Prevention. (2006f). CDC HIV/AIDS fact sheet: HIV/AIDS among men who have sex with men. Atlanta, Georgia: U.S. Department of Health and Human Services, Centers for Disease Control and Prevention (July 2006). Last accessed October 1, 2006; Available at http://www.cdc.gov/hiv/resources/factsheets/msm.htm

Fields, S. D., Wharton, M. J., Marrero, A. I., Little, A., Pannell, K., & Morgan, J. H. (2006). Internet chat rooms: connecting with a new generation of young men of color at risk for HIV infection who have sex with other men. *Journal of the Association of Nurses in AIDS Care, 17(6)*, 53–60.

Glynn, M., & Rhodes, P. (2005). Estimated HIV prevalence in the United States at the end of 2003. Presented at the *National HIV Prevention Conference*, June 2005, Atlanta, Georgia [Abstract T1-B1101].

Grieco, E. M., & Cassidy, R. C. (2001). Census 2000 brief: overview of race and hispanic origin. Washington, D.C.: U.S. Department of Commerce, U.S. Census Bureau (March 2001). Last accessed October 1, 2006; Available at http://www.census.gov/prod/2001pubs/c2kbr01-1.pdf

Halkitis, P. N., Wilton, L., Wolitski, R. J., Parsons, J. T., Hoff, C. C., & Bimbi, D. S. (2005). Barebacking identity among HIV-positive gay and bisexual men: Demographic, psychological, and behavioral correlates. *AIDS, 19*(Suppl 1), S27–S35.

Harawa, N. T., Greenland, S., Bingham, T. A., Johnson, D. F., Cochran, S. D., & Cunningham, W. E., et al. (2004). Associations of race/ethnicity with HIV prevalence and HIV-related behaviors among young men who have sex with men in 7 urban centers in the United States. *Journal of Acquired Immune Deficiency Syndromes, 35(5)*, 526–536.

Health Resources and Services Administration. (2003). Reaching men of color who have sex with men. *HRSA CAREAction*, 2003, June, 1–8. Rockville, MD: U.S. Department of Health and Human Services, HRSA. Last accessed September 29, 2006; Available at http://hab.hrsa.gov/publications/june2003/

Health Resources and Services Administration. (2006a). Men of color who have sex with men and HIV/AIDS in the United States [fact sheet]. Rockville, MD: U.S. Department of Health and Human Services, HRSA (June 2006). Last accessed September 29, 2006; Available at http://hab.hrsa.gov/history/MenOfColor/

Health Resources and Services Administration. (2006b). Men who have sex with men and HIV/AIDS in the United States [fact sheet]. Rockville, MD: U.S. Department of Health and Human Services, HRSA (June 2006). Last accessed September 29, 2006; Available at http://hab.hrsa.gov/history/MSM/

Henry J. Kaiser Family Foundation. (2006a). HIV/AIDS policy fact sheet: the HIV/AIDS epidemic in the United States. Menlo Park, CA: The Henry J. Kaiser Family Foundation (November 2006). Last accessed December 7, 2006; Available at http://www.kff.org/hivaids/upload/3029-071.pdf

Henry J. Kaiser Family Foundation. (2006b). HIV/AIDS policy fact Sheet: Black Americans and HIV/AIDS. Menlo Park, CA: The Henry J. Kaiser Family Foundation (December 2006). Last accessed January 4, 2007; Available at http://www.kff.org/hivaids/upload/6089-04.pdf

Henry J. Kaiser Family Foundation. (2006c). HIV/AIDS policy fact sheet: Latinos and HIV/AIDS. Menlo Park, CA: The Henry J. Kaiser Family Foundation (December 2006). Last accessed January 4, 2007: Available at http://www.kff.org/hivaids/upload/6007-04.pdf

Jimenez, A. D. (2003). Triple jeopardy: targeting older men of color who have sex with men. *Journal of Acquired Immune Deficiency Syndromes, 33*(Suppl 2), S222–S225.

Molitor, F., Waltermeyer, J., Mendoza, M., Kuenneth, C., Aguirre, A., & Brockmann, K. et al. (2006). Locating and linking to medical care HIV-positive persons without a history of care: Findings from the California Bridge Project. *AIDS Care, 18(5)*, 456–459.

Parsons J. T., Kutnick, A. H., Halkitis, P. N., Punzalan, J. C., & Carbonari, J. P. (2005). Sexual risk behaviors and substance use among alcohol abusing HIV-positive men who have sex with men. *Journal of Psychoactive Drugs, 37(1),* 27–36.

Winiarski, M. G., Beckett, E., & Salcedo, J. (2005). Outcomes of an inner-city HIV mental health programme integrated with primary care and emphasizing cultural responsiveness. *AIDS Care, 17*(6), 747–756.

Chapter Eight
HIV/AIDS in Cleveland: A Case Study of One Community

David Bruckman

Introduction

Measurement of the progression of HIV/AIDS among African Americans in United States relies on prompt, accurate, and complete reporting of incident HIV and new AIDS diagnoses through CD4 levels. The City of Cleveland, Ohio has been fortunate in several factors: three large teaching medical systems, each with centralized centers of excellence having highly competent infectious disease departments; neighborhood clinics that report cases responsively though their internal laboratories or their contracted agencies; and the existence of a centralized HIV/AIDS surveillance database within the public health system that has collected cases reported since the early 1980s. These three factors have allowed the Cleveland Department of Public Health (CDPH), the central reporting agency for all cases reported by agencies in Cuyahoga County, to provide its citizens with quarterly prevalence and exposure reports and detailed annual epidemiological summaries that report incidence rates and temporal trends among groups by race/ethnicity, age, and exposure history to HIV. This chapter describes the social and economic context of HIV transmission in the Cleveland area and provides an epidemiological analysis of HIV/AIDS among Black/African Americans in Cleveland.

Demographic and Economic Context

Cleveland lies on the northern coast of Ohio against Lake Erie, the second largest city in the state behind Columbus, the state capital. Since 1980, the proportion of Black/African Americans in Cleveland has grown each decade from 43.8%, 46.6% and then 51.0%, while the overall population has decreased

David Bruckman
Cleveland Department of Public Health, Cleveland, OH

S. Loue (ed.), *Health Issues Confronting Minority Men Who Have Sex with Men.*
© Springer 2008

from 573,822 to 478,403 in 2000 (US Bureau of the Census, 2005a). According to the Population Estimate Program of the US Census, there were 452,208 residents in Cleveland at midyear 2005, with 41.5% White and 1.4% Asian/ Pacific Islanders (US Bureau of the Census, 2005b). While 7.3% of surveyed residents are Hispanic, these residents tend to be underrepresented, especially among children (West, Robinson, & Knavery, 1998).

With Lake Erie setting the northern border, Cleveland is surrounded by some 50 other municipalities within Cuyahoga County. Fewer than 1.4 million residents live in the County, where 27.7% are Black/African American overall. Most Black/African Americans in Cleveland reside in the eastern and central neighborhoods or statistical planning areas. (See map.)

African Americans constitute the majority population within 17 of 36 neighborhoods, reflecting majority presence from Downtown to North Collinwood to the northeast and to Lee-Miles to the southeast. Cleveland was, and by many still is, considered by many to be heavily segregated, and this disparity has prompted legal action. In 1976, the federal district court under Judge Frank J. Battisti ordered Cleveland public schools to be desegregated (*Reed v. Rhodes*, 1976, 1978, 1979, 1980). The resulting mandated busing of students contributed to a 34% drop in student enrollment during the first 4 years of implementation and the

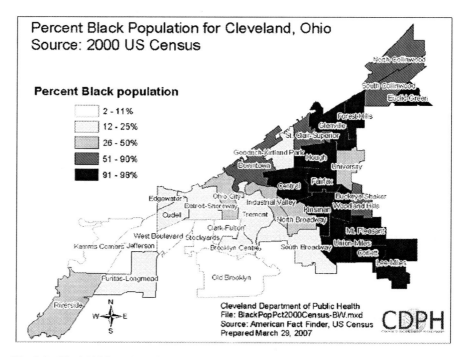

Fig. 8.1 Black/African American Population Distribution across Statistical Planning Areas of Cleveland, 2000 (US Bureau of the Census, 2000).

migration of families out of Cleveland. With a lower student population and smaller tax base, funding for schools dropped precipitously (Ohio Historical Society, 2005).

The out-migration of White and Black residents was hastened by the economic decimation resulting from oil shortages and inflation of the 1970s and a wide contraction of the heavy steel, automotive, and large-scale manufacturing base that has lasted to this current day. Currently, the largest employers in Cleveland are hospitals and direct medical care, local universities, and government. Cleveland serves as the headquarters of two major banks and several financial agencies due to the location of 1 of the 12 Federal Reserve Banks.

During the past decade, poverty has gripped the city and the region. In 2003, Cleveland's poverty rate was 31.1%, nearly twice the rate of Columbus (16.5%), the capital city, and national levels (12.7%). Lower economic prosperity, unmitigated deterioration of the tax base and quality schools, and fewer job opportunities have contributed to Cleveland's ranking as one of the three poorest major cities in the United States, with the ignomious title of "Nation's Poorest Major City" for the years 2003 and 2005 (Smith & Davis, 2004; Webster & Bishaw, 2006). A study by the Center for Community Solutions determined that approximately two-thirds of African American and Hispanic youth live in severely distressed areas, and three-quarters of youths living in predominately African American neighborhoods were in homes in poor condition (Salling, 2006).

Foreclosure rates in Cleveland during the first four months of 2006 were third highest in the nation with 95 per 100,000 residents, surpassed only by Detroit and Dallas–Fort Worth (Fitch, 2006). Nationally, the annual foreclosure rate was 29 per 100,000 residents. Compounding these problems has been a spate of predatory lending throughout Ohio. Poor enforcement of existing laws and agreements between government and banks has allowed predatory lending firms a relatively open field. With the recent change in gubernatorial leadership in 2006, the state attorney general Marc Dann has made predatory lending a priority of his 2006–2009 term (Dann, 2007).

African Americans in Cleveland and throughout major Ohio cities have been victims of housing bias. Almost one-third of all reports of housing discrimination in Northeast Ohio during 2002–2004 relate to minority populations (The Housing Research and Advocacy Center, 2003). In January 2004, the United States Department of Housing and Urban Development awarded $1.3 million in grants to Ohio agencies that investigate allegations of housing discrimination and work closely with citizens, area development corporations, and government to promote fair housing. Two of the seven Ohio agencies receiving such awards were located in Cleveland and work specifically in areas with low–moderate income and minority representation (US Department of Housing and Urban Development, 2004). However, in the past two decades, segregation of African Americans in Cleveland and Cuyahoga County has only marginally improved despite the efforts of many municipalities to enact fair housing laws (Dillman, Pleasants, Roskilly, & Farmby, 2006).

Health Indicators

In the midst of these economic pressures, African Americans experience reduced access to medical care and services. Two-thirds of Cleveland neighborhoods with predominately African American populations lie in areas that lack a threshold number of primary care physicians. Based on Health and Human Service Department regulations, much of eastern Cleveland can be officially designated as Health Professional Shortage Areas (HPSA). In fact, a majority of African Americans in all of Cuyahoga County reside in these HPSA areas (Lenahan, 2005). The incidence of low-birth weight babies and higher infant mortality are greater among African American mothers compared with both White non-Hispanic and Hispanic mothers (Cuyahoga County Board of Health, 2004; Lenahan, 2005). Low birth weight infants (under 2,500 grams) and infant mortality are associated with maternal health factors such as maternal smoking, morbid obesity, diabetes, less than 12 years education, poor nutrition, and lack of prenatal care (David & Collins, 1997; Goldenberg & Culhane, 2007).

African American teens in Cleveland appear to be more sexually active and take greater risks during and among sexual encounters. First, 2003 birth rates to teens aged 15–19 in Cleveland are twice as high as rates for Cuyahoga County and Ohio. Sixty-nine percent of these births were to African American teen mothers. Second, the impact of sexually transmitted disease (Chlamydia, gonorrhea, and syphilis) cannot be understated as a sentinel marker for risky sexual behavior. Chlamydia is the most frequently reported sexually transmitted disease (STD) infection in the United States, Ohio, and Cleveland (Centers for Disease Control and Prevention, 1996; Cleveland Department of Public Health, 2007; Ohio Department of Health, 2007). Many studies have shown that the presence of STDs increases the risk of acquiring HIV, either by physiological, sociological, or assortive and probabilistic means (Centers for Disease Control and Prevention, 2001; Fleming & Wasserheit, 1999; Halfors, Iritani, Miller, & Bauer, 2007; Laumann & Youm, 1999; Wasserheit, 1992). Administration of the Youth Risk Behavioral Survey at several middle and high schools in Cleveland during 2004 revealed earlier initiation of sex, more binge drinking, and marijuana use among African American students than their White and Hispanic counterparts. Seventy-one percent of students had ever engaged in sexual intercourse. Almost half were currently sexually active within the month of the survey. Most disturbing, only 40% of all students regardless of race and ethnicity did not use a condom during their last sexual intercourse at the time of the survey (Center for Adolescent Health, 2006).

Most cases of Chlamydia and gonorrhea reported for Cuyahoga County occur among those at 15–29 years of age at the time of diagnosis. At least 75% of Chlamydia and gonorrhea incident cases reported in 2005 were among Cleveland residents. In Cleveland, African Americans experience the highest annual incidence rates for Chlamydia and gonorrhea compared with White non-Hispanic and Hispanic residents. Chlamydia is now endemic among African American teen females (aged 15–19). On average, one in ten young girls in Cleveland were reported as infected with Chlamydia in 2005 (10,775 per 100,000 group population), a level that has not substantially changed since in-depth analysis began in 2005 with testing for 2002–2003. For African American males and females aged 20–29, Chlamydia infection incidence rates were 5,083 and 3,384 per 100,000, from 3 to 11 times higher than their Hispanic and White non-Hispanic counterparts.

The third and most pressing factor rests entirely on new HIV/AIDS surveillance results identified and reported by CDPH. More African Americans have HIV/AIDS than any other race or ethnic group in Cuyahoga County and Cleveland. Fifty-nine percent (1,543) of some 2,622 Cleveland residents reported and living with HIV as of December 31, 2006 are African American (CDPH, 2007). Their prevalence of 692.6 per 100,000 (African American) population is second to only 1,039 Hispanics per 100,000 living with HIV. With Hispanics making up slightly over 7% of the population, the 333 cases reflect a greater prevalence rate; however, the absolute burden on the African American community is far greater.

In 2006, the CDPH reported that new HIV infections were appearing in middle- and high school-age adolescents (Cleveland Department of Public Health, 2006). In 2004–2005, 19 incidence cases of HIV were reported among teens aged 15–19 in Cuyahoga County, a majority of whom were African American males, most of whom reported male–male (MSM) sexual exposure risk. Twelve cases were Cleveland residents at the time of diagnosis. One of 19 was later diagnosed as an incident AIDS case (i.e., being an incident AIDS case as having been initially diagnosed with HIV within the previous 12 months). In 2003, there were five incident HIV cases in Cleveland. Prior to 2003, HIV cases among teens were very rare. In fact, 60–65% of all incident diagnoses of HIV (only) and AIDS over all ages for Cleveland are African American. In 2006, 45% of all new HIV/AIDS cases were attributable to African American males. In retrospect, it was fortunate that these adolescents were reported so soon, as studies have shown an increase in the incidence of HIV-positive young gay Black males, many of whom were unaware of infection and not seeking routine (annual) HIV screening (Centers for Disease Control and Prevention, 2002; MacKellar et al., 2005; Valleroy et al., 2000). In light of these cases, CDPH initiated a Rapid Assessment and Response Evaluation with the assistance of an Epidemiological Investigation Service intern from the Centers for Disease Control and Prevention (CDC). The project targeted youth to determine perceptions, behaviors, and barriers to seeking screening and treatment. Based on the initial findings, CDPH encouraged several of its funded agencies to work more closely with lesbian, gay, transsexual and bisexual adolescents and young adults to encourage HIV testing, prevention education, and esteem building.

Additionally, relevant to the startling STD incidence rates is a sustained increase in HIV and AIDS incidence among 20- to 29-year-old residents in the past decade. Since January 2004, 25% of new HIV cases and 20% of new AIDS cases are among residents aged 20–29 at the time of diagnosis. The chart below shows that more than 25% of incident AIDS cases among African Americans were in this age group. This differs substantially from 10 years ago, where slightly over 3% of incident HIV and AIDS cases in 1995–1996 were aged 20–29 at the time of diagnosis. Sixteen of 21 (76%) Black males aged 20–29 at the time of diagnosis of HIV or AIDS in 2006 reported MSM behavior, with another 4 (19%) reporting bisexual behavior. Only one male reported solely high-risk heterosexual contact as the primary route of HIV exposure. In the previous year, 64% of new HIV/AIDS cases among Black males aged 20–29 reported MSM and 18% reported bisexual behavior.

Finally, maps developed by CDPH and presented to Cuyahoga County health officials showed a diffusion of high Chlamydia and gonorrhea incidence rates beyond those municipalities directly adjacent to the eastern and southern Cleveland borders. Therefore, both by age and geography, the possibility of undetected cases of HIV and STDs in adolescent and young adults throughout the entire county has never been greater.

High rates of unsafe sexual activity, high birth rates to teens, and a potential for HIV to spread among middle and high school students amidst the endemic transmission of Chlamydia and gonorrhea among teens led CDPH Director Matt Carroll and Mayor Frank G. Jackson, in 2006, to take the progressive action of establishing a new sexual health curriculum for the Cleveland Municipal School District (CMSD), one that built off of a 2002 plan to deliver a comprehensive health plan (City of Cleveland, 2006; Cleveland Municipal School District, 2006). Waves of layoffs of Cleveland school teachers, guidance counselors, nurses, social workers, and physical education staff have curtailed many supplemental programs including personal health education (Catalyst Cleveland, 2006; Okoben & Reed, 2005).

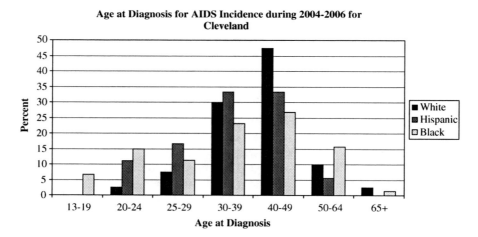

Age at Diagnosis for AIDS Incidence during 2004-2006 for Cleveland

Fig 8.2 Age Distribution (Percent) of White, Non-Hispanic, Black/African American-Non-Hispanic and Hispanic Persons from Cleveland at Time of Initial AIDS Diagnosis. Cases reported in 2004, 2005, and 2006. (Cleveland Department of Public Health, 2007).

The new comprehensive sexual health curriculum was jointly developed by city and county health agencies alongside CMSD. Cuyahoga County Health Commissioner Terry Allan secured critical TANF funding from county commissioners to support development and implementation of the curriculum. Messages are age/grade appropriate. When fully completed, the curriculum will extend from grades K through 12. (For example, personal cleanliness and appropriate touching would be applied in K–6 school levels.) Abstinence plus comprehensive health education is stressed, with materials that include information about condom use and contraceptives. Parents can opt out, removing their children from the curriculum. Prevention information is based on CDC, National Institutes of Health and Ohio Department of Health information. All 7th, 8th, 11th, and 12th grade students were the first to receive the curriculum in 2006. Other grades are being included with each year.

A presentation of this curriculum by curriculum leaders from CDPH and CMSD at the Ohio Health Coalition meeting in Columbus, Ohio in April 2007 drew a near-capacity attendance (in the largest conference room at the meeting.) Representatives of other major municipal school systems in Ohio and at least six other states have contacted the CDPH HIV Prevention Unit office, whose office at CDPH leads the initiative, for additional information. According to David Merriman, Project Coordinator of the CDPH HIV Prevention Unit, most parents with whom he has spoken and those contacting curriculum instructors have expressed their encouragement and support for the initiative. Very few parents have opted out and removed their children from the program.

HIV/AIDS in Cleveland

On a larger scale, the HIV/AIDS epidemic is a mature chronic disease in that HIV appeared in Cuyahoga County early in the 1980s with racial and exposure distributions that were similar to many major East Coast cities that have a large African American presence. Based on CDPH HIV data, 90% of HIV/AIDS cases reported in the early 1980s in Cleveland were male and mostly White non-Hispanic. By 1986, Hispanic and African American males accounted for 53% of the reported cases, although the combined population of Hispanics and African Americans represented 51% of the Cleveland population in 1990 (United States Bureau of the Census, 1990). Of these, 50% of the men reported having sex with men (MSM), 16.5% self-identified as bisexual, and 20% reported having engaged in injection drug use (IDU). Only 4% reported high-risk heterosexual contact as the primary route of HIV transmission. The mean age among males was 32 years at the time of diagnosis. However, these data from the 1980s and 1990s may be confounded by secular changes related to HIV and AIDS surveillance, treatment, counseling, and disease definition (Centers for Disease Control, 1992).

No longer could HIV/AIDS in Cleveland be called "a gay white man's disease" (Greeley, 1995; Mundell, 2007). Since 1997, African Americans have accounted for a near constant 60–65% of incident HIV and AIDS reports. African American males have represented from 40 to 48% of incident HIV and AIDS cases annually since 1997, while African American females represented 11–24% of incident cases, exceeding 20% in 1998 and 2003. For 2006, more than three-quarters (76.1%) of the 161 incident HIV (non-AIDS) and AIDS cases in Cleveland in 2006 were male. Sixty-five percent were African American non-Hispanic, 18.0% White non-Hispanic, and 6.8% Hispanic.

Since 2004, a greater proportion of younger (13–29) and older (50–64) adult African Americans are appearing as incident HIV and AIDS cases. Most cases are males. (See previous figure.) The increase has been slow but steady in percentage and absolute numbers. Most of the older men have reported high-risk heterosexual behavior, with some MSM and lesser IDU activity. None reported bisexuality in 2006 incidence reports. Whether this increase is due to more screening, awareness of STDs, availability of drugs for erectile dysfunction or random chance, more time and investigation are needed to determine if the trend continues.

Transmission reported by IDU was and still is highest among Hispanic persons; however, nearly 25% of all HIV/AIDS cases during the first two decades of the epidemic. HIV exposure through IDU was reported to be as high as 61% of incident HIV/AIDS Hispanic cases. By the end of 2006, only 11% of prevalent cases were attributable to IDU, and IDU use is currently reported in only 20% of Hispanic males with HIV/AIDS. Any history of IDU was reported by 12% of those African Americans currently living with HIV (CDPH, 2007) but was reported in as many as a quarter of annual incident cases two decades ago, mostly among older males. No IDU has been reported in the past 5 years among incident HIV and AIDS cases among African American adolescents and young adults aged 15–29.

Surveillance

Reporting of new cases has significantly improved since the early 1990s. Because diagnoses of new HIV seroconversion, CD4 levels, and AIDS diagnoses are reported to the CDPH through passive surveillance, greater efforts were established by 1985 by Dr. John Neill at CDPH to begin tracking suspected cases. A refinement of AIDS diagnosis in 1992 for 1993 surveillance changed the landscape of surveillance, allowing for a clearer case definition and encouraging more states to establish surveillance (Centers for Disease Control and Prevention, 1992). Reporting of these HIV and AIDS diagnoses is mandated by law (Ohio Department of Health, 2005). Viral loads are also often reported by primary care medical centers and laboratories; this marker is often tested alongside CD4 lymphocyte counts, the sentinel marker for progression to AIDS. The viral load is just one biomarker useful in monitoring compliance with highly active antiretroviral therapy (HAART) (Kojima et al., 1993; Levine, 1988; Little et al., 1999). Some active surveillance is performed by the Office of Biostatistics at CDPH. On request, CDPH has received completed audits of all HIV-positive patients who have been treated at specific clinics in Cleveland. Data base records are updated and reconciled and new information on patients is shared among HIV state and federal surveillance offices of the Ohio Department of Health and the CDC.

Reporting from local medical centers, clinics, and laboratories has been reliable and prompt. Since 2000, an average of 19% of incident cases reported to CDPH lack risk factor information. For reports on males, the average is 21%. This is significantly fewer missing data than occurs at the national level, where more than one-third of all reports to the CDC lack risk factor information (Centers for Disease Control and Prevention, 2006). Because there are under 200 incident diagnoses of HIV and AIDS annually for Cleveland (and under 300 for Cuyahoga County), having complete information is key to provide accurate surveillance and valid estimates.

Obtaining prevalence rates through passive surveillance presents many challenges. Rates may be biased positively (overestimated) due to the lack of information relating to migration, changes in addresses, and death. Deaths are difficult to track and access to official death records from the Ohio Department of Health (ODH) lags by approximately 2 years. Although the Vital Statistics Office of ODH rigorously processes and reconciles death certificates with other state and national offices, the process is resource-intensive. By February 2007, CDPH had received only the official 2003 death records in electronic format. Receipt of the 2004 death records is anticipated shortly, but this delay in reconciling deaths among HIV/AIDS patients hampers accurate adjustment and confers a positive bias. The overall negative bias in rates occurs from underreporting and lack of testing among persons at high risk of acquiring HIV.

Biases due to lack of reporting information has been greatly reduced through the efforts of the Disease Intervention Specialists (DIS). DIS agents receive reports from CDPH and directly from several health and testing agencies. DIS agents contact individuals with incident HIV and AIDS diagnoses to encourage partner notification, provide educational and supportive messages, and assist in referral to appropriate services. The skilled, compassionate, and well-trained agents are at the frontline of initiating care and networks for newly diagnosed persons. They are directly involved in counseling and cases tested at the CDPH health centers and encourage those who were tested anonymously to be retested confidentially. Only those testing positive through confidential testing (providing name, address, and other personal health identifiers) are eligible to receive support from state and federal services. Such diligence in contacting newly diagnosed HIV-positive persons and notifying partners vastly improves surveillance reporting for cases of HIV/AIDS among African Americans and Hispanics. Most homeless in Cleveland are African American, and obtaining stable addresses and residence information is difficult. Many have a long history of potential exposure to HIV, and recall bias is inevitable. Distrust of medical and government officials exists. In addition, among Hispanics, a language barrier may hamper the delivery of service, contact, or education. Successful enumeration and description of cases leads to more accurate surveillance that can ultimately lead to more funding for prevention and care.

Those infected with HIV in both African American and Hispanic communities battle stigmatization at home, in the church, and in receiving medical care. Fortunately in Cleveland, federal aid is widely available through Ryan White Acts and other entitlements for services, medical care, and housing. Agencies such as the Free Clinic of Greater Cleveland have become national models for the provision of free or reduced-price care to the community. More agencies have been hiring and training bilingual case workers and staff. Their efforts to care for and refer HIV-positive patients to some of the many services in Cleveland have led to the common knowledge among the national gay community that Cleveland is one of many resource-rich cities for people suffering with HIV/AIDS in the nation.

Surveillance data culled and analyzed to produce quarterly and annual reports and to monitor potential trends among groups at risk. Statistical analyses and mapping of incident cases of HIV and AIDS are analyzed for trends among new cases, while monitoring of prevalent cases provides ample evidence of the potential burden of existing cases on social, governmental, and medical systems. Age is a major factor, as younger persons contract HIV through unsafe behavior, compounded by the lack of experience to the high mortality rate of AIDS prior to combination therapy. Maps of incident cases are developed through specialized mapping software (e.g., ArcGIS, ESRI International, Inc.). These maps provide the Unit with critical information where outreach may be needed. Together, behavior patterns, location, and age are the primary determinants for groups at risk.

The CDPH HIV Prevention Unit is responsible in Cuyahoga County for disbursing approximately $2.1 million dollars annually in federal and state aid earmarked for HIV/AIDS-related services, prevention education, and screening. The Unit uses guidance from the CDC that directs funding to be based on behavior groups rather than on racial or ethnic groups. Agencies are invited to submit proposals in response to a formal request for proposal (RFP) announcement. CDPH receives over 30 proposals for Community Development Black Grant and housing for people with AIDS funding. Every 3 years, this number nearly doubles in response to the federal HIV funding cycle. The proposals submitted by individual agencies are graded based on merit, efficacy of behavior-based intervention, appropriateness of target population served, outcomes evaluation, and measurement of those served through some form of formal project evaluation. This has been a difficult task for many agencies since they often do not have staff with formal training in project evaluation. Some do not have adequate computing resources. Proposal grading is provided by a select group of representatives from academia, medical and service agencies, governmental officials, and prevention specialists. Experts are chosen from these fields having multiple skill sets. These experts must lack a fiduciary or underlying association with the applicants, or recuse themselves from grading proposals where a conflict of interest may arise. Numeric grades are generated, ranked, and proposals reevaluated against the principal aims of the aims delineated in the RFP guidelines.

This process has been streamlined through the use of an internal evaluation process. For several years, the Unit has hired an academician expert in evaluation to review the funded agencies for the breadth and scope of their efforts. An outcome evaluation was included in the most recent report (Smith, 2007). Agencies are asked to provide comments of their experience to improve future performance. CDPH HIV Prevention Unit uses these evaluations to recalibrate its RFP process, provide feedback to the agencies, and inform local and state officials.

Agencies that recently applied for funding were encouraged to address specific groups not formally reached and to study evidence-based methods for effective interventions (Center on AIDS & Community Health, 2007). For example, those groups reaching youth can access non-traditional venues (e.g., hip-hop events, clubs, recreation centers, barbershops, beauty salons, jails, and shelters) where younger persons and those at the margins of society may congregate. To youth, context is as important as message and those agencies effective in reaching these groups have greater success in diffusing complex prevention messages into straight talk. For the 2007–2008 CDPH funding cycle, more than $250,000, some 14% of the annual federal funding, will go to interventions that target youth as their primary or secondary populations. All six programs funded will reach minority youth.

Nearly 8% of disbursed funding will go to four interventions that target African American females as a primary or secondary population. This population is the target of a CDC social marketing campaign launched in October 2006 in Cleveland and Philadelphia. "Take Charge, Take the Test" targets African American females aged 15–34 in Cleveland and surrounding suburbs to seek routine and regular HIV testing, reduce stigma, encourage partners to be screened, and avoid risk behaviors. Abstinence is encouraged, and methods of protection from STD and HIV infection are similarly recommended. Handbills, posters, billboard, transit advertising, and radio spots blanketed a large portion of zip code areas in Cuyahoga County as a test demonstration. The CDPH Office of Biostatistics is working directly with the CDC and Research Triangle Institute, Inc (RTI, Inc., Triangle Park, NC) to evaluate the efficacy of the messages based on testing patterns and calls to a toll-free HIV hotline advertised in campaign material. Preliminary results of this pilot project were favorable. Increases in HIV testing were registered at the two CDPH health clinics and the Free Clinic of Greater Cleveland.

Conclusions

Local health departments (LHDs) in other cities are encouraged to consider several avenues to expand surveillance. Since most state-level agencies only report overall counts or rates for STDs and HIV/AIDS at the county or major city level, trends in incidence among target populations can easily be missed. Lack of incidence and subgroup analysis is detrimental to funding organizations, LHDs, and citizens.

For example, CDPH requested STD data from the Ohio Department of Health in late 2004 and 2006 to analyze underlying trends among teens and young adults. Reported incident rates for Chlamydia infections in Cleveland peaked in 2002–2003 at 1,081 per 100,000 only to drop 4.8% for 2004–2005. Regrettably, infection rates for African American males aged 15–19 and 20–24 increased by 26.5% and 76.9%, respectively. Without secondary analysis, these opposing trends among groups at highest risk would not have been uncovered. Therefore, LHDs should consider acquiring assistance in quantitatively and qualitatively examining surveillance data obtained from their state STD and HIV/AIDS surveillance units.

LHDs lacking staff who are trained in data analysis can partner with local academic centers to extend resources, leverage experience and knowledge, and expand surveillance activities (Covich, Parker, & White, 2005; Livingood, Goldhagen, Little, Gornto, & Hou, 2007). Academic experts from schools of public health (epidemiology and biostatistics) programs, medical education, sociological, psychological, and anthropological programs are ideal partners. Research, student internship, and potential job placement opportunities often arise from these partnerships. LHDs can vet student interns as potential hiring candidates, while academics can widen their research base and community service.

Many successful synergies have been applied to interventions with urban African American communities (Levine et al., 2003; VanDevanter, et al., 2002). Once a joint plan has been developed, a letter of proposal, memorandum of understanding, data sharing agreements, and possibly contracts for consulting can be used to formalize and make operational the partnership. Privacy rules concerning the use of public health information should be reviewed between agencies to ensure that all participants are aware of privacy and confidentiality concerns (Thacker, 2003). Due to the sensitive nature of STD and HIV surveillance data, state health departments may be deeply involved in the arrangement depending on the proposed activities.

One major issue is the final reporting of the results, whether those results will be part of an internal process to improve the activities and public service within the public health agencies or if reporting will be peer reviewed and reported as research. This issue of the definition of research is contentious, as the interpretation of the Common Rule of research when applied to public health activities relying on iterations to inform quality improvement or provide feedback is not always clear (Bromley, 1991; Code of Federal Regulations, 2005; Doezema & Hauswald, 2002; Lynn, 2004). Since surveillance data is collected as part of a legal and social contract to prevent and control the spread and impact of disease through surveillance and other relevant activities, data are collected on the public without direct consent. Consent is implied as part of this social compact and analysis and public reporting of surveillance is to be routinely performed as a business activity of the public health agency (United States Department of Health and Human Services, 2005a). If the academic/LHD relationship involves the potential for direct contact with the public (e.g., surveys, interviewing, focus groups, etc.) often with the intent to publish the findings as research, then involvement with an Institutional Review Board (IRB) or Human Rights Board may be necessary or recommended by university or state statues and officials, respectively. If the involvement does not span into research but remains in the realm of the mandates, process, or service improvement as a routine internal activity of the public health agency, IRB involvement may not be necessary (United States Department of Health and Human Services, 2005b).

Therefore, LHDs and their academic contacts should document their shared objectives with care and foresight. Established partnerships may be leveraged beyond surveillance, reporting, internal process improvement, and research. Partnerships are ideal candidates for federal funding for collaborative interventions requiring analysis of outcomes related to proposal aims and objectives.

Second, LHDs should consider analysis of surveillance data using some form of geographic information system that generate maps or spatial presentation. Maps can display patterns hidden in mere tables and charts. Maps may be used internally to provide exact location of cases, or be generalized to the census tract or neighborhood to provide a greater measure of confidentiality. In our experience, maps using the residence location of incident cases were highly useful to target areas where interventions may be critically needed. These maps provided greater equity and determination for funding recommendations in the CDPH RFP process.

Most LHD officials can generate basic epidemiological measures from initial data exploration, and most surveillance analysis can be performed without a background in advanced statistics. However, a background in epidemiological measures is recommended for those performing data analysis. Widely available programs such as Microsoft Excel (Microsoft Corporation, Bellvue, WA) can be used to sort and identify cases, generate counts of groups (e.g., by area) and subgroups (e.g., by age, race/ethnicity). Many websites exist that walk users of Excel through the steps and pitfalls in using Excel as a primary analysis tool (Last, 2007; University of Kansas, 2003). The number of new cases occurring annually (as a numerator) along with appropriate census data (denominator) can provide annual incidence rates (Gordis, 2004). Depending on the time range of the data, existing cases can be used to generate point or period prevalence. Prevalence is a useful indicator of the burden of HIV and AIDS on the local medical, social, and governmental systems. Persons new to data analysis should employ epidemiologists or biostatisticians for initial guidance and validation of results. Expert users in sophisticated statistical programs such as SAS (SAS Institute, Cary, NC), SPSS (SPSS Inc., Chicago, IL), R (R Foundation for Statistical Computing, Vienna, Austria), or EpiInfo (CDC, Atlanta, GA) can more easily perform data preparation and analysis to generate categorical counts and rates.

Qualitative analyses can range from surveys and response cards to focus groups and interviews. Because of the nature of direct contact and requirement for consent, IRB involvement will be required. Skills for survey construction, data coding, appropriate discourse, and facilitation of focus group participants are advanced and well-documented. LHD staff considering use of qualitative analysis should seek expert advice as early as possible in the development stage (Miles & Huberman, 1994; Rea and Parker, 2005).

Third, community agencies should take a more open approach in seeking the advice of LHDs in determining how to best identify populations in need of outreach, testing, and service (Meyer, Armstrong-Coben, & Batista, 2005). Too often, agencies only make contact with LHDs in response to funding opportunities. Each party can quickly lose track of priorities, many of which are shared. This is especially important for those agencies involved with minority populations. A community agency can drive the need for additional surveillance of populations when no surveillance analyses may exist. In our experience, the uncovered risk for cross transmission of HIV into the youngest populations where STDs are endemic was a major catalyst for action. Focus groups with adolescents at higher risk of acquiring STDs and HIV were critical in promoting specific outreach initiatives and developing effective prevention messages (Keagy, 2006).

Lastly, it has been our experience that progress towards reducing the spread of HIV and STDs begins with the quantitative recognition of the problem and determining progressive, community-driven, and evidence-based solutions. These solutions can be achieved by any community—government, LHD, health delivery, and service organizations and community groups—dedicated to the task.

References

Bromley, D.A. (1991). Federal policy for the protection of human subjects: Notices and rules (Part II). Federal Register, *56*(118), 28001–18102.

Catalyst Cleveland. (2006). Report Card On Reform. September/October 2006. Last accessed April 22, 2007; Available at http://www.catalyst-cleveland.org/assets

Center for Adolescent Health, Case Western Reserve University (2006). 2004 Cleveland Municipal School District YRBS (Youth Risk Behavioral Survey) Report. Last accessed February 6, 2006; Available at http://www.case.edu/

Centers for Disease Control and Prevention. (1992). 1993 revised classification system for HIV infection and expanded surveillance case definition for AIDS among adolescents and adults. *Morbidity and Mortality Weekly Report, Recommendations and Reports*, 41(RR-17). Last accessed February 4, 2007; Available at http://www.cdc.gov/mmwr/preview/mmwrhtml/00018871.htm

Centers for Disease Control and Prevention (CDC) (1996). Ten leading nationally notifiable infectious diseases—United States, 1995. *Morbidity and Mortality Weekly Report*, 45, 883–884.

Centers for Disease Control and Prevention (2001). *HIV Prevention Strategic Plan Through 2005*. Last revised January 2001; Last accessed April 18, 2007; Available at CDC National Prevention Information Network website, http://www.cdcnpin.org/scripts/hiv/connect.asp

Centers for Disease Control and Prevention (2002). Unrecognized HIV infection, risk behaviors, and perceptions of risk among young black men who have sex with men, six U.S. cities, 1994–1998. *Morbidity & Mortality Weekly Report*, *51*, 733–736.

Centers for Disease Control and Prevention (2006). AIDS cases, by geographic area of residence and metropolitan statistical area of residence, 2004. *HIV/AIDS Surveillance Supplemental Report*, *12*(2), 11, 16 (Tables 3b, 4b). Available at http://www.cdc.gov/hiv/topics/surveillance/resources/reports

Center on AIDS & Community Health (2007). DEBI, diffusion of effective behavioral interventions. Last accessed April 25, 2007. Available at http://www. effectiveinterventions.org/

City of Cleveland Office of the Mayor (2006). Mayor Jackson, CMSD and County announce Responsible Sexual Behavior program, present sample lesson as part of Comprehensive Health Plan. Last revised October 23, 2006; Last accessed February 24, 2007; Available at http://www.city.cleveland.oh.us/pdf/ press/2006102377.pdf

Cleveland Department of Public Health (CDPH) (2006). Findings among Cleveland residents living with HIV/AIDS: Provisional results for cases reported through December 31, 2005. Last updated June 15, 2006; Last accessed April 24, 2007;Available at http://www.clevelandhealth.org/Assets/AcrobatFiles/HealthStatistics/

Cleveland Department of Public Health (CDPH) (2007). Cleveland (Only) HIV/AIDS prevalence report: Reported persons living with HIV/AIDS as of December 31, 2006 by selected characteristics, Cleveland resident cases, and prevalence per 100,000. Last updated March 27, 2007; Last accessed April 24, 2007. Available under Health Division, HIV/AIDS at http://www.clevelandhealth.org/

Cleveland Municipal School District, (2006). Responsible sexual behavior curriculum delivery. Last accessed February 24, 2007; Available at http://www.cmsdnet.net/students/HealthFactSheets/sexual_behavior.htm

Code of Federal Regulations. (2005). Title 45, Part 46, sections 46.101(a, b). Protection of human subjects.

Covich, J. R., Parker, C. L., & White, V. A. (2005). The practice community meets the ivory tower: A health department/academic partnership to improve public health preparedness. *Public Health Reports*, *120*(Suppl. 1), 84–90.

Cuyahoga County Board of Health (2004). Child and Family Health Services (CFHS) *Community health indicators profiles, Phase IV, Vol. 2*. Last revised September 2004; Last accessed April 21, 2007; Available at http://www.ccbh.net/ cfhs/indicator.pdf

Dann, M. (2007) State of Ohio Attorney General Inaugural Address, Jan. 8, 2007. Last accessed February 4, 2007; Available at http://www.ag.state.oh.us/press/07/01/pr070108d.asp

David, R. J. & Collins, J. W. (1997). Differing birth weight among infants of U.S.-born Blacks, African-Born Blacks, and U.S.-Born Whites. *New England Journal of Medicine*, *337(17)*, 1209–1214.

Dillman, J. D., Pleasants, C. B., Roskilly, A. B., & Farmby, H. K. (2006). The state of fair housing in Northeast Ohio: April 2006. Housing Research and Advocacy Center, Cleveland. Last accessed April 24, 2007; Available at http://www. thehousingcenter.org/

Doezema D, & Hauswald M. (2002). Quality improvement or research: A distinction without a difference? *Ethics & Human Research*, 24, 9–11.

Fitch, S. (2006). Home foreclosure hot spots. *Forbes Magazine Online*. Last updated June 1, 2006; Available at http://www.msnbc.msn.com/id/13086712/

Fleming, D. T. & Wasserheit, J. N. (1999). From epidemiological synergy to public health policy and practice: The contribution of other sexually transmitted diseases to sexual transmission of HIV infection. *Sexually Transmitted Infections, 75*, 3–17.

Goldenberg, R. L. & Culhane, J. F. (2007) Low birth weight in the United States. *American Journal of Clinical Nutrition, 85*(suppl.), 584S–590S.

Gordis, L. (2004). *Epidemiology*, 3rd edition. W.B. Saunders Co.

Greeley, A. (1995) Concern about AIDS in minority communities. *FDA Consumer Magazine* Last accessed April 21, 2007; Available at http://www.fda.gov/fdac/features/095_aids.html

Halfors, D. D., Iritani, B. J., Miller, W. C., & Bauer, D. J. (2007). Sexual and drug behavior patterns and HIV and STD racial disparities: The need for new directions. *American Journal of Public Health, 97(1)*, 125–132.

The Housing Research and Advocacy Center. (2003). Analysis of lending patterns in the City of Cleveland. Last accessed January 6, 2007; Available at http://www.thehousingcenter.org/

Keagy, J. (2006). Cleveland youth RARE project & social marketing campaign for HIV, STD, and teen pregnancy reduction. Cleveland Department of Public Health, Cleveland, Ohio. Last revised September 2006. Last accessed May 19, 2007. Available at http://www.clevelandhealth.org/Assets/AcrobatFiles/RareProject Reports/YouthRAREReport.pdf

Kojima, E., Shirasaka, T., Anderson, B., Chokekijchai, S., Sei, S., & Yarchoan, R., et al. (1993). Monitoring the activity of antiviral therapy for HIV infection using a polymerase chain reaction method coupled with reverse transcription. *AIDS, 7*(suppl 2), S101–S105.

Laumann, E. O. & Youn, Y. (1999). Racial/ethnic group differences in the prevalence of sexually transmitted diseases in the United States. *Sexually Transmitted Diseases, 29*, 13–19.

Last, D. (2007). Audience Dialogue: Using Excel for survey analysis (1). Last accessed May 19, 2007. Available at http://www.audiencedialogue.org/excel1.html

Lenahan, T. (2005). Shortage areas of primary medical professionals. *Public Health GIS and Information, 63*, 19–21. Last accessed April 21, 2007; Available at http://www.cdc.gov/nchs/data/gis/cdcgis63.pdf

Levine, A. (1998). Antiretroviral therapy: Adherence. *Medscape HIV/AIDS eJournal*: 4(2). Last accessed April 21, 2007; Available at http://www.medscape.com/viewarticle/408212

Levine, D. M., Bone, L. R., Hill, M. N., Stallings, R., Gelber, A. C., & Barker, A., et al. (2003). The effectiveness of a community/academic health center partnership in decreasing the level of blood pressure in an urban African-American population. *Ethnicity & Disease, 13*(3), 354–61.

Little, S. J., McLean, A. R., Spina, C. A., Richman, D. D., & Havlir, D. V.(1999). Viral dynamics of acute HIV-1 infection. *Journal of Experimental Medicine, 190*, 841–850.

Livingood, W. C., Goldhagen, J., Little, W. L., Gornto, J., & Hou, T. (2007). Assessing the status of partnerships between academic institutions and public health agencies. *American Journal of Public Health, 97*(4), 659–666.

Lynn J. (2004). When does quality improvement count as research? Human subject protection and theories of knowledge. *Quality and Safety in Health Care, 13*, 67–70.

Miles, M.B & Huberman, A. M. (1994). *Qualitative data analysis*, 2nd rev. ed. Thousand Oaks, California: Sage.

MacKellar, D. A., Valleroy, L. A., Secura, G. M., Bel, S., & Bingham, T., et al. (2005). Unrecognized HIV infection, risk behaviors, and perceptions of risk among young men who have sex with men: opportunities for advancing HIV prevention in the third decade of HIV/AIDS. *Journal of Acquired Immune Deficiency Syndrome, 15*, 603–14.

Meyer, D., Armstrong-Coben, A., & Batista, M. (2005). How a community-based organization and an academic health center are creating an effective partnership for training and service. *Academic Medicine, 80*(4), 327–333.

Mundell, E. J. (2007). Advances, failures mark AIDS' first 25 years. Last revised June 5, 2007; Last accessed April 25, 2007; Available at http://www.drkoop.com/newsdetail/93/533060_2.html

Ohio Department of Health (2005). Ohio Administrative Code and Ohio Revised Code, Content applicable to communicable disease, Sections 3701—3–02 and 3701-3-13. Last revised April 2005; Last Accessed February 4, 2007; Available at http://www.odh.ohio. gov/pdf/IDCM/sect2a.pdf

Ohio Department of Health (2007). Data information warehouse. Last updated March 1, 2007; Last accessed April 24, 2007; Available at http://dwhouse.odh.ohio.gov/ datawarehousev2.htm

Ohio Historical Society (2005). *Reed v. Rhodes,* Ohio history central: An online encyclopedia of Ohio history. Last accessed at January 7, 2007; Available at http://www.ohiohistory.org

Okoben J. & Reed, E. (2005). Nearly 500 teachers will be cut-Cleveland schools to send pink slips next week in first wave of layoffs .*Cleveland Plain Dealer*, April 23. Last accessed April 22, 2007; Available at http://www.cleveland.com/clevelandschools/ index.ssf?/clevelandschools/more/1114248889275150.html

Rea, L. M. & Parker, R. A. (2005). *Designing and conducting survey research: A comprehensive guide*, 3rd ed. Jossey-Bass, San Francisco, CA.

Reed v. Rhodes, 422 F. Supp. 708, 793 (N. D. Ohio 1976), *remanded per curiam*, 559 F.2d 1220 (6th Cir. 1978), *supplemental opinion on remand*, 455 F. Supp. 569 (N. D. Ohio 1978), *aff'd in relevant part and remanded on other grounds*, 607 F.2d 714 (6th Cir. 1979), *cert. denied*, 455 U.S. 935 (1980).

Salling, M. (2006). Children living in severely distressed neighborhoods and poor housing. *Public Health GIS and Information*. (68), 19–22. Last accessed April 21, 2007; Available at http://www.cdc.gov/nchs/data/gis/cdcgis68.pdf

Smith, R. L. & Davis, D. (2004). Cleveland No.1 in big-city poverty/Nearly half of children among the poor. *Cleveland Plain Dealer*. Last updated August 27, 2004; Last accessed April 24, 2007; Available at http://www.cleveland.com (archived) and UrbanOhio.com archives, http://www.urbanohio.com/forum2/index.php?topic = 978.0

Smith, M. K. (2007). Evaluation report of the HIV/AIDS Prevention Initiative and the HOPWA program 2005–2006, City of Cleveland (Year VII). Cleveland, OH: Cleveland State University.

Thacker, S. B. (2003). HIPAA privacy rule and public health. Guidance from the CDC and the U.S. Department of Health & Human Services. *MMWR*, 52, 1–12. Last revised 4/11/ 2003. Last accessed May 25, 2007. Available at http://www.cdc.gov/mmwr/preview/ mmwrhtml/m2e411a1.htm

United States Bureau of the Census. 1990 decennial census for Cleveland, Ohio. Last accessed December 29, 2007; Available at http://factfinder.census.gov

United States Bureau of the Census. 2000 census of population, general population charac-teristics, Cleveland, Ohio, Summary File (SF1). Available at http://factfinder.census.gov

United States Bureau of the Census. 2005 American community survey, general population characteristics, Cleveland, Ohio. Available at http://factfinder. census.gov

United States Bureau of the Census (2005a). 2005 Population Estimates, Population Estimates Program, Table T1. Available at http://factfinder.census.gov

United States Department of Housing and Urban Development (2004). Bush Administration awards $17.6 million in fair housing grants to continue fight against housing bias. News release HUD No. 04-0001OH. January 12, 2004. Last accessed May 19, 2007. Available at http://www.hud.gov/local/oh/news/2004-01-12.cfm

United States Department of Health & Human Services (2005a). Office for Human Research Protections. Secretary's Advisory Committee on Human Research Protections (SACHRP) Appendix 1. Last revised February 59, 2005. Last accessed May 19, 2007. Available at http://www.hhs.gov/ohrp/sachrp/appendixi.html

United States Department of Health & Human Services (2005b). Office for Human Research Protections. Code of Federal Regulations, Title 45 Public Welfare, Part 46 Protection of Human Subjects. Last revised June 23, 2005. Last accessed May 19, 2007. Available at http://www.hhs.gov/ohrp/humansubjects/guidance/45cfr46.htm

University of Kansas, Academic Computing Center (2003). Functions & data analysis tools. Last revised Feb. 14, 2003. Last accessed May 19, 2007. Available at http://www.techdocs. ku.edu/docs/excel_2000_functions.pdf

Valleroy, L. A., MacKellar, D. A., Karon, J. M., Rosen, D. H., McFarland, W., & Shehan, D. A., et al. (2000). HIV prevalence and associated risks in young men who have sex with men. Young Men's Survey Study Group. *Journal of the American Medical Association, 284,* 198–204.

VanDevanter, N., Hennessy, M., Howard, J. M., Bleakley, A., Peake, M., & Millet, S., et al. (2002). Developing a collaborative community, academic, health department partnership for STD prevention: the Gonorrhea Community Action Project in Harlem. *Journal of Public Health Management and Practice, 8*(6), 62–68.

Wasserheit, J. N. (1992). Epidemiologic synergy: Interrelationships between human immunodeficiency virus infection and other sexually transmitted diseases. *Sexually Transmitted Diseases, 9,* 61–77.

Webster, Jr., B. H. & Bishaw, A. (2006). American community survey reports, ACS-02, income, earnings, and poverty data from the 2005 American Community Survey. Washington, DC: United States Bureau of the Census. Last revised August 2006; Last accessed January 6, 2007; Available at http://www.census.gov/prod/2006pubs/acs-02.pdf

West, K., Robinson, J. G. & Knavery, A. (1998). What do we know about the undercount of children?, Presentation at the Annual Meeting of the Southern Demographic Association, Annapolis, Maryland, October 29–31.

Part VI
HIV, Multiple Minority Status, and Stigma

Chapter Nine
Why Tell? Serostatus Disclosure and HIV Stigma among HIV Seropositive Asians and Pacific Islander Men who have Sex with Men in New York City

Ezer Kang and Bruce D. Rapkin

Introduction

Many persons living with HIV wrestle with the dilemma of whether or not to disclose their serostatus. The benefits of being supported by a network of confidants are weighed against the risks of being rejected and ostracized by family and peers. As such, many persons living with HIV/AIDS continually struggle to fulfill competing needs to share information about their illness and to preserve privacy or maintain control over who, what, and when to disclose their serostatus (Derlega, Lovejoy, & Winstead, 1998). The timing of selective serostatus disclosure can be influenced by disease progression (Mansergh, Marks & Simoni, 1995), length of HIV diagnosis (Emlet, 2006), cultural norms (Simoni et al., 1995; Mason, Marks, Simoni, Ruiz, & Richardson, 1995), relational commitment (Perry et al., 1994), and the number of sexual partners (Marks, et al., 1992).

Decisions regarding serostatus disclosure pose a unique challenge for Asian and Pacific Islander (A&PI) men who have sex with men (MSM) largely because of cultural proscriptions against homosexuality and HIV. Lye Chng, Wong, Park, Edberg, & Lai, (2003) highlighted how prescribed social scripts and roles influence relationships and social exchanges among A&PI MSM. Consideration of how personal decisions reflect upon one's family reputation and the value of passing on the family lineage are two notable social scripts that complicate intentional disclosure of HIV or sexual identity among A&PI MSM.

This chapter focuses on our findings from a cross-sectional study initiated to further our understanding of the relationship between five dimensions of HIV stigma and factors related to decisions about serostatus disclosure among HIV-seropositive A&PIs receiving services at community organizations in New York City (NYC). It is important to note that although the aggregate term "A&PI" is referenced in this study, the authors acknowledge significant

Ezer Kang
Columbia-Presbyterian Center of New York Presbyterian Hospital; Harlem Hospital Center, New York State Psychiatric Institute, New York, NY

S. Loue (ed.), *Health Issues Confronting Minority Men Who Have Sex with Men.*   197
© Springer 2008

differences in cultural traditions and values, language, dialects, migration history, and acculturation among A&PIs. As such, the implications of findings from this study are limited to specific groups represented in the sample and may not necessarily apply to all APIs.

A&PI MSM and HIV: Epidemiological Profile

In the United States, 7,317 cumulative adult AIDS cases were reported among A&PIs through 2004 (CDC, 2005). In NYC, a cumulative of 1,088 (0.8 %) adult cases of AIDS was reported among A&PIs through December 2004 (NYCMH, 2006). The majority of A&PIs newly diagnosed with HIV in 2004 were foreign-born, with Asia accounting for 69% of new diagnoses among foreign-born (NYCDOH, 2006). HIV continues to spread nationally and locally at alarmingly high rates among MSM of color. In the USA, 72% ($n = 2,445$) of estimated A&PI males living with AIDS in 2004 were among MSM, compared with 52% among Hispanic, 57% among American Indian/Alaska Native, and 44% among Blacks (CDC, 2006). In NYC, MSM accounted for 80% of new HIV diagnosis among A&PI males. Although the rate of AIDS among A&PIs (4.0 per 100,000 population) was low compared with other racial/ethnic groups in the USA, the estimated number of HIV/AIDS cases has increased among A&PIs between 2000 and 2003 at rates comparable with Whites and Hispanics, and far faster than African Americans, American Indians, and Alaska Natives.

Despite low HIV/AIDS incidence rates among A&PIs in the USA, numerous studies have highlighted specific trends that warrant concern including higher rate of HIV risk behavior and depressive symptoms among A&PI MSM compared with other racial/ethnic groups (MacFarland, Chen, Weide, Kohn, & Klauser, 2004; Yoshikawa, Wilson, Chae, & Cheng, 2004), lower rates of HIV testing (Wong, Campsmith, Nakamura, Crepaz, & Begley, 2004), perceived invulnerability to a HIV infection (Choi et al., 1995), delay in accessing medical and supportive services (Chin, Kang, Kim, Martinez, & Eckholdt, 2006; Pounds, Conviser, Ashman, & Bourassa, 2002; Eckholdt & Chin, 1997), and difficulties adhering to their antiretroviral regimen (Kang & Rapkin, 2003).

Decision to Disclose Serostatus

Disclosure is a "strategic social behavior" that is influenced by conscious or unconscious motivation to achieve specific social goals (Omarzu, 2000). Individuals' strategic decisions to disclose can be influenced by a need to fulfill specific personal or interpersonal needs. Sheon and Crosby's (2004) qualitative study of MSM in San Francisco found that eagerness to disclose their serostatus to casual sexual partners was largely attributed to relinquishing personal responsibility for transmission and engaging in barebacking or unprotected sex. Serovich's (2001) consequences theory of HIV disclosure contends that the decision to inform others is a process of weighing the costs and benefits of disclosure. Individuals therefore disclose their serostatus if there are substantial emotional, physical, and social benefits from others knowing about their illness, and conversely conceal their serostatus when they anticipate negative social consequences. Previous studies have identified various benefits of serostatus disclosure that include receiving forms of social support and reaffirmation of self-worth (Parsons, VanOra, Missildine, Purcell, & Gomez, 2004). However, these anticipated benefits of serostatus disclosure are weighed against shifting the blame and worry of living with the illness to others and fear of discrimination (Petrak, Doyle, Smith, Skinner, & Hedge 2001). Applications of Serovich's consequence theory of HIV disclosure are largely influenced by gender, sexual identity, social and family networks, and culture. Higher rates of serostatus disclosure, for example, have been found among more acculturated Latino gay or bisexual men (Hays, Turner, & Coates, 1992; Mason et al., 1995), English-speaking Latinas (Simoni, et al., 1995), and documented Asian immigrants (Kang, Rapkin, Springer, & Kim, 2003).

Decisions to disclose one's serostatus can be motivated by a need to release internalized feelings and anxiety over living with a stigmatized illness (Holt et al., 1998). Among Asian undocumented immigrants with HIV/AIDS, for example, living a double life in order to maintain one's serostatus a secret can be physically and emotionally draining and affects how they manage and reorient their lives (Kang et al., 2003). Decisions to disclose one's serostatus can also be influenced by one's sense of duty to protect the well-being of their casual sex partners in order to reinforce protective sexual practices or to encourage partners to get tested for HIV (Gorbach et al., 2004; Serovich & Mosack, 2003). In a study of HIV-seropositive African American MSM, one's felt obligation to disclose, coupled with their fear of rejection, discouraged participants from pursuing sexual relationships (Harawa, Williams, Ramamurthhi, & Bingham 2006). Decision to conceal one's serostatus is largely influenced by a perceived fear that others will inadvertently or intentionally breach confidence and disclose their serostatus to others. In a study of 54 A&PIs living with HIV in NYC, Kang, Rapkin, Remien, Mellins, & Oh, (2005) found that fear of inadvertent serostatus disclosure by others heightened psychological distress. Reservations about serostatus disclosure area could also be heightened by a pervasive sense of self-blame for contracting the virus (Derlega, Winstead, Greene, Serovich, & Elwood, 2002). One bears the immense psychological consequences of living with HIV and construes disclosure as a means of garnering support from others—a resource they perceive as undeserving.

Numerous studies have shown that different types of relationships influence how HIV-seropositive persons weigh the costs and benefits of disclosing their diagnosis (Kalichman, DiMarco, Austin, Luke & DiFonzo, 2003). Disclosure to sex or injecting drug using partners, for example, is motivated by an intention to protect the well-being of others (Schnell et al., 1992), while one's decision to disclose to family members is largely determined by a personal need for support, or a desire to alleviate possible relational strains of concealing one's diagnosis (Simoni et al., 1995). In Zea, Reisen, Poppen, Bianchi, & Echeverry, (2005) study of 155 HIV-seropositive gay Latino men in the USA, participants' decision to disclosure their serostatus to select members of their social networks (parents, close friends, and primary sexual partners) was motivated by different factors. Emotional closeness, for example, was associated with disclosure to parents and awareness of participants' sexual activity with other men was associated with higher likelihood of disclosure to parents and friends (Zea, Reisen, Poppen, Echeverry, & Bianchi 2004).

The consequences of voluntary serostatus disclosure have been also widely considered in the literature, particularly its influences on health-related quality of life (Chandra, Deepthivarnma, & Thomas, 2003) and mental health outcomes. Although many persons with HIV understandably anticipated the negative impact of disclosing their serostatus, studies indicate surprisingly positive responses. A recent study of 76 HIV-seropositive MSM reported that participants did not report regret about disclosing their illness to family or friends (Serovich, Mason, Bautista, & Toviessi, 2006). Similarly, among a sample of acculturated A&PI gay men, disclosing their serostatus and sexual identity to family members resulted in positive outcomes (Nemoto, et al., 2003).

A&PI and HIV Stigma

Scrambler and Hopkins (1990) defined felt stigma as one's fear of being discriminated against solely on the grounds of one's perceived unacceptability or inferiority and the feeling of shame associated with having a stigmatized illness. This phenomenon was described by a number of A&PI MSM in the study who were ashamed that they contracted HIV because they felt that they "should know better." They feared being discriminated against by the mainstream A&PI community and shunned by HIV-negative MSM (A&PIs and non-A&PIs) because of their perceived unacceptability. In Courtenay-Quirk, Wolitski, Parsons, & Gomez' (2006) cross-sectional study of 205 MSM living with HIV, perceived HIV-related stigma within the gay community were associated depressive markers, maladaptive ways of coping, and serostatus disclosure to potential friends and sexual partners.

Stigma is explained to a large extent by both individual perceptions of HIV/AIDS and the attitudes confronted in one's social network and reference groups. Alonzo & Reynolds (1995: 305) noted that stigma is "intrinsically entwined with the disease course but is uniquely tied to the responses of the broader society, family, peers, strangers, health professionals, and the identity of the individual." Felt stigma is perpetuated by multiple minority status based on ethnicity, sexual identity, and immigration status. Being marginalized for one's HIV serostatus in addition to one's racial/ethnic identity and sexual orientation creates further ambiguity about whether discriminatory events occur as a result of any particular group membership. As such, gay A&PI men might encounter different forms of racism and anti-immigration and homosexual sentiment across different social milieus. In Wilson and Yoshikawa (2004) study of A & PI gay men, for example, participants reported most frequent race-based discrimination within the White gay community.

AIDS stigmatization has been recognized as one of the major impediments to timely diagnosis of HIV (Eckholdt & Chin, 1997; Wong et al., 2004), utilization of medical care (Kang et al., 2003; Pounds et al., 2002), serostatus disclosure (Chin & Kroesen, 1999; Yoshioka & Schustack, 2001), and medical treatment adherence (Kang & Rapkin, 2003) among A&PIs living with HIV/AIDS. In a precursor to the present study examining 54 HIV-seropositive A&PIs living in the USA, various dimensions of stigma related to negative self-worth and compromised quality of interpersonal relationships were associated with heightened level of psychological distress (Kang et al., 2005). A follow-up to the study found that encounters with HIV-related stigma carry long-term detrimental consequences to one's psychological well-being in two specific areas of functioning. First, A&PIs' perceived or actual rejection by others on account of one's HIV status lowered their self-esteem at follow-up even after controlling for measures of baseline self-esteem and physical symptomatology at follow-up (Kang, Rapkin, & DeAlmeida, 2006). Second, financial insecurity heightened by HIV stigma and fear of inadvertently disclosing one's serostatus contributed to A&PIs' pessimistic view of their future and sense of dread.

It is also important to consider the immediate social context and the meaning the stigmatized ascribes to it. Crocker (1999: 89), for example, argued that the consequences of stigma are not simply "internalized, stable distortions of personality that individuals carry with them." Rather, it varies as a function of collective representations, situational cues, and individual differences. A&PIs' fear of being shunned is largely shaped by firmly held views of HIV within the Asian immigrant community. Collective beliefs of casual contagion and discriminatory attitudes towards homosexuals, intravenous drug users, and undocumented immigrants shape A&PIs' experiences of their illness and trigger fears of being overtly ostracized by others.

Stigma and Serostatus Disclosure

Numerous studies have considered how HIV stigma influences serostatus disclosure (Courtenay-Quirk et al., 2006). AIDS-related stigma among A&PIs is a "persistent predicament" that is perpetuated by self-attribution and blame for acquiring HIV, and is recognized as one of the major impediments to serostatus disclosure among A&PIs living with HIV illness, due to pervasive cultural proscriptions against homosexuality and injection drug use within A&PI communities. The behavior and personal decisions that result in HIV infection often carry a stigma independent of HIV. In Chin and Kroesen's (1999) study of HIV-seropositive A&PI women, the stigma of pre-marital sex as well as HIV were carefully weighed in decisions to disclose. In a study of 605 Chinese participants in rural China, the intention to disclose one's serostatus was negatively associated with felt stigma (Liu et al, 2006).

Regardless of how the virus was acquired, participants' decision to disclose to whom and when is largely influenced by intrinsic fears of public marginalization. In Yoshioka & Schustack's (2001) qualitative study of 16 HIV-positive Asian men, it was found that serostatus disclosure is further complicated for gay men because of implicit disclosure of one's sexual orientation. Decisions to withhold or delay disclosure within the family network were largely influenced by a desire to protect them from the inherent stigma of HIV and homosexuality. In collectivistic cultures, individual decisions are framed within a broader social context, such that HIV stigma extends to one's family and community (Chin & Kroesen, 1999). Within the Chinese community, for example, stigma associated with homosexuality is perpetuated by the cultural primacy of preserving the family unit and maintaining social status, perceptions of homosexuality as immoral or abnormal, and social constructs of masculinity (Liu & Choi, 2006). Many A&PIs decide to disclose their serostatus when their health deteriorates—leaving them with an overwhelming sense of obligation to disclose their illness to family members (Yoshioka & Schustack, 2001). In contrast, underlying decisions to disclose one's serostatus to friends are often influenced by a desire to garner emotional support (Choi, Kumekawa, Dang, Kegeles, Hays, & Stall 1999).

Fear of social exclusion after disclosure may by attributed to HIV-related stigma, but also to other forms of stigma perpetuated by social biases based on gender (Anderson & Doyal, 2004; Chin & Kroesen, 1999), sexuality (Keogh, Henderson, & Dodds 2004), ethnicity (Körner, 2007), acculturation (Simoni, et al., 1995), and immigration status (Kang et al., 2003). As such, disclosure decisions are often informed by illness stigma compounded by social scripts ascribed to specific groups. In Simoni et al.'s (1995) study of disclosure patterns among HIV-seropositive Spanish-speaking Latinas, findings of low disclosure rates compared with English-speaking Latinas suggested that cultural denunciation of homosexuality based on religious beliefs heighten pre-existing HIV stigma, thereby discouraging serostatus disclosure.

Methods

Procedure

Individual 2–3-hour semi-structured interviews were conducted with a non-random convenience sample of 56 HIV-seropositive A&PIs referred by two AIDS service organizations. Eligible clients were identified and contacted by caseworkers regarding participation in the study. A written informed consent form approved by a university- and research-based institutional review board was reviewed and signed by all participants prior to each interview. Upon completion of the interview, they were reimbursed for their involvement in the study and asked for consent to be contacted for future studies. A follow-up study was funded 2 years later, during which the research team contacted participants from the baseline study ($n = 54$) regarding participation in the current study. Forty-four participants were recruited from the baseline study and 12 were new participants.

Trained bilingual, bachelor-level interviewers and the principal researcher conducted the interviews in English, Cantonese, or Mandarin. Although we recognized the tremendous diversity of racial and ethnic groups among A&PIs, it was beyond the scope of this study to translate the instrument battery into multiple A&PI languages. Interview instruments were therefore translated into Chinese because they were the largest Asian group, representing nearly half of all Asians in NYC (Scott, 2001). The interview battery was translated into written Chinese by: (1) discussing the content equivalence and sensitivity of the instruments to Chinese with bilingual colleagues; (2) translating the instruments into Chinese by one translator; (3) back-translating instruments into English by another independent translator with conceptual, rather than literal, meaning as the goal; (4) holding a meeting with the translator, back-translator, and the principal researcher, who was tri-lingual (English, Cantonese, and Mandarin), to examine and resolve differences that emerged from the back-translation (Chang, Chau, & Holroyd, 1999).

Dependent Variables

Reasons For and Against Serostatus Disclosure. The Reasons for Disclosure Questionnaire (Derlega, et al., 2002) included 21 items measuring how much specific reasons accounted for decisions to disclose or not one's HIV serostatus. A principal components analysis with varimax rotation resulted in a five-component solution that accounted for 70% of the total variance (see Appendix A). The five components included three reasons for serostatus disclosure: (1) Duty to inform (e.g., "I felt a sense of duty to tell my friend/ family member"); (2) Desire to protect others (e.g., "I didn't want my friend/ family member to have to worry about me"); and (3) Supportive relationships (e.g., "My friend/family member would be able to support me"). The two reasons for non-disclosure included (4) Negative self-concept (e.g., "I felt ashamed for being HIV-positive"); and (5) Privacy (e.g., "information regarding the diagnosis is my own private information"). Participants were asked to rate the extent to which specific reasons accounted for their decision to disclose or not disclose their HIV serostatus, using a five-point Likert scale ranging from 0 (Not at all important) to 5 (Extremely important). The internal consistencies for the subscales were derived from this study (Cronbach $\alpha = 0.63–0.87$).

Independent Variables

HIV-Related Stigma. Perception of being stigmatized was measured using a 24-item instrument, Social Impact Scale (Fife & Wright, 2000). A principal components analysis with varimax rotation resulted in a six-component solution that account for 69% of the total variance (see Appendix B). The five components included: (1) Social Rejection; (2) Financial Insecurity; (3) Secrecy; (4) Self-blame; (5) Secrecy; and (6) Negative Self-Worth. Participants were asked to rate the extent to which they agreed with experiences of being stigmatized by selecting responses scored 1 (strongly disagree) to 4 (strongly agree). Total scores ranged from 24 to 96, with a highest score indicating the strongest sense of feeling stigmatized (Cronbach $\alpha = 0.75$–0.92).

Sociodemographic Information. Sociodemographic variables included age, ethnicity, country of birth, sexual orientation, language preference, education and employment history, housing, marital status, medical insurance coverage, and immigration status.

Medical Information. Participants self-reported CD4 lymphocyte cell count, HIV/RNA viral load, date of and reason for HIV-antibody test, and HIV disclosure information.

Statistical Methods

Prior to conducting the major analyses to determine the relationship between HIV-related stigma factors and reasons for and against disclosure, we examined the bivariate relationships between sociodemographic variables and disclosure. Independent sample *t*-tests were also conducted to compare mean group differences on outcome variables between documented and undocumented participants, and homosexual and heterosexual orientations. In order to obtain an independent measure of each stigma and disclosure factor, exact-weighted scores were obtained based on the principal components solution after varimax rotation. Exact weighted scores effectively isolated variance related to major aspects of stigma onto different summary scales that were constrained to be orthogonal. The five orthogonal stigma variables summarize 69% of the total variance among 19 items, and six orthogonal disclosure variables summarized 70% of the total various among 18 items. As such, they were included in the regression analyses without concern for multicollinearity.

Hierarchical forward multiple regression analyses were performed to determine main effects of HIV-related stigma factors (Social Rejection, Financial Insecurity, Secrecy, Self-Blame, Social Isolation, and Negative Self-Worth) on reasons for or against disclosure while controlling for demographic confounding variables. Given the small sample size, six sets of forward stepwise regressions were preformed separately for each of the reasons for or against disclosure. Only those independent variables that met criteria for forward stepwise selection were retained at each step. Given the small sample size, the significance level for entry was set at $p<0.10$. Exact weighted scores were used in these regressions. Thus, all scores were created with a mean of 0, effectively "centering" variables for this multiplicative treatment. Centering of scores reduces multicollinearity effects between components included in the same regression model.

Results

Description of the Sample

The ages of the 56 participants ranged from 31 to 67 years ($M=44$ years, $SD=8.35$)—47 men, 8 women, and 1 unknown gender. The ethnic composition of the sample varied as follows: 37 were Chinese (66%), 4 were Filipino (7%), 6 were Southeast Asian (the 12% included Cambodian, Laotian, Malaysian, and Thai), 4 were Japanese (7%), and 5 were mixed-race/other (8%). The majority of participants were born in Asia or the Pacific (94%), and only 8 (14%) spoke primarily English. The most common primary language reported was Chinese, with 25% of respondents speaking primarily Mandarin and another 25% speaking primarily Cantonese. Twenty (36%) participants self-identified as homosexual, 30 (54%) as heterosexual, 2 (4%) as bisexual, and 4 (7%) declined to respond about their sexual orientation. Twenty-eight (50%) participants were single, never married, and 19 (34%) were married (58% of whom were living with their spouse).

   There were 31 (55%) legally documented immigrants or US citizens, and 25 undocumented (45%) who entered the USA illegally or overstayed their visas. The majority of participants were not born in the USA ($n=53$, 95%) but had been living in the USA for a mean of 16 years ($SD=9.75$) and completed a mean of 11 years of school in the USA and/or abroad ($SD=5.72$). The majority of the participants were unemployed ($n=23$, 41%) and lived in rental apartments ($n=43$, 77%). Many received health insurance coverage from the AIDS Drug Assistance Program (ADAP; $n=30$, 54%) and/or Medicaid ($n=26$, 46%).

   The mean length of post-HIV/AIDS diagnosis was 7 years ($SD=4.45$, range$=1$–18 years), and the majority of participants self-reported stable immune functioning with 87% reporting undetectable HIV/RNA viral load, and 95% reporting CD4 lymphocyte cell counts greater than 200 cells/mm^3.

Associations Between Stigma and Reasons For or Against Disclosure

Bivariate correlations indicated significant positive correlation between social support reasons for disclosure and demographic variables including years living in the USA ($r = 0.29$, $p<0.05$), MSM status ($r = 0.50$, $p<0.001$), and years of education completed ($r = 0.47$, $p<0.001$). Duty to protect others was positively correlated with stigma-related self-blame ($r = 0.32$, $p<0.05$). Non-disclosure due to difficulty accepting HIV serostatus was positively correlated with stigma-related Secrecy ($r = 0.32$, $p<0.05$).

Independent sample t-tests showed that A&PIs who self-identified as MSM completed more years of education, lived in the USA longer, and has been diagnosed with HIV longer that A&PIs who self-identified as heterosexual. MSM in this cohort also endorsed lower levels of stigma-related social rejection than Asians who self-identified as heterosexuals ($t(52) = -2.32$, $p<0.05$). In addition, self-identified MSM endorsed receiving support as the reason to disclose their serostatus more frequently than heterosexual participants ($t(52) = 3.86$, $p<0.001$) (see Table 9.1). Hierarchical regression analyses further indicated sexual risk practice (MSM/heterosexual), years of education, and length in the USA accounted for 32% of the variance in serostatus disclosure to receive support (Adjusted $R^2 = 0.321$, $p<0.001$). When simultaneously entered into the equation sexual risk practice ($t(52) = -2.20$, $p<0.05$) and years

Table 9.1 Means and standard deviations of predictor and outcomes variables for participants who self-identified as MSM or heterosexual

	MSM (n = 22)	Heterosexual (n = 30)
Demographic variables		
Age	44 (8.51)	42 (9.13)
Years of education completed	14 (4.96)	8 (4.84)***
Length of HIV diagnosis	9 (4.25)	6 (4.13)*
Years living in the US	22 (9.63)	11 (5.71)***
Stigma		
Social Rejection	2.26 (0.846)	2.68 (0.476)*
Financial Insecurity	2.56 (0.756)	2.72 (0.618)
Secrecy	2.63 (0.813)	2.74 (0.657)
Self-Blame	2.80 (0.722)	2.74 (0.577)
Social Isolation	2.63 (0.71)	2.60 (0.48)
Negative Self-Worth	2.56 (0.726)	2.74 (0.493)
Reasons for or against disclosure		
Reasons to disclosure		
Duty to inform	2.84 (1.02)	2.56 (0.964)
Duty to protect others	3.00 (1.06)	2.65 (0.792)
Supportive relationship	3.45 (0.816)	2.47 (1.02)***
Reasons to not disclose		
Difficulty accepting HIV serostatus	2.50 (1.32)	2.79 (1.05)
Privacy	3.44 (1.12)	3.26 (0.932)

*$p<.05$ (two-tailed); ***$p<.001$ (two-tailed)
Note: Higher scores indicate stronger indicators of illness stigma and endorsement of reasons for disclosure or non-disclosure. Four cases of non-reported sexual identity were excluded from this analysis.

of education ($t(52) = 2.08$, $p<0.05$) significantly predicted serostatus disclosure to receive support.

Hierarchical forward stepwise regression analyses were conducted to determine whether the stigma factors were independently associated with motivating factors for serostatus disclosure, controlling for MSM status and years living with HIV—both were significant variables in the bivariate analyses. As shown in Table 9.2, MSM status and length of HIV diagnosis at Steps 1 and 2, respectively, were not significantly associated with negative self-concept as reason for non-disclosure. Entry of stigma-related Secrecy at Step 3 added significantly to the regression equation (Adjusted R^2 = 0.123, with a significant R^2 Change = 0.120, $p<<0.05$). When stigma-related negative self-worth was added at Step 4, the equations remained significant (Adjusted R^2 = 0.25, with R^2 Change = 0.070, $p<<0.05$). Overall, stigma-related social isolation did not add significantly to the model. The overall model explained 21% of the variance in not disclosing due to difficulty accepting one's HIV status ($F(5,46) = 3.75$, $p<0.01$).

Table 9.2 Hierarchical forward stepwise regression predicting non-disclosure due to difficulty accepting HIV serostatus

	R^2	Adj R^2	$R^2\Delta$	β	t
Step 1	0.050	0.031			
MSM				−0.223	−1.62
	0.055	0.055	0.005		
MSM				−0.202	−1.40
Length of HIV diagnosis				−0.073	−0.502
	0.175	0.123*	0.120*		
MSM				−0.245	−1.78
Length of HIV diagnosis				0.69	0.470
HIV Stigma—Secrecy				0.373	2.65*
	0.245	0.181**	0.070*		
MSM				−0.231	−1.74
Length of HIV diagnosis				0.065	0.456
HIV Stigma—Secrecy				0.381	2.80**
HIV Stigma—Negative Self-Worth				0.265	2.09*
	0.290	0.213**	0.045		
MSM				−0.264	−2.00
Length of HIV diagnosis				0.047	0.338
HIV Stigma—Secrecy				0.370	2.77**
HIV Stigma—Negative Self-Worth				0.240	1.92
HIV Stigma—Social Isolation				0.217	1.71

*$p<0.05$; **$p<0.01$, ***$p<0.001$
Note: β, standardized regression coefficients

Discussion

The decision to intentionally conceal or disclose one's serostatus is a process of weighing the costs and benefits of revealing or maintaining one's illness a guarded secret within family and peer networks. Determination of the risks and value of disclosure can be influenced by gender, cultural identity, medical condition, or discriminatory attitudes toward persons living with HIV/AIDS (Kang et al., 2003, 2006). This cross-sectional study highlighted specific dimensions of stigma that weighed upon A&PI MSM's decision to disclose their serostatus. Specifically, HIV stigma-related secrecy was associated with non-disclosure due to difficulty accepting one's serostatus, after controlling for sexual risk behavior and length of HIV diagnosis. Moreover, MSM in this study reported less stigma-related social rejection and were more likely to disclose their serostatus based on need for social support, compared with heterosexuals in the study. Based on these findings, several considerations for clinical practice and research are noteworthy.

First, regardless of sexual risk behavior, self-identified A&PI MSM and heterosexuals both held reservations about disclosing their serostatus due to shame and difficulty accepting the reality of their illness. Perceived stigma that heightened fear of public ostracism and rejection swayed A&PIs toward concealing their HIV status. It is noteworthy that the length of HIV diagnosis did not necessarily facilitate acceptance of illness, nor did it mitigate the negative consequences of stigma. Self-imposed shame and passive denial of HIV influenced personal decisions to conceal one's serostatus, even years after learning about their diagnosis (mean length of HIV diagnosis was 7 years). Moreover, as the epidemic approaches its third decade, it is unsettling that perceived and actual HIV stigma continue to significantly influence A&PI's disclosure decisions and relationships. Studies have also suggested that MSM in the USA continue to contend with HIV stigma within gay communities in form of discriminatory attitudes, thereby creating a divide between HIV-seropositive and negative men (Collins, 1998; Courtenay-Quirk et al., 2006).

Both dimensions of HIV stigma and reasons for non-disclosure were related to internalized processes of maintaining secrecy, shame, and denial of illness. This underscores the importance of considering how multiple layers of stigma might heighten the overwhelming task of preserving one's serostatus a secret. Perceptions of marginalization and social rejection could be perpetuated by virtue of one's serostatus, risk behaviors associated with HIV transmission, undocumented immigration status, gender, or sexual orientation. A&PI MSM, for example, further contend with race-based stigma within the gay community that compounds their overall sense of marginalization—specifically perceived stereotypes of A&PIs adopting a submissive or feminized role in sexual relationships (Nemoto et al., 2003). Disentangling the multiple layers of stigmatizing attributes is crucial to informing effective policies and interventions that mitigate the effects of HIV stigma on disclosure and other quality of life outcomes (Reidpath & Chan, 2005).

Previous studies with a similar cohort of A&PIs found that felt stigma and perceived repercussions of public disclosure are shaped by both individual perceptions of HIV/AIDS and the dominant attitudes in one's community (Kang, et al., 2003, 2005). The interplay of individual and social forces that shape illness stigma underscores the importance of challenging A&PIs' misperceptions of HIV transmission and risk behaviors, and discriminatory attitudes towards homosexuality and bisexuality in order to promote greater understanding of the illness and wider acceptance of persons living with HIV.

Second, educated A&PI MSM in this study were inclined to disclose their serostatus for purposes of receiving support from others, highlighting the importance of establishing and sustaining supportive relationships, at the risk of possible rejection. Previous cross-sectional studies had found that serostatus disclosure was associated with greater quality of social support from target groups (Zea, et al., 2005; Simoni, Demas, Mason, Drossman, & Davis 2000). It is noteworthy that the source and type of support one hopes to receive as a result of serostatus disclosure are speculative from the current findings. Previous studies, however, have highlighted various support networks available to and utilized by MSM. Friendships with other gay men, for example, helped to mitigate the effects of homophobia among A&PI MSM (Wilson & Yoshikawa, 2004), and interaction with other HIV-seropositive A&PIs alleviated feelings of isolation (Chin et al., 2006).

However, perceived available social support and received social support are distinct dimensions (Schwarzer, Dunkel-Schetter & Kemeny, 1994; Derlega, Winstead, Oldfield, & Barbee, 2003). Previous studies on Asian American women with breast cancer, for example, highlighted the important distinction between wanting support and acknowledgment of need that will lead to actual solicitation of support (Wellisch et al., 1999; Kagawa-Singer & Wellisch, 1997). Josephson's (1997) study of 163 persons with HIV found that both actual and perceived social were associated with decisions to disclose serostatus. The extent to which A&PI MSM possibly underutilize available forms of support should be considered, particularly if serostatus disclosure is perceived as a relational requisite for soliciting support from others.

Although previous studies have consistently highlighted the importance of social networks and providing a venue for A&PI MSM to safely garner support, further work is needed to assist A&PI MSM solicit specific forms of support. Taylor et al., (2004), for example, highlighted Asians and Asian American's proclivity to underutilize social support for coping because of fear that imposing one's problems on others will undermine group harmony, overly burden others, resulting in critical judgment by others. Moreover, cultural scripts sway individuals to bear the responsibility of personal decisions rather than to place that burden on others. It is noteworthy that findings from this study are based on a convenience sample of HIV-seropositive A&PIs who are engaged in services at a community-based organization that provides an array of peer-oriented supportive programs. As such, the importance of social support networks may be understated or overstated, given that the sample is biased towards those receiving support.

Further studies are needed to clarify specific forms and utility of social support among A&PI MSM when considering their motives for serostatus disclosure. Although social networks can buffer against disruptive life events, the costs and benefits of social support are not equally shared across groups (Kawachi & Berkman, 2001; Smith & Rapkin, 1996). For women with low resources, for example, Belle (1987) found that participation in social networks might be more harmful than helpful because they face greater demands from their support networks. Moreover, particular A&PI groups place value on their ability to cope with problems independently and differentiate between the support received from "in-group" (e.g., family and intimate friends) and "out-group" members (e.g., service providers; Matsudaira, 2003). Some HIV-seropositive A&PIs, for example, garner mutual support from other APIs living with the illness who function as a proxy for family (Eckholdt et al., 1997), while others minimize their contact with other A&PIs in fear that suspicions of their illness will circulate within their community (Yoshikawa et al., 2001). This underscores the importance of clarifying how APIs define and utilize supportive networks and identifying specific aspects of social support that buffer against psychological distress.

Clinical interventions perhaps should move beyond helping A&PI MSM consider whether or not to disclosure their serostatus, to begin addressing issues that potentially curtail the benefits of disclosure to specific social networks. What factors possibly interfere with the process of garnering support from targets of disclosure or fulfilling a sense of relational duty and responsibility? Findings from this study suggest that perceived HIV stigma within one's personal social network (defined by sexual orientation, ethnicity, immigration status, social class, and gender) and internalized shame and non-acceptance of personal serostatus pose significant challenges for A&PI MSM and heterosexual men when considering decisions to disclosure. However, serostatus disclosure is not a static event; rather, it is a dynamic process by which A&PIs continue to wrestle with issues that rendered their initial disclosure decision difficult. It cannot be presumed that internalized denial of HIV and isolation, for example, would be immediately resolved following the disclosure event. Interventions that focus on A&PI's adjustment to post-disclosure should address how these transitory issues unravel in the context of a "new relationship." Moreover, the uncertainly of whether the potential relational benefits of disclosure may dissipate or be sustained over time warrant longitudinal studies that will clarify our understanding of the impact on disclosure mental health and quality of life indices (Zea, et al., 2004).

Study Limitations and Future Directions

This study has several limitations that could affect its generalizability and interpretation. First, this study did not specify how types of relationships influence disclosure decisions. Previous studies have consistently found that

MSM were more inclined to disclose their serostatus to friends or sexual partners than to family members (Kalichman et al., 2003; Zea et al., 2005). Given that decisions to disclose to various targets are influenced by an appraisal of potential benefits, further studies are needed to specifically examine common and distinctive reasons that inform serostatus disclosure to sex partners, friends, and family among A&PI MSM. Moreover, efforts to clarify the relational consequences of disclosure necessitate examining the content of disclosure. Omarzu (2000), for example, highlighted the importance of considering the dimensions of breadth, duration, and depth in theoretical models of self-disclosure. Given the influence of stigma on disclosure decisions, describing one's HIV diagnosis as a "chronic blood disease" rather than being "HIV-positive" to family members bear different relational consequences.

Second, findings from this study focused on illness-specific stigma without considering the different "layers" of HIV-related stigma that influence serostatus disclosure (Reidpath & Chan, 2005). Perceptions of marginalization and social rejection could be perpetuated by virtue of one's serostatus, risk behaviors associated with HIV transmission, immigration status, or sexual orientation. It is conceivable that A&PI MSM's reluctance to disclose their serostatus is largely influenced by their avoidance of revealing their sexual practices or identity, and less by fear of discrimination on the basis of their HIV illness.

Third, the findings and implications of this study cannot be generalized to the experiences of all Asians and Pacific Islanders living with HIV/AIDS in the USA. The findings are limited to a small convenience sample of HIV-seropositive APIs receiving supportive services from community-based AIDS organizations, 66% of whom were ethnic-Chinese. The majority of A&PIs in this sample were also in medically stable conditions (87% reported undetectable HIV/RNA viral load). These self-selection biases limit the generalizability of the current findings to those similarly situated individuals and may not be relevant to those who are not accessing or utilizing supportive services as well as other A&PI groups with more significant immunocompromise. Notwithstanding these limitations, findings from this study demonstrate that decision-making regarding serostatus disclosure is a complex and multifaceted process that continues to be influenced by HIV stigma—a pernicious social phenomena that perpetuates internalized secrecy, shame, and denial of illness. Efforts to mitigate the influence of stigma on A&PI MSM's disclosure decisions must recognize that HIV stigma encompasses formidable social biases based on sexual orientation, ethnicity, immigration status, and country of origin—that persists even as the epidemic approaches its third decade

Acknowledgment This research was supported by the Office of AIDS Research, National Institute of Mental Health, and the HIV Center for Clinical and Behavioral Studies at the New York State Psychiatric Institute and Columbia University (P50/P30 MH43520; Principal Investigator: Anke A. Ehrhardt, Ph.D.) The authors thank the Asian and Pacific Islander Coalition on HIV/AIDS, Inc. and Chinese American Planning Council, Inc., for supporting this study and tirelessly advocating for the needs of A&PIs.

Appendix A

Factor 1: Duty to Inform (Five Items)[a]

I didn't want to have to carry this information about me all by myself.
I felt obligated to tell my friend/family member.
This person had the right to know what is happening to me.
I felt a sense of duty to tell my friend/family member.
I wanted to make sure that my friend knew how serious this disease is.

Factor 2: Duty to Protect Others (Five Items)[b]

I felt bad about myself.
I didn't know how to start telling my friend/family member about the diagnosis.
I was concerned that my friend/family member wouldn't understand what I was going through.
I didn't want my friend/family member to worry about me.
I didn't want my friend/family member to have to make sacrifices for me.

Factor 3: Supportive Relationship (Four Items)[c]

I wanted to prepare my friend/family member for what might happen to me.
I trusted my friend/family member.
My friend would be able to provide support.
My friend would provide me with assistance.

Factor 4: Difficulty Accepting HIV serostatus (Two Items)[d]

I had difficulty accepting that I was HIV-positive.
I felt ashamed about being HIV-positive.

Factor 5: Privacy (Two Items)[e]

My friend/family member might tell other people.
Information about the diagnosis is my own private information.

Excluded Items

I didn't want to risk any health problems for my friend/family member; I wanted to see how my friend would react when I told them the information; I didn't feel my friend/family member would be supportive.

---

[a] Five items; $\alpha = 0.833$; eigenvalue $= 6.41$; percent of the variance explained $= 30.53$

[b] Five items; $\alpha = 0.838$; eigenvalue $= 3.61$; percent of the variance explained $= 17.22$

[c] Four items; $\alpha = 0.877$; eigenvalue $= 1.72$; percent of the variance explained $= 8.20$

[d] Two items; $\alpha = 0.841$; eigenvalue $= 1.65$; percent of the variance explained $= 7.85$

[e] Two items; $\alpha = 0.632$; eigenvalue $= 1.21$; percent of the variance explained $= 5.79$

Appendix B

Social Impact Scale

Factor 1: Social Rejection (Seven Items)[f]

I feel that I have been treated with less respect than usual by others.
I feel others are concerned they could "catch" my illness through contact like a handshake or eating food I make.
I feel others avoid me because of my illness.
Some family members have rejected me because of my illness.
I feel some friends have rejected me because of my illness.
I encounter embarrassing situations as a result of my illness.
Due to my illness others seem to feel awkward and tense when they are around me.

Factor 2: Financial Insecurity (Three Items)[g]

I have experienced financial hardship that has affected how I feel about myself.
My job security has been affected by my illness.
I have experienced financial hardship that has affected my relationship with others.

Factor 3: Secrecy (Three Items)[h]

I do not feel I can be open with others about my illness.
I fear someone telling others about my illness without my permission.
I feel I need to keep my illness a secret.

Factor 4: Self-Blame (Two Items)[i]

I feel others think I am to blame for my illness.
I feel I am at least partially to blame for my illness.

Factor 5: Social Isolation (Two Items)[j]

I feel lonely more often than usual.
Due to my illness, I have a sense of being unequal in my relationship with others.

Factor 6: Negative Self-Worth (Two Items)[k]

Due to my illness, I sometimes feel useless.
Changes in my appearance have affected my social relationships.

---

[f] Seven items; $\alpha = 0.923$; eigenvalue = 10.37; percent of variance explained = 43.22
[g] Three items; $\alpha = 0.866$; eigenvalue = 2.20; percent of variance explained = 9.19
[h] Three items; $\alpha = 0.869$; eigenvalue = 1.74; percent of variance explained = 7.28
[i] Two items; $\alpha = 0.768$; eigenvalue = 1.62; percent of variance explained = 6.76
[j] Two items; $\alpha = 0.757$; eigenvalue = 1.28; percent of variance explained = 5.34
[k] Two items; $\alpha = 0.774$; eigenvalue = 1.07; percent of variance explained = 4.46

Excluded Items

My employer/co-workers have discriminated against me because of my illness; Some people act as though I am less competent than usual; I feel set apart from others who are well; I have a greater need than usual for reassurance that others care about me; I feel less competent than I did before my illness.

References

Alonzo, A. A. & Reynolds, N. R. (1995). Stigma, HIV, and AIDS: An exploration and elaboration of a stigma trajectory. *Social Science and Medicine, 41*, 303–315.

Anderson, J. & Doyal, L. (2004). Women from Africa living with HIV in London: A descriptive study. *AIDS Care, 16*, 95–105.

Belle, D. (1987). Gender differences in the social moderators of stress. In R. C. Barnett, L., Biener, & G. K. Baruch (eds.). *Gender and stress* (pp. 257–277). New York: The Free Press.

Chandra, P. S., Deepthivarma, S., & Manjula, V. (2003). Disclosure of HIV infection in south India: Patterns, reasons and reactions. *AIDS Care, 15*, 207–15.

Chang, A. M., Chau, J. P., & Holroyd, E. (1999). Translation of questionnaires and issues of equivalence. *Journal of Advanced Nursing, 29*, 316.

Centers for Disease Control and Prevention. Cases of HIV infection and AIDS in the United States, by race/ethnicity, 2000–2004 (2006). *HIV/AIDS Surveillance Supplemental Report, 12*(1).

Centers for Disease Control and Prevention (2005). HIV/AIDS surveillance report, 2004. Vol. 16. US Department of Health and Human Services, Centers for Disease Control and Prevention.

Chin, J., Kang, E., Kim, H. J., Martinez, J., & Eckholdt, H. (2006). Service delivery for Asians and Pacific Islanders living with HIV/AIDS: Challenges and lessons learned. *Journal of Health Care for the Poor and Underserved, 17, 910–927*.

Chin, D. & Kroesen, K. W. (1999). Disclosure of HIV infection among Asian/Pacific Islander women: Cultural stigma and support. *Cultural Diversity and Ethnic Minority Psychology, 5*, 222–235

Choi, K. H., Salazar, N., Lew, S., & Coates, T. J. (1995). AIDS risk, dual identity, and community response among gay Asian and Pacific Islander men in the United States. In G. M. Herek, & B. Green (Eds.), *AIDS, identity and community: The HIV epidemic and lesbians and gay men* (pp. 115–134). Thousands Oaks, CA: Sage.

Choi, K., Kumekawa, E., Dang, Q., Kegeles, S., Hays, R. B., & Stall, R. (1999). Risk and protective factors affecting sexual behavior among young Asian and Pacific Islander men who have sex with men: Implications for HIV prevention. *Journal of Sex Education and Therapy, 24*, 47–55.

Collins, R. L. (1998). Social identity and HIV infection: The experiences of gay men living with HIV. In V. J. Derlega & A. P. Barbee (Eds), *HIV & social interaction*. Thousand Oaks, CA: Sage Publications.

Courtenay-Quirk, C., Wolitski, R. J., Parsons. J. T., & Gomez, C. A. (2006) Is HIV/AIDS stigma dividing the gay community? Perceptions of HIV-positive men who sex with men. *AIDS Education and Prevention, 18*, 56–67.

Crocker, J. (1999). Social stigma and self-esteem: Situational construction of self-worth. *Journal of Experimental Social Psychology, 35*, 89–107.

Derlega, V. J., Lovejoy, D., & Winstead, B. A. (1998). Personal accounts of disclosing and concealing HIV-positive test results: Weighing the benefits and risks. In V. J. Derlega & A. P. Barbee (Eds), *HIV & social interaction*. Thousand Oaks, CA: Sage Publications.

Derlega, V. J., Winstead, B. A., Greene, K., Serovich, J., & Elwood, W. N. (2002). Perceived HIV-related stigma and HIV disclosure to relationship partners after finding out about the seropositive diagnosis. *Journal of Health Psychology, 7*(4), 415–432.

Derlega, V. J., Winstead, B. A., Oldfield, E. C., & Barbee, A., (2003). Close relationship and social support in coping with HIV: A test of sensitive interaction systems theory. *AIDS and Behavior, 7*, 119–129.

Eckholdt, H. & Chin, J. (1997). Pneumocystis carinii Pneumonia in Asians and Pacific Islanders. *Clinical Infectious Disease, 24*, 1265–1267.

Eckholdt, H. M., Chin, J. J., Manzon-Santos, J. A., and Kim, D. D. (1997). The needs of Asians and Pacific Islanders living with HIV in New York City. *AIDS Education and Prevention, 9*, 493–504.

Emlet, C. A. (2006). A comparison of HIV stigma and disclosure patterns between older and younger adults living with HIV/AIDS. *AIDS Patient Care and STDs, 20*, 350–358.

Fife B,L., & Wright E. R. (2000). The dimensionality of stigma: a comparison of its impact on the self of persons with HIV/AIDS and cancer. *Journal of Health Social Behavior, 41*, 50–67.

Gorbach, P. M., Galea, J. T., Amani, B., Celum, C., Kerndt, P., & Golden, M. R. (2004). Don't ask, don't tell: Patterns of HIV disclosure among HIV positive men who have sex with men with recent STI practicing high risk behavior in Los Angles and Seattle. *Sexually Transmitted Infections, 80*, 512–517.

Harawa, N. T., Williams, J. K., Ramamurthhi, H. C., & Bingham, T. A. (2006). Perceptions towards condom use, sexual activity, and HIV disclosure among HIV-positive African American men who have sex with men: Implications for heterosexual transmission. *Journal of Urban Health: Bulletin of the New York Academy of Medicine, 83*, 682–694.

Hays, R. B., Turner, H. A., & Coates, T. J. (1992). Social support, HIV symptoms, and depression among gay men. *Journal of Consulting and Clinical Psychology, 60*, 463–469.

Holt, R., Court, P., Vedhara, K., Nott, K. H., Holms, J., & Snow, M. H. (1998). The role of disclosure in coping with HIV infection. *AIDS Care, 10*, 49–60.

Josephson, S. B. (1997). Correlated of HIV/AIDS disclosure: Psychosocial stresses; demographics; social support; coping; and quality of life. *Dissertation Abstracts*.

Kalichman, S., DiMarco, M., Austin, J., Luke. W., & DiFonzo, K. (2003). Stress, social support, and HIV-status disclosure to family and friends among HIV-positive men and women. *Journal of Behavioral Medicine, 26*(4), 315–323.

Kang, E., Rapkin, B. D., & DeAlmeida C. (2006) Are psychological consequences of stigma enduring or transitory? A longitudinal study of HIV stigma and psychological distress among Asians and Pacific Islanders living with HIV illness. *AIDS Patient Care and STDs, 20(10)*, 712–723.

Kang, E., Rapkin, B. D., Remien, R. H., Mellins, C. A., & Oh, A. (2005). Multiple dimensions of HIV stigma and psychological distress among Asians and Pacific Islanders living with HIV illness. *AIDS & Behavior, 9(2)*, 145–154.

Kang, E., Rapkin, B., Springer, C. & Kim, H. J. (2003). The "demon plague" and access to care among undocumented Asian immigrants living with HIV disease in New York City. *Journal of Immigrant Health, 5*(2), 49–58.

Kang, E & Rapkin, B. (2003). Adherence to antiretroviral medication among undocumented Asians living with HIV disease in New York City. *The Community Psychologist, 36*(2), 35–38.

Kagawa-Singer, M., & Wellisch, D. (1997). Impact of breast cancer on Asian American and Anglo American women. *Culture Medicine, Psychiatry, 21*, 449–480.

Kawachi, I. and Berkman, L. F. (2001). Social ties and mental health. *Journal of Urban Health, 78*, 458–467.

Keogh, P., Henderson, L., & Dodds, C. (2004). *Ethnic minority gay men: Redefining community restoring identity*. London: Sigma Research.

Körner, H. (2007). Negotiating cultures: Disclosure of HIV-positive status among people from minority ethnic communities in Sydney. *Culture, Health & Sexuality, 9*(2), 137–152.

Liu, H., Hi, Z., Li, Xiaoming, L., Stanton, B., Naar-King, S., & Tang, H. (2006). Understanding interrelationships among HIV-related stigma, concern about HIV infection, and
intent to disclose HIV serostatus: A pretest-posttest study in a rural area of eastern China.
AIDS Patient Care and STDs, 20(2), 133–142.
Liu, J. & Choi, K. (2006). Experiences of social discrimination among men who have sex with
men in Shanghai, China. *AIDS and Behavior, 10*, S25–S33.
Lye Chng, C., Wong, F. W., Park, R. J., Edberg, M. C., & Lai, D. S. (2003). A model for
understanding sexual health among Asians American/ Pacific Islander men who have sex
with men (MSM) in the United States. *AIDS Education and Prevention, 15*(Suppl. A), 21–38.
MacFarland, W., Chen, W., Weide, D., Kohn, R., & Klauser, J. (2004). Gay Asian men in
San Francisco follow the international trend: Increases in rates of unprotected anal
intercourse and sexually transmitted diseases, 1999–2002. *AIDS Education and Prevention,
16*, 13–18.
Mansergh, G., Marks, G., & Simoni, J. M. (1995). Self-disclosure of HIV infection among
men who vary in time since seropositive diagnosis and symptomatic status. *AIDS, 9*, 639.
Marks, G., Bundek, N. L., Richardson, J. L., Ruiz, M. S., Maldanoado, N., & Mason, H. R. C.
(1992). Self-disclosure of HIV infection: Preliminary results from a sample of Hispanic
men. *Health Psychology, 11*, 300–306.
Mason, H. R. C., Marks, G., Simoni, J. M., Ruiz, M. S., & Richardson, J. L. (1995).
Culturally sanctioned secrets? Latino men's nondisclosure of HIV infection to family,
friends, and lovers. *Health Psychology, 14*, 6–12.
Matsudaira, T. (2003). Cultural influences on the use of social support by Chinese immigrants
in Japan: "Face" as a keyword. *Quality of Health Research, 13*, 343–357.
Nemoto, T., Operario, D., Soma, T., Bao, D., Vajrabukka, A, & Crisostomo, V. (2003). HIV
risk and prevention among Asian/ Pacific Islander Men Who Have Sex With Men: Listen
to Our Stories. *AIDS Education and Prevention, 15*(Suppl. A), 7–20.
New York State Department of Health (2006, April). New York State HIV/AIDS surveil-
lance semiannual report: For cases diagnosed through December 2004. Bureau of HIV/
AIDS Epidemiology.
New York City Department of Health and Mental Hygiene, HIV Epidemiology Program
(February 2006). *HIV/AIDS in New York City, 2004: Asians/ Pacific Islanders.*
Omarzu, J. (2000). A disclosure decision model: Determining how and when individuals will
self-disclose. *Personality and Social Psychology Review, 4*, 174–185.
Parsons, J. T., VanOra, J., Missildine, W., Purcell, D. W., & Gomez, C. A. (2004). Positive
and negative consequences of HIV disclosure among seropositive injection drug users.
AIDS Education and Prevention, 16, 459–475.
Perry, S., Card, A. L., Moffatt, M., Ashman, T., Fishman, B., & Jacobsberg, L. (1994). Self-
disclosure of HIV infection to sexual partners after repeated counseling. *AIDS Education
and Prevention, 6*, 403–411.
Petrak, J. A., Doyle, A-M., Smith, A., Skinner, C., & Hedge, B. (2001). Factors associated
with self-disclosure of HIV serostatus to significant others. *British Journal of Health
Psychology, 6*, 69–79.
Pounds, M. B., Conviser, R.., Ashman, J. J., & Bourassa, V. (2002). Ryan White CARE Act
service use by Asian/Pacific Islanders and other clients in three California metropolitan
areas (1997–1998). *Journal of Community Health, 27*, 403–417.
Reidpath D. D. & Chan, K. Y. (2005). A method of the quantitative analysis of the layering of
HIV-related stigma. *AIDS Care, 17*, 425–432.
Schwarzer, R., Dunkel-Schetter, C. & Kemeny, M. (1994). The multidimensional nature of
received social support in gay men at risk of HIV infection and AIDS. *American Journal of
Community Psychology, 22*, 319–339.
Schnell, D., Higgins, D., Wilson, R., Goldbaum, G., Cohn, D., & Wolitski, R., (1992). Men's
disclosure of HIV test results to male primary sex partners. *American Journal of Public
Health, 82*, 1675–1676.

Scott, J. (2001, July). In population ranks, an ascent of Asians, *New York Times*.

Scrambler G. & Hopkins, A. (1990). Generating a model of epileptic stigma: The role of qualitative analysis. *Social Science and Medicine, 30*(11), 1187–1194.

Serovich, J. M., (2001). A test of two HIV disclosure theories. *AIDS Education and Prevention, 13*, 355–364.

Serovich, J. M. & Mosack, K. E. (2003). Reasons for HIV disclosure or nondisclosure to casual sexual partners. *AIDS Education and Prevention, 15*, 70–80.

Serovich, J. M., Mason, T. L., Bautista, D., & Toviessi, P. (2006). Gay men's report of regret of HIV disclosure to family, friends, and sex partners. *AIDS Education and Prevention, 18*(2), 132–138.

Simoni, J., Mason, H., Marks, G., Ruiz, M., Reed, D., & Richardson, J. (1995). Women's self disclosure of HIV infection: Rates, reasons, and reactions. *Journal of Consulting and Clinical Psychology, 63*, 474–478.

Simoni, J. M., Demas, P., Mason, H. R. C., Drossman, J. A., & Davis, M. L. (2000). HIV disclosure among women of African American descent: Associations with coping, social support, and psychological adaptation. *AIDS and Behavior, 4*, 147–158.

Sheon, N. & Crosby, M. (2004). Ambivalent tales of HIV disclosure in San Francisco. *Social Science and Medicine, 58*, 2105–2118.

Smith, M. Y. & Rapkin, B. D. (1996). Social support and barriers to family involvement in caregiving for persons with AIDS: implications for patient education. *Patient Education Counseling, 27*, 85–94.

Taylor, S. E., Sherman, D. K., Kim, H. S., Jarcho, J., Takagi, K., & Dunagan, M. S. (2004). Culture and social support: Who seeks it and why? *Journal of Personality and Social Psychology, 87*, 354–362.

Wellisch, D., Kagawa-Singer, M., Reid, S. L., Lin, Y. J., Nishikawa-Lee, S., & Wellisch, M. (1999). An exploratory study of social support: A cross-cultural comparison of Chinese-Japanese-, and Anglo-American breast cancer patients. *Psycho-Oncology, 8*, 207–219.

Wilson, P. A., & Yoshikawa, H. (2004). Experiences of and responses to social discrimination among Asian and Pacific Islander gay men: Their relationship to HIV risk. *AIDS Education and Prevention, 16*, 68–83.

Wong, F. Y., Campsmith, M., Nakamura, G., Crepaz, N., & Begley, E. (2004). HIV testing and awareness of care-related services among a group of HIV-positive Asian Americans and Pacific Islanders in the United States: Finding from a supplemental HIV/AIDS surveillance project. *AIDS Education and Prevention, 16*, 440–447.

Yoshikawa, H., Wilson, P, A.D, Chae., D. H., & Cheng, J. F. (2004). Do family and friendship networks protect against then influence of discrimination on mental health and HIV risk among Asian and Pacific Islander gay men. *AIDS Education and Prevention, 16*(1), 84–100.

Yoshikawa, H., Kang, E., Wilson, P., Hseuh, J., Rosman, E., and Park, T. (2001). HIV prevention needs assessment of API MSMs in New York City. Report submitted to the New York City Department of Health.

Yoshioka, M. R., Schustack A. (2001). Disclosure of HIV Status: Cultural issues of Asian patients. *AIDS Patient Care & STDs, 15*, 77–82.

Zea, M. C., Reisen, C. A., Poppen, P. J., Echeverry, J. J., & Bianchi, F. T. (2004). Disclosure of HIV-positive status to Latino gay men's social networks. *American Journal of Community Psychology, 33*, 107–116.

Zea, M. C., Reisen, C. A., Poppen, P. L., Bianchi, F. T., & Echeverry, J. J. (2005). Disclosure and HIV status and psychological well-being among Latino gay and bisexual men. *AIDS and Behavior, 9*, 15–26.

Chapter Ten
Disclosure of HIV Status and Mental Health among Latino Men who have Sex with Men

Maria Cecilia Zea

Early in the HIV/AIDS epidemic, I had two personal experiences that made me acutely aware of the difficulty of disclosing seropositive status, which at the time was very highly stigmatized, to other people—even friends and relatives. The first experience was 2 years after I had left Bogota to come to the University of Maryland at College Park. My best friend, who still lived in Bogota, died of AIDS without having disclosed to anyone, not even his partner, that he was infected. At that time, in 1987, there had been few cases of HIV/AIDS in Colombia. To this day, I wonder what consequences of disclosing he feared, and it saddens me that he did not feel it was safe to tell anyone, despite his being openly gay.

The second experience was a few years later; one of my colleagues from clinical internship, a young African American man from the South, called a friend from his college years and informed him that he was hospitalized, but that no one was to know. He died a couple of days later, and his death caught his family and all of his friends, including his partner, by surprise. Although it must have been very frightening for my colleague to realize that he was dying of AIDS, the prospect of his family's discovery that he was HIV-positive and gay must have been even more terrifying. Therefore, he chose to die alone. For both these men, the psychological toll of keeping their serostatus a secret must have been very high, particularly for the latter, who had such a lonely death. Neither family members nor friends were able to support and comfort him during his hospitalization, which proved devastating to his partner, friends, and family.

Another personal experience made me aware of the importance of the target of disclosure, with disclosure to people within the gay community being easier than to non-gay friends and relatives. This experience took place years later, when there was a great deal of activism in the gay community, including the Latino gay community. One strong advocate of HIV/AIDS prevention in the community was Manuel Sandoval, a gay man from Panama. When I visited Manuel at the George Washington University Hospital, so many of his friends

Maria Cecilia Zea
Gerorge Washington University, Washington, D.C.

S. Loue (ed.), *Health Issues Confronting Minority Men Who Have Sex with Men.*   219
© Springer 2008

were present that they had filled up his room and spilled out into the corridor. Manuel had been out as a gay man and as HIV-positive in the Washington, DC area, and he died surrounded by friends. Paradoxically, despite years of using his own HIV status as a platform to prevent the spread of AIDS among other Latinos, Manuel had not told his mother that he was HIV-positive. Manuel died before his mother and siblings arrived from Panama, and many of his friends had to take care of his family. We watched his mother and siblings deal with the fact that Manuel was dead, and that they had not arrived in time because Manuel had instructed his friends not to tell his family. His family members suffered greatly; not only had they lost a loved one, but they had been unable to say goodbye to him, because he had not revealed that he was dying of AIDS.

A few years later, when I participated in the Minority Collaborative Research Program that Barbara Marin directed at the Center for AIDS Prevention Studies at the University of California in San Francisco, I knew I wanted to study and understand disclosure of serostatus among Latino gay men. The stories mentioned above inspired me to look deeper into the phenomenon of non-disclosure or selective disclosure of positive serostatus. Even though I consider sexual risk behavior a fundamental public health issue, and I believe that disclosure supports individual decision-making about sexual activities, I was more intrigued by the mental health consequences of disclosure. This chapter focuses mainly on the mental health aspects of disclosure. Although HIV is no longer considered a death sentence, HIV-positive Latino men who have sex with men (MSM) continue to face complex mental health issues. Throughout the years, I have seen that many HIV-positive gay men, when faced with their diagnosis, demonstrate resilience, optimism, and the ability to be emotionally close to others. At some point, these men disclose their serostatus to their loved ones. I have also encountered, however, some depressed men who fear the consequences of being found out and who live with anxiety. Facing the stigma of HIV and stressors of a chronic illness is difficult for any individual. This burden is compounded by the stigma of homosexuality. Any balanced portrayal of the mental health issues of Latino gay and bisexual men must take into account both positive and negative aspects of disclosure.

Consequences of disclosing to others can range from extremely positive to extremely negative. Recipients of disclosure may react in ways that convey acceptance and understanding. They may offer various types of help, which can range from giving nurturance to providing financial and emotional support, taking the person living with HIV to see physicians, and encouraging adherence to medication regime. Conversely, recipients of disclosure may react with anger and rejection; the consequences can include risks to life and severe losses, e.g., jobs, health insurance, and friends (Derlega, Winstead, & Folk-Barron, 2000; Derlega, Winstead, Oldfield, & Barvee, 2003). Many individuals anticipate negative consequences of disclosure, whereas others anticipate positive outcomes.

This chapter presents findings from several studies conducted with four samples of Latino MSM. The first study includes findings from an unpublished qualitative study for which I interviewed HIV-positive Latino MSM (Zea, 1999). This chapter also includes findings from two separate samples in a quantitative study funded by the National Institute of Mental Health (R01 MH60545) and a sample of a study funded by the National Institute of Child Health and Human Development (R01 HD046258).

Qualitative Study

The goal of the first study was to conduct in-depth interviews to find out whether participants had disclosed their serostatus to other members of their social network, and to inquire about the types of experiences they had when they disclosed to others, or the feelings associated with withholding disclosure from others. In 1998, I interviewed 21 HIV-positive Latino gay men from the Washington, D.C. Metropolitan area. These men were recruited by HIV-positive Latino gay activists or referred by caseworkers and health care providers from HIV/AIDS Clinics. All participants who were referred attended the interviews, which took place in Spanish. Each interview lasted between 1 and 2 hours, and participants were compensated $50 for their time and transportation costs. A limitation of this study was that the most reticent non-disclosers would not be likely to participate in such face-to-face interviews and, therefore, were probably underrepresented. However, I know that some reticent individuals did participate. In one instance, a man who had great difficulty disclosing was encouraged to meet with me by his case worker, who had taken an interest in him. In another instance, a young man was referred by a physician who was aware that this man had not disclosed his serostatus to anyone.

Reasons to Disclose or Withhold Information

Some men felt they had reasons to disclose to their loved ones, whereas others felt they had reasons to avoid disclosure. For instance, Juan Carlos[1], an Argentine man, decided to reveal his serostatus to his mother because he could not bear the thought that she would find out when he died. He felt that waiting until he died would have been a bigger blow than telling her while he was alive. On the other hand, Tomás, a Puerto Rican man, who had disclosed to his main partner and to many friends, felt that the news "would kill" his mother,

---

[1] From here on, names are fictitious to protect the privacy of participants.

and therefore preferred not to disclose to her. The argument Tomás used was that even if he were to live for only 10 years, he would spare her pain and suffering during that time and, moreover, he hoped to outlive her. Although both of these men expressed a rationale to protect their mothers from suffering, the outcomes were completely opposite, with one having disclosed to his mother whereas the other had not. Both of these men's attitudes reflect the importance of the mother in Latino culture, which is consistent with the value that is known as familism.

The perception of mothers as strong individuals is highlighted in the experience of Carlos, a Salvadoran man, when he tested positive for HIV. Carlos reported that his mother had shown strength and was capable of dealing with his seropositive status. Carlos recalled his mother's probing about his serostatus by telling him about an acquaintance who was infected and showing great compassion towards this acquaintance:

> Carlos—"and then she noticed I was crying, and she asked why I was crying, and so I said to her 'because I am just as [sick] as he is', but she is a very strong person and does not let things get to her; she is not too sentimental".
> Interviewer—"And how did you feel after telling her"?
> Carlos—"Calm. . . because I had someone I could trust and rely on."

When he found out that he had AIDS, another Salvadoran man, José, recalled his feelings of loneliness and isolation, which were exacerbated by the difficulty of disclosing to his mother, who was the person towards whom he felt the closest. He described his experience in this way:

> José—It was such sadness, I was so lonely, I didn't have the courage to tell even my own mother. The truth is that I started doing crack, I felt like the world had fallen on my shoulders... And I started doing drugs, I didn't even check the oil in my car... I became careless about everything.

Consequences of Disclosure

It is not uncommon that for some men, disclosure generates a great relief. For instance, Miguel, a Salvadoran man, recalls his experience disclosing to his sister:

> Miguel—"I felt like a great weight lifted off my shoulders. I got in the car, and I felt like I was flying in the car. I felt free, free from that pressure, from that secret. Because it was a secret I needed to share. I felt like a bird, I tell you, flying. And it wasn't that I was speeding, but that I felt free. . ."

This quote illustrates that disclosure can bring about great relief and euphoria. The discomfort of keeping HIV status secret is alleviated after the disclosure.

Participants anticipated different reactions from different members of their social network. Carlos, who experienced his mother as supportive, felt he would lose his job if he disclosed to his boss, and that he would lose his friends if he disclosed to them. Moreover, he felt his life would be in danger if he disclosed his seropositive status to his partner of 3 years. Carlos preferred to abandon his partner when he himself started presenting symptoms of Kaposi's sarcoma, because that meant he could no longer keep his serostatus secret. Carlos disclosed selectively, because he felt that he would be safe with his mother but very unsafe with his partner. Like Carlos, many men seem to have mixed feelings regarding disclosure of serostatus, and these feelings often include fear, anxiety, and depression. In contrast, feelings may be positive—such as relief, greater intimacy, and even a passion for a newly discovered mission as AIDS activist.

Disclosure of Seropositive Status as an Indirect Disclosure of Sexual Orientation

Being seropositive is a stigmatized condition in itself, which is compounded by the stigma of sexual orientation. José, mentioned earlier, illustrates a segment of the MSM population who experience being gay as extremely stigmatizing. He related

> José—"...I've been *escondido* (closeted); today I am talking to you like this, but I feel very ashamed if people find out about...."
> "Well, the truth is that nobody knows..."
> Interviewer—"Nobody knows. . ."
> José—"About me. For me it is a shame if my family finds out...."
> Interviewer—"Finds out. . ."
> José—"Yes."
> Interviewer—"Your family knows that you are HIV-positive but they think that. . ."
> José—"Yes. They think I am a man."

As this and the earlier quote illustrated, for José being HIV-positive was very difficult and depressing, but being gay was even worse. Homosexuality was perceived as a serious threat to his manhood and generated extreme feelings of shame. José was so concerned about people finding out that he had sex with men, that he admitted in the interview that he had sex with women so that nobody would suspect his sexual orientation or, as he defined it, that he was not a man.

Quantitative Study 1

Disclosure of Serostatus and of Sexual Orientation

Although much less extreme than José's concern, the possibility of being "outed" remains an issue for some men. The purpose of the first quantitative study was to examine the relationship between disclosure of serostatus and sexual orientation in a more systematic way. We hypothesized that there would be different levels of disclosure towards different members of the social network, and that one of the strongest predictors of disclosure of serostatus to specific individuals in the social network would be whether those individuals knew the gay or bisexual sexual orientation of the person living with HIV. Furthermore, we hypothesized that emotional closeness to the target would also be related to disclosure of serostatus. For this purpose, we considered individual targets, such as mother, father, main partner, closest friend, as well as group targets, which encompassed family as well as Latino and non-Latino friends. We controlled for acculturation to US culture as well as time since HIV diagnosis in all analyses (Zea, Reisen, Poppen, Echeverry, & Bianchi, 2004).

For this study, we relied on a sample of 155 HIV-positive Latino gay and bisexual men from New York City and Washington, DC. The majority (140) of the participants were immigrants who had come to the United States to improve their financial situation (46%), live a homosexual life more openly (34%), and get HIV medication (26%). Participants ranged from 18 to 67 years of age.

To assess disclosure of HIV status to parents, we first ascertained whether the specific individual was alive or part of the participant's life at the time of the diagnosis. If the parent was alive, we asked: "Does your mother know that you are HIV-positive?" Choices were *yes*, *no*, or *she suspects it, but I am not sure she knows*. If the target knew, then we asked how she found out; we treated as disclosure those instances in which the participant told her directly or asked somebody to tell her. We treated as non-disclosure situations in which the mother acquired the information some other way, as well as situations in which she was unaware of the person's HIV status. We repeated this pattern with fathers, closest friend, main partner, and with two target groups: family members and friends. We followed each HIV disclosure question with question: "Does your mother (father, closest friend, family, etc.) know that you have sex with men?"

To assess emotional closeness, we asked separate questions relating to each target relationship at the time of diagnosis. The question asked was, "How would you describe your emotional relationship with your mother/father/closest friend/main partner at the time of your HIV diagnosis?" Responses ranged from 1 (*very distant*) to 4 (*very close*).

Our findings indicated that when these men were not out as gay or bisexual to their parents, friends, or other family members, they would not share with them the fact that they were living with HIV. Emotional closeness was also an important predictor, but it was less strongly associated with disclosure than knowledge of sexual orientation. We found that disclosure to mothers occurred more frequently than to fathers, and that men who were more acculturated into US culture were more likely to disclose to fathers than those who were less acculturated. Participants were more likely to disclose to close friends and sex partners than to parents (Zea et al., 2004).

The in-depth interviews and study 1 findings highlight the dual stigma of seropositive status and sexual orientation among Latino gay men across their social network. When participants perceive their sexual orientation in a negative light or when they anticipate a negative reaction, they may be less likely to disclose sexual orientation. José's interview was a powerful example of fear of disclosing sexual orientation. José's interview also suggested that lack of disclosure was stressful and anxiety provoking. Conversely, Miguel's feelings of exhilaration when he was finally able to disclose to his sister reveal a connection between disclosure and positive emotions and mental health in general. Consequently, to further explore the relationship between disclosure of HIV status and mental health outcomes, we conducted quantitative study 2. This study is reported below.

Quantitative Study 2

Disclosure and Mental Health

For this subsequent study on disclosure of serostatus and mental health outcomes, we collected data on 301 HIV-positive Latino gay and bisexual men who were part of a larger study on disclosure. Findings from study 2 have been published elsewhere (Zea, Reisen, Poppen, Bianchi, & Echeverry, 2005), and therefore below is a summary. The aim of this study was to examine the relationship between disclosure of HIV status and mental health outcomes, controlling for education and income. We assessed disclosure in the same way as in study 1, described above (Zea et al., 2004).

Mental health indicators were assessed with the short form of the Beck Depression Inventory (Beck, Steer, & Garbin, 1988), the Quality of Social Support Scale (QSSS; Goodenow, Reisine, & Grady, 1990), and the Single-Item Self-Esteem Scale (Robins, Hendin, & Trzesniewski, 2001). These measures were previously translated into Spanish and back-translated into English to ensure that they had equivalent meaning that had not been lost in translation. An invited panel of Spanish-speaking experts from different Spanish-speaking countries ensured that the Spanish version was equivalent and applicable to individuals from various countries. Participants could choose their preferred language, Spanish or English.

As in study 1, disclosure of serostatus differed depending on the target. Disclosure to the closest friend was more frequent (84.7% of those who had a closest friend), and significantly higher than disclosure to main partner (77.5%) for the 187 men who had a male main partner. Twenty men who had a female partner had only disclosed to 65% of their female partners. For those with living parents, 37.1% had disclosed to their mothers, which was significantly higher than the 23.2% who had disclosed to their fathers (Zea et al., 2005). We also examined the proportions of the target groups (friends and family) to whom participants had disclosed. More than one-third reported that they had disclosed to most of their friends, while 15% had disclosed to none. A similar proportion had disclosed to most of their family members, but a larger proportion (29%) had disclosed to no family members.

Using the set of outcomes (social support, depression, and self-esteem), we conducted separate multivariate analyses of covariance for each target: mother, father, main partner, and closest friend. Disclosure to father was not significant, so this member of the social network was dropped for the remaining analyses. We found that, for all targets, disclosure of serostatus was associated with increased quality of social support (Zea et al., 2005). That is, higher levels of disclosure to specific targets and target groups were related to higher quality of social support. Thus, across the board, there was a positive association between disclosure and social support, a finding that is consistent with previous studies (Kadushin, 2000; Simoni, Demas, Mason, Drossman, & Davis, 2000). Because this was a cross-sectional study, we could not infer causality. It is possible that disclosure increases social support, but it is also possible that having a supportive social network provides a context in which people feel comfortable disclosing. It is also possible that there is a bidirectional relationship between social support and disclosure: those who disclose receive support, which encourages them to disclose even more, which in turn is a feedback loop into an increase in supportive networks.

We also examined the relationship between disclosure and depression and self-esteem. These findings were not as consistent across all specific targets and target groups as the relationships between social support and disclosure. Disclosing seropositive status to mothers and to the main male partner was directly related to less depression. This finding suggests that withholding a secret of such a magnitude from two highly valued individuals can lead to negative mood and depression. Disclosure to family members as a group, to friends as a group, and to the closest friend was not related to depression. It is possible that these components of the social network are less emotionally close, and therefore withholding a secret from them may not be as burdensome.

The main male partner was the only individual target for whom disclosure was related to self-esteem. It is possible that concealing information that can place a sex partner at risk would have a negative impact on opinion of self and, conversely, that being able to share this information helps respondents feel like better individuals. Disclosure to groups such as family and friends was also related to increased self-esteem, but it is also possible that high self-esteem facilitates disclosure to these groups.

Because disclosing seropositive status to mothers and main male partners was directly related to less depression, we were able to further examine whether social support was a mediator through which this relationship occurred. We found that disclosure resulted in greater social support, which in turn decreased depression.

We also examined whether social support mediated the relationship between disclosure to main male partner and self-esteem. Disclosure to main male partner increased social support, which in turn resulted in higher self-esteem. The same mediational mechanism operated for family and friend networks.

The in-depth interviews from the qualitative study had suggested a relationship between disclosure of serostatus and psychological well-being, which was corroborated by a number of findings from the quantitative data. These findings allow us to acknowledge that disclosure and mental health are linked, although with this cross-sectional design causal direction remains unclear. Longitudinal studies are needed to elucidate a causal direction.

Thus, this chapter has examined ongoing, more sustained effects of disclosure of serostatus. Short-term effects, such as mood, are worth examining. A separate and much larger study, which did not focus on disclosure, allowed us to gather data on specific sexual encounters of Latino MSM and examine whether openness regarding HIV status was related to the mood during the specific sexual encounter. Below are unpublished findings of a set of variables from the larger study.

Quantitative Study 3

Disclosure in the Context of a Sexual Encounter

The study described here is part of a larger study on contextual factors of sexual risk (R01 HD 046258, Zea, Principal Investigator, Paul Poppen and Carol Reisen, Co-Investigators). As part of this study, we used self-administered computer-based interviews with an audio-component. We used a mixed serostatus sample, which consisted of 482 Brazilian, Colombian, and Dominican MSM in New York City. For this chapter, we include a subsample of those people for whom the most recent sexual encounter occurred within the last week, i.e., 354 MSM. We also dropped those who did not know their own serostatus, which left us with a sample of 311 MSM.

We asked participants to answer questions at multiple levels, which included person- and encounter-level questions. Person-level questions included demographic information (country of birth, income, education) and HIV status. Of the subsample who had a sexual encounter within the last week, 146 were Brazilian, 169 Colombian, and 167 Dominican. About 27% were HIV-positive, 62% HIV-negative, and the remaining 11% did not know their serostatus. Although 72% had some college education and above, 42% made less than $800 a month.

For the encounter-level questions, we instructed participants as follows: "First, we would like to ask about the LAST TIME you had sex. Take a moment to think about it—where it happened, when it happened, with whom it happened, and what happened. To help you remember, please think about the time of year, the time of day, or anything else that brings the occasion into your mind more fully. Think carefully about this occasion and recall, as well as you can, what happened. We will ask a lot of questions about this encounter". Then we asked "When was THE LAST TIME that you had sex?", followed by "How did you feel that day you had sex?" Participants could say "yes," "no," or "I do not remember" to several questions regarding mood. We used this mood variable as an indicator of depression, our dependent variable. For the findings presented here, the question was "Did you feel depressed?" We also asked whether participants knew the serostatus of their sex partner(s) in the last sexual encounter. Possible answers were "I know he/she is positive," "I think he/she is positive," "I know he/she is negative," "I think he/she is negative," and "I don't know". We then asked whether the sex partner knew the participant's serostatus, to which the respondent could answer "yes," "no," and "I don't know". The frequencies with which each of these alternatives were endorsed were: "I know he/she is positive," 5.8%; "I think he/she is positive," 1.7%; "I know he/she is negative," 38%; "I think he/she is negative," 19%; and "I don't know," 35%. When asked "Does your partner know your serostatus?," participants said "yes" in 48% of the cases, "no" in 40% of the cases, and "I don't know [if he or she knows]" in 11% of the cases.

Using multiple regression, we predicted depression from country of birth, income, education, respondent serostatus, and whether the sex partner in last encounter knew the respondent's serostatus, as well as the interaction between serostatus of respondent and sex partner's knowledge of respondent's serostatus, which in this case is similar, though not equivalent, to disclosure. Controlling for income ($F = 3.66$, $p < 0.06$), we found that HIV-positive respondents were more depressed than HIV-negative respondents ($M = 1.79$ and 1.57, $F = 5.61$, $p < 0.02$), but if the sex partner knew the participant's serostatus, he was less depressed than if the sex partner did not ($M = 1.57$ and 1.71, $F = 4.62$, $p < 0.05$). There was a trend in the interaction, which showed greater depression among HIV-positive participants whose partner did not know their serostatus than among those whose partner knew their serostatus ($M = 1.93$ and 1.64, $F = 2.76$, $p < 0.10$). It must be noted that the question participants were responding to was knowledge of serostatus, which is not identical to disclosure of serostatus, as sometimes people can find out some other way, such as when individuals use their HIV-positive status as the basis of activism, or if someone else disclosed.

These findings suggest that having a sexual encounter with someone who does not know the participant's serostatus can be burdensome for HIV-positive individuals and, therefore, the mood in the last sexual encounter is depressed. In contrast, an HIV-negative individual's mood is not affected if the sex partner does not know the HIV-negative status of the respondent, because there is no burden associated with not disclosing seronegative status. This interaction may also suggest that individuals who are HIV-positive and depressed may be less able to disclose their HIV status to their sex partners.

Conclusions

The studies reported above are cross-sectional, and therefore not indicative of causality; these findings, however, suggest a connection between disclosure of HIV status and mental health. Participants' narratives provided a rich description of the difficulty of disclosing when the expected reaction is negative, and how depressed and isolated individuals feel when they cannot disclose their seropositive status to somebody else. The narratives also showed that many participants felt free and exhilarated after disclosing and no longer carrying the burden of a secret. Moreover, in many instances, participants' loved ones received their disclosure with love and support.

Latino MSM disclose at different rates to their main male partner, their closest friend, their parents, and friends and family in general. Participants whose social networks know about the participants' sexual orientation are also more likely to be able to disclose seropositivity. A connection between disclosure of serostatus and mental health is also evident, and also varies according to the target of the disclosure. Moreover, having a sexual encounter with someone who does not know the positive serostatus of a participant is related to a depressed mood during the encounter.

Clinical work with Latino HIV-positive MSM should include a careful evaluation of the degree to which these men have disclosed their serostatus to members of their social network, and whether efforts to conceal a gay sexual orientation or an HIV-positive diagnosis are emotionally taxing for the individual. A discussion about the persons that are important to Latino MSM might guide an intervention. Such intervention could help identify whether it is safe to disclose, to whom a disclosure should be made, and how the disclosure will take place if it is in the MSM's best interest to disclose. Counselors and educators might benefit from understanding the connection between disclosure of seropositive status and psychological well-being. Moreover, keeping in mind that there are different consequences depending on the target of the disclosure might help prioritize to whom an individual might disclose first.

Future Directions

Given how limited cross-sectional studies are in establishing causality, the next logical step in the study of disclosure of HIV status is to conduct longitudinal follow-up studies of individuals living with HIV. Ideally, these studies could begin immediately after an individual's diagnosis, to examine the process of disclosure, and the trajectory of the mental health outcomes associated with disclosure. The ability to make causal inferences can also guide the development of interventions to promote disclosure of seropositive status.

It is unclear whether these findings apply to non-Latino groups, but much of the research on disclosure suggests similar trends with different levels of intensity. That is, White MSM are more likely to disclose than Latino MSM, but Latino MSM are more likely to disclose to close friends and male partners than to parents. Future studies should target transgender individuals, as they deal with additional layers of stigma and discrimination.

References

Beck, A. T., Steer, R. A., & Garbin, M. G. (1988). Psychometric properties of the Beck Depression Inventory: Twenty-five years of evaluation. *Clinical Psychology Review, 8,* 77–100.

Derlega, V. J., Winstead, B. A., & Folk-Barron, L. (2000). Reasons for and against disclosing HIV-seropositive test results to an intimate partner: A functional perspective. (pp. 53–69). In S. Petronio (Ed.), *Balancing the secrets of private disclosures.* Mahway, NJ: Lawrence Erlbaum.

Derlega, V. J., Winstead, B. A., Oldfield, E. E. III, & Barvee, A. P. (2003). Close relationships and social support in coping with HIV: A test of sensitive interaction systems theory. *AIDS and Behavior, 7,* 119–129.

Goodenow, C., Reisine, S. T., & Grady, K. E. (1990). Quality of social support and associated social and psychological functioning in women with rheumatoid arthritis. *Health Psychology, 9,* 266–284.

Kadushin, G. (2000). Family secrets: Disclosure of HIV status among men with HIV/AIDS to the family of origin. *Social Work in Health Care, 30,* 1–17.

Robins, R.W., Hendin, H. M., & Trzesniewski, K. H. (2001). Measuring global self-esteem: Construct validation of a single-item measure and the Rosenberg Self-Esteem Scale. *Personality and Social Psychology Bulletin, 27,* 151–161.

Simoni, J. M., Demas, P., Mason, H. R. C., Drossman, J. A., & Davis, M. L. (2000). HIV disclosure among women of African descent: Associations with coping, social support, and psychological adaptation. *AIDS and Behavior, 4,* 147–158.

Zea, M. C. (November, 1999). *Latino HIV-positive gay men's narratives on disclosure of serostatus.* Paper presented at the 127th American Public Health Association Annual Meeting. Chicago, IL.

Zea, M. C., Reisen, C. A., Poppen, P. J., Bianchi, F. T., & Echeverry, J. J. (2005). Disclosure of HIV status and psychological well-being among Latino gay and bisexual men. *AIDS & Behavior, 9,* 15–26

Zea, M. C., Reisen, C. A., Poppen, P. J., Echeverry, J. J., & Bianchi, F. T. (2004). Disclosure of HIV-positive status to Latino gay men's social networks. *American Journal of Community Psychology, 33,* 107–116.

Part VII
Building Community

Chapter Eleven

The Beyond Identities Community Center: A Community-Focused, Rights-Based Program to Address HIV/AIDS and Sexual Health Among Young Men Who have Sex with Men of Color in Cleveland, Ohio

Tracy Jones and Earl Pike

> *"... it is a simple fact that telling the truth, making simple statements of fact about your identity and beliefs—particularly when they don't match up with existing social prejudices—can get people attacked, maligned, or murdered."*
>
> —Dorothy Allison, *Skin: Talking About Sex, Class & Literature*

"Gonna pass me a law
that night last longer.
Gonna pass me a law
Larry come home from Vietnam,
wherever that is.
Gonna pass me a law
no woman can be my age
and not know enough
to read a map.
Gonna pass me a law
that my heathen daughter
don't never get hurt
nor learn how to mind me,
nor learn how to mind
nobody cept herself.
Gonna pass me a law
say Nat King Cole
gotta come over my house
come over my house
come over every night
and stroke my soul."

—Caroline, in, *Caroline, or Change* (Tony Kushner)

For many, the modern HIV/AIDS epidemic has grown in soil, on a landscape, already marred with enormous threat and peril. The persistent realities of poverty, racism, homophobia, gender inequality, structural and interpersonal violence, and inequitable distribution of health care resources have collectively

---

Tracy Jones
MNO, AIDS Taskforce of Greater Cleveland, Cleveland, OH

S. Loue (ed.), *Health Issues Confronting Minority Men Who Have Sex with Men.*
© Springer 2008

provided fertile ground for an expanding epidemic marked by staggering imbalances in access to care, and the menu of care available. For lesbian/gay/ bisexual/transgender (LGBT) youth of color in the USA, we can add to those larger realities more particular conditions: in many cities, the public education system is crumbling and no longer prepares youth for the future; the supposed zone of safety for youth—the family—may actually be dangerous because of family's reaction to disclosure of sexual identity. Even the streets, for those youth whose gender expressions do not conform to expected norms, pose enormous risk—sometimes from others in the neighborhood, sometimes from the very individuals and institutions, such as the police, who are charged with protecting individuals from harm. Telling the truth about who you are—being open and un-self-censoring about identity—can get you murdered. Not telling the truth, as has been reinforced throughout this volume, can increase your risk of other harms, including mental illness, substance abuse, and HIV/AIDS.

For too long, the standard response to the growing crisis of HIV/AIDS ignored the terrain that helped it grow, and instead offered only this: education. In time, the shared commitment to implement education was modified by the condition that such education be culturally competent, which meant everything from the shallow adoption of a particular vernacular believed to prevail among target audiences, to more sophisticated (and necessary) interventions that understood "culture" and its endless permutations and combinations to be a complex and dynamic reality. But the notion that simple instruction in risk reduction strategies, or conveyed comprehension of how HIV is and is not transmitted has only limited effectiveness. Even now, a frightening naivety persists: we are HIV/AIDS educators, and only that; this is the part we do (instruction, experiential learning); others will do the rest of what needs doing (addressing poverty, racism, structural violence, and so on). Somehow it will all come together, and make a difference.

More recently, public health officials, academicians, and ground-level edu- cators and service providers alike have begun to embrace a more multidimen- sional approach, one that does more than simply acknowledge the rough terrain. The challenge of HIV/AIDS prevention, they have said, is a process of engaging individuals in their cultural/community contexts, and cultures/ communities in their individual representations, in a manner that fully recog- nizes—and indeed, openly contests—an inequality of rights in all its facets. Put that way, the evolving perspective is developmental: our task, as advocates of health against disease, is to build communities that can, on their own, advocate for and secure the rights that will promote health, and that can, on their own, foster intrapersonal states and interpersonal/behavioral norms that are known to support health and well-being.

This perspective is long-term: it proposes that we will be most successful if we work to strengthen communities in a way that will outlast the epidemic, rather than focusing on the duration and dynamics of the epidemic itself. To do so, this perspective is predicated on the belief that the factors affecting individual/ community ability to respond to the specific crisis of HIV/AIDS may and most likely do include those that do not directly relate to HIV/AIDS, but nevertheless condition the spread of the disease, such as education, socioeconomic inequality, the local availability of fair-wage jobs, the condition of local housing stock, and many others. This is the broad tapestry of situational conditions and needs that speak to the more fundamental desires of human existence: not merely to live absent one disease (among many), but to have life "stroke my soul."

Some models have recently emerged that reflect the multidimensionality of the epidemic, and that define as a locus of impact communities themselves, rather than merely individuals within those communities. The Centers for Disease Control and Prevention (CDC) evidence-based Mpowerment program, for example, combines structured interventions with community-building, and further acknowledges, through its encouragement of the use of the Internet, that "community" is not confined to geographic space, but rather clusters around shared narrative and experience. But we need more.

One example of a model intended to build nurturing community to support healthy behavior in a rights-based context is the Beyond Identities Community Center (BICC) in Cleveland, Ohio. The remainder of this chapter will explore the genesis and evolution of BICC, its characteristic features and program offerings, its successes and failures, and its limitations.

Community/Organizational Context

As reported by Bruckman in this volume, Cleveland is a poor, economically struggling city in a rust-belt region of northeast Ohio. It has suffered an alarming out-migration of residents over the past 50 years, a steadily shrinking tax base, financially strapped and academically challenged schools, deteriorating housing, and a loss of decent jobs that include health insurance. Recently, the city has been challenged by one of the highest foreclosure rates in the country—a telling indicator of poverty—and by inadequately regulated predatory lending, which has only made the poor poorer. Paradoxically, Cleveland is also a home to some of the best health care institutions in the USA, with the Cleveland Clinic, MetroHealth Hospital, and University Hospitals (which houses an AIDS Clinical Trials Unit engaged in significant research on HIV treatment and the development of effective microbicidal agents). Cleveland is a minority–majority city, and in a significant numbers of neighborhoods, over 90% of residents are African American. Geographic segregation of communities—White, African American, and Hispanic/Latino—is high.

The AIDS Taskforce of Greater Cleveland is the region's largest and most comprehensive HIV/AIDS service, prevention education, and advocacy organization, with a current budget of just over $4 million and a staff of 64 full- and part-time staff. Because of Cleveland's endemic poverty, the overwhelming majority of clients are not merely poor, but many would be termed destitute:

90% of the AIDS Taskforce of Greater Cleveland's (ATGC's) nearly 2,000 clients report an annual income of less than $10,000 when first seeking services, and 60% report an annual income of less than $3,000 a year. Just over 60% of all clients are African American and 15% are Latino, and nearly one-third are women (up from 11% a decade ago). Because of poverty, homelessness, and hunger, the ATGC provides an array of services that address simple "survival," including an extensive food bank, housing services, and direct transportation to and from medically necessary appointments.

ATGC staff are diverse, and broadly reflect the racial and sexual orientation demographics of clients served. In recent years, the ATGC, like the city itself, and like many other AIDS Service Organizations (ASOs) in the United States, has struggled to preserve programs and services. Since 1999, a number of ASO mergers have occurred in Cleveland: nutrition services (provided by a separate organization), the AIDS Housing Council, the Open House, and Stopping AIDS is My Mission have all merged into the ATGC; in three of those cases, the merger was engendered by acute financial crisis. These structural alliances have permitted HIV/AIDS nonmedical core services to survive in Cleveland, but barely: most recently, the ATGC has undergone a painful period of expense reductions and program curtailments.

It is against this backdrop that the creation and evolution of the BICC should be viewed.

Origins of BICC

The origins of the BICC rest with three community programs designed to serve adult men of color who have sex with men (MSM): BlackOut Unlimited, a social networking organization that hosted a 3-day educational/social weekend for African American members of the LBGT community; the Brother's Circle of Greater Cleveland, a social support group for African American same gender-loving men; and the AIDS Taskforce of Greater Cleveland's Brother to Brother program, a prevention education program for men who have sex with men between the ages of 18 and 44. All the three programs were active, to varying degrees, in the mid-1990s, operating at times in competition with each other, and at times collaboratively.

After several years, the difficulty of maintaining several programs with largely overlapping goals and missions led to a merger between Brother's Circle and BlackOut, with the latter serving as the surviving legal entity. With moderate funding from the Cleveland Department of Public Health, BlackOut elected to focus its educational activities on youth. Concerned about the numbers of young gay boys of color whose first "coming out" experiences involved intergenerational dating, and whose introductions to the gay community took place in bar settings that included underage drinking, BlackOut launched a social group for young men who have sex with men (YMSM).

Named "Club 1722" (for youth between the ages of 17 and 22), the new social/educational group developed a significant following via word of mouth and telephone chat lines. A number of youth began to attend the program on a regular basis and program organizers quickly realized the need to collaborate with other community programs, such as the AIDS Taskforce of Greater Cleveland.

The program began to gain further interest after organizing social events, such as "Houseballs," for youth. But growth was also accompanied by challenges: space was limited and there were too few adults to help manage events and groups.

Parallel to the launch of Club 1722, the AIDS Taskforce began to identify the need to nurture the "next generation" of peer leadership in the local community of young MSM of color, and subsequently launched a Youth Drop-In Center that could serve as an informal training and peer leadership development venue. That Center quickly adopted a training model that incorporated HIV/AIDS knowledge, decision-making and conflict management skills, and emotional regulation to increase self-esteem and self-efficacy.

In 2001, the AIDS Taskforce and BlackOut Unlimited combined their efforts, and jointly applied for CDC funding to carry out HIV prevention programs for MSM of color between the ages of 13 and 24.

The CDC YMSM Initiative

The newly funded YMSM program was based on a youth development model that required significant input and decision-making from participant youth, and that endeavored to address, on both individual and community levels, the wide ranges of issues that impacted HIV/AIDS risk behavior. It included several key elements:

1. the focused development of peer leadership to carry out structured interventions and the more subjective tasks of community-building for the target population;
2. street- and venue-based outreach (including condom distribution), conducted by peer leadership, to other youth in the target community;
3. programming designed to address the array of needs identified by participant youth, on topics such as relationship violence, the risks of intergenerational dating, LGBT identity, and others;
4. social events designed to both build community and attract other youth to programming; and
5. ongoing provision of primary and ancillary supports, such as HIV and sexually transmitted disease (STD) testing and screening, mental health counseling, referrals for spiritual support, assistance in meeting basic needs such as food and housing, homework assistance and tutoring, job referrals, and more.

Fourteen youth were selected, through a highly competitive process, to serve as Peer Educators, and underwent an extensive, 2-year training program that covered basic facts about HIV history, transmission, epidemiology, illness and its management, and the psychosocial aspects; general theory and practice in community needs assessment; and federal and local "HIV systems," such as Community Planning Groups, the Ryan White Planning Council, the Title II Consortia, and nonprofit agencies. Peer leadership positions were treated as jobs and participating youth received a stipend for their work. Later, additional training components were added, including HIV test counseling, social marketing, and HIV/AIDS behavior change theory. A new cohort of Peer Educators was hired each year. The basic concept was simple and has been carried out elsewhere: peers would receive high-level training and then implement an array of interventions in community settings. In the case of the YMSM program, there was one significant and important difference: Peer Leaders who successfully completed the 2-year work/training program would be eligible to receive a $1,000 scholarship for post-high school education, to a school of their choice. By so doing, the AIDS Taskforce sought not merely to train leadership within a community, but also to nurture broader, long-term leadership in the community as a whole—in other words, to support the development of Cleveland community leadership for the future, leadership that would more accurately reflect the identities of those most severely impacted by the local HIV/AIDS epidemic.

During the first year, the ATGC hired L. Michael Gipson (LMG Consulting Partnerships, Ltd) to strengthen the curriculum and to more thoroughly ground the program in a youth development model. Out of that first year of development and experimentation, a comprehensive training schedule took form and youth began developing and delivering a menu of prevention interventions.

Youth-Led Interventions

One example of how interventions were developed and implemented might illustrate the degree of youth involvement and control.

All Peer Leaders hired under the grant were provided with extensive training in the theory and practice of models designed to impact HIV transmission and acquisition. One of those models was social marketing for behavior change or, as it has been called elsewhere, cause-related marketing.

Beginning the second year of the grant, Peer Leaders were divided into two teams and underwent extensive instruction in social marketing theory and practice, including the use of consumer feedback—focus groups and interviews—to craft effective behavior-change messages. Training included program design, management, and budgeting. Upon completion of training, the two teams were charged with developing a social marketing campaign designed to positively change the behavior of YMSM of color in the Greater Cleveland region, and each team was allocated an "up to" budget, ranging from $10,000 to 20,000, to cover campaign costs.

At the end of this development phase, the two teams presented their "proposed campaign" to a community panel composed of HIV service consumers, HIV/AIDS educators and service providers, YMSM of color, and local HIV/AIDS administrators and funders. In those presentations, each team "pitched" their proposal to the panel, outlining the theoretical basis for their campaign, actual campaign strategy, management and financial requirements, and expected outcomes.

Panel members, through a deliberative process, selected one of the two proposals for implementation and allocated the requested funds. Valuable elements from the unfunded proposal were integrated into the successful campaign, and both teams reunited for implementation.

Through this process, Peer Educators have, over the last 5 years, launched a number of effective social marketing campaigns, including a full-length CD of music and spoken word poetry (emphasizing community, relationships, and safer sex) that was distributed free of charge to area youth and club DJs; a poster campaign emphasizing self-worth and the importance of testing and safer sex that was mounted in youth venues and on city bus kiosks; and a full-length movie written and performed by youth, and produced and directed by a professional videographer (and distributed, as in the case of the CD, free of charge to area youth). The movie—*Destinies Fulfilled*—addressed the invisibility of YMSM of color in a dramatic format, and portrayed youth taking positive steps, with the support of peers, to maintain sexual health.

The Birth and Growth of BICC

Despite the success of the CDC YMSM program in its first several years, it gradually became apparent that long-term viability and success would depend on securing a physical space—a center—that could draw more youth to programming and build community and sustainable culture among participating youth. A critical need was "community space" that would be affiliated with the AIDS Taskforce of Greater Cleveland, but separate, with its own identity and expression.

In April 2004, the AIDS Taskforce opened the BICC in shared warehouse space about ten blocks from the ATGC's main administrative offices. Youth wishing to "join" BICC were required to complete a confidential registration form; within its first month, 138 members, of whom 94 were YMSM of color of 13–22 years old, had joined (as of the summer of 2006, that number had reached nearly 800). Each member received a referral for HIV testing at BICC. In addition, new members completed a risk assessment to identify direct HIV risk behavior and situational risks strongly correlated to HIV infection, such as substance abuse, mental illness, poverty, and homelessness or unstable housing.

In its first 2 months of operation, BICC staff provided 138 HIV testing referrals, conducted 21 HIV tests, offered 40 HIV prevention education referrals, and provided 24 referrals for employment, housing, counseling, and other services. In addition, BICC also began its first support group for youth of color infected or affected by HIV.

One-on-one Prevention Case Management services were added, provided by a licensed social worker and monitored by a licensed independent social worker (LISW). Street- and community-level outreach continued on a weekly basis to ensure that the target population was being effectively reached through the street team's efforts. (The street team supervisor, BICC's manager, and the peer leader mentors conducted occasional surprise spot checks based on the street teams' outreach calendar to ensure the integrity of the reported outreach and the appropriateness of the street team's outreach techniques; and we contracted with an independent evaluator to develop a rigorous evaluation tool to determine actual program outputs and outcomes for the target population.) An ongoing Friday Night social event was added, which regularly attracted between 70 and 140 youth.

Membership at BICC continued to rise throughout 2004 and 2005. In that period, BICC partnered with an array of other organizations to supplement existing BICC programming and reduce duplication of youth services in Cleveland.

The aforementioned social marketing campaigns played a critical role in the promotion of BICC and its service offerings, and in the subsequent rise in membership. Copies of the DVD *Destinies Fulfilled*, for example, were distributed to 500 YMSM and youth agencies throughout the Cleveland metropolitan area, drawing additional youth to the Center. The poster campaign announced area DVD showings, while simultaneously raising HIV awareness for the target population. The campaign also placed movie posters in 16, three-sided kiosks strategically located in areas known to be gathering places for target community youth. Based on data received from the contracted marketing firm, the combined market viewer exposure rate average was 35,000 views per week, per kiosk.

BICC members also promoted BICC awareness through a range of community outreach events that included distribution of over 3,200 safer sex kits, with information about HIV testing, at clubs, bars, targeted street locations, and community-level outreach events. Community-level outreach events included a Youth Poetry Slam, a youth booth at the annual Gay Pride Festival, a Mini-Ball, a Black Pride Celebration Family Picnic, and a Back-to-School Picnic Jam. In addition, BICC received considerable exposure and positive press coverage in the *Gay People's Chronicle*, *Scene Magazine*, and the Cleveland *Plain Dealer*.

The rapid growth rate and high demand for youth services required new strategies and creative use of existing resources—and, more than anything else, additional space. More recently, the ATGC found and secured a larger, more inviting center a few blocks from the previous location. Continuation (and increased) funding from the CDC facilitated the transition, and by the end of 2006, the full menu of available services included mental health counseling, Internet and computer access, educational or social service referrals, sexual health small group interventions, HIV and STD testing, a library, parent outreach programming, a young women's support/discussion group, and targeted programs addressing HIV cofactors and youth development issues such as sexual abuse, domestic violence, gender identity, employment, leadership, tobacco use prevention, and literacy. On Friday evenings, BICC continues its tradition of social gatherings.

Lessons Learned

In its goal of building a rights-based community that can nurture positive behavior change, BICC has been enormously successful: membership has grown steadily; there is strong evidence that BICC has helped foster new behavioral norms among participating youth; and BICC members continue to develop and display growth and leadership skills that have strengthened the specific community of young MSM of color, and the larger Cleveland community as well. A number of youth who started involvement with youth programming 5 years ago have gone on to higher education, are successfully employed at the AIDS Taskforce, or have moved on to program leadership positions at other agencies across the country. The mark of their efforts has rippled outward and is being felt.

But arriving at that point—a successfully operating youth program/center that can sustain both services and community cohesion—required years of effort and more than a few mistakes. Several lessons, from that experience, are now clear.

1. Youth involvement and decision-making is critical and must be intrinsic to the very fabric of the program. Throughout the history of BICC, conscious efforts were made to solicit youth perspectives, promote youth leadership, and highlight youth achievements. When faced with a challenge or dilemma, informal and formal consultation with BICC members nearly always pointed toward the effective resolution, and once decided, a course of action was "owned" by BICC members, rather than imposed from above.
2. Provision of a wide array of support services was, and remains, essential, since BICC members bring to the Center an astonishing variety of challenges. Youth problems, in all their forms, must be addressed *parallel* to efforts to reduce HIV risk, in a manner that integrates programming. Constant assessment, to learn "what's going on" with current members, is required, and must be followed up with appropriate programming or referral protocols.

3. Maintaining a relatively low public profile has helped BICC grow (membership growth is largely word-of-mouth), since many young MSM of color are unlikely to visit a center with too much public visibility. At the same time, public promotion (such as social marketing campaigns) has sometimes been necessary in order to "spread the message" of community health. Striking a balance between the two has not always been easy. Recently, BICC staff have developed more formal procedures to harvest BICC member input on decisions regarding public visibility, especially as it relates to media coverage, in order to give BICC members the "final say" on community representation.

4. Many of the challenges one might typically associate with a large youth center—relationships and relationship break-ups among members, the development of cliques, interpersonal conflict that sometimes erupted into fights, and so on—have been present at BICC since the beginning, and will probably never disappear. It has been critical to give youth the power and responsibility to develop and promote normative standards that everyone can agree on, but it has also been necessary, at times, for adult staff to take more decisive action by temporarily barring a member from the Center or implementing other disciplinary action. These steps are, however, viewed as a last resort, and every effort is made to reintegrate struggling youth back into BICC as soon as possible. In that sense, BICC has, from the outset, made an important commitment: BICC staff will not attempt to generate positive outcome data by "creaming" membership, but will invite all youth, with diverse problems and challenges, to become members.

5. Finally, the implementation of the CDC YMSM program, and BICC as its successor, created one tension that was entirely unexpected. The growing addition of a large number of youth to the "family" of services offered by the AIDS Taskforce proved difficult for some adult professionals among ATGC staff, who found a more formal working environment both changed and challenged by the addition of "youth energy." In retrospect, more preparation and planning could have helped prevent the problem. The provision of training for all staff on youth issues and youth development helped, at later points in time, to integrate the older staff and younger Peer Leaders and BICC members. Now, the two groups mingle well together—helped, to a large degree, by the fact that a number of BICC Peer Leaders have moved up to full-time staff positions at the AIDS Taskforce.

Shortly after the opening of BICC at its initial location, a BICC member—a young transgender African American male—was murdered in a random act of street violence. It was a devastating blow to BICC members, who reacted as a community: on their own, with only back-up support from staff, BICC members worked with the victim's family to organize a memorial service in which over 140 youth poured into the Center and down the hallway. (Letters written by BICC members in response to this violence, as well as the eulogy by L. Michael Gipson, appear earlier in the volume.) Later, BICC members organized a silent march from the Center to the main AIDS Taskforce offices to draw attention to the fragile lives of young, African American adults—especially when they are gay, lesbian, bisexual, or transgender.

In the 2 years following two other murders of BICC-associated youth would take place. There is no evidence that any of the three might have constituted a hate crime, though to our knowledge, no arrests have yet been made and the cases remain unsolved.

These events have served as the ultimate and tragic expression of the fragility of "life on the streets," and the multiple vulnerabilities—only one of which is HIV/AIDS—that young MSM of color face every day. To be successful, efforts to reduce HIV must address all of those vulnerabilities, or as many as possible, in an integrated community context and empower the community—however superficial that word has become—to develop its own resources to respond, to fight back.

Several months ago, one of us was in attendance at BICC during the early evening. As the Center closed, around 8:00 p.m., BICC members began spilling out the door and heading—by bus, on foot—home (whatever home was). Soon there were only about 25 youth remaining, standing at the bus stop, waiting for the bus, laughing and joking.

Suddenly, a car careened around the corner and screeched to a halt about a half-block up. Several young, White men jumped out of the car, and reports vary, but it is believed that one of them was brandishing a gun. These young men began screaming threats and racial epithets at the BICC members.

One of the BICC Peer Leaders immediately dialed police on his cell phone, and quite literally within seconds (an unusually rapid response time), police sirens could be heard, and a patrol car could be seen heading toward the intersection. The threatening young men jumped into their car and sped away, the police right after them.

A few minutes later, the Peer Educator who had made the phone call turned and said, "See, this is what we deal with every day."

Within 10 minutes, the excitement had worn off and a bus showed up. The remaining youth climbed aboard, and BICC staff headed toward their cars to go home.

Telling the truth can get you murdered. This is the soil, the terrain. Only community, and leadership of our own, can protect us.

Portrait Six
For Jayla

L. Michael Gipson

For almost 3 years, I've known the beautiful, talented and charismatic young man whose life has us all gathered together in his name. In life, Jay was one of the most respectful and kindhearted young people who ever walked through our doors. It doesn't seem possible to many of us, myself included, that we'll never see his smile, or experience his dancing talents, or witness his latest designer creation (because nobody could rock an outfit quite like Jay!). Having to write something this week that honors someone who died so young and filled so many of us with warmth has been one of the most difficult experiences of my life; especially given some of the circumstances surrounding his death. I've spent this week haunted by the hugs and sweet words Jay had for me every time, we saw one another and his willingness to show up week after week to do something positive and uplifting with his life and for the youth in this community. And to know that I won't have that experience again, that I won't witness him constantly striving to be a better person, breaks me up inside.

All this week, I've talked with many of you about honoring Jay's death and ensuring that his death was not in vain. But what does that mean exactly, when so much about his death seems so senseless and unnecessary? How can you make this young man's death not be in vain? I believe you do that by honoring Jay's morals and values in your daily walk, but avoid some of the choices, people and situations that can place you in harms way. In life, Jay was a teacher and I think in his death, he has taught us all many lessons, some that I am still learning.

Jay was a complete person with many amazing qualities, he was also, like many of us, a flawed young person still trying to understand what kind of adult he wanted to be and trying to find ways to be that person. With Jay, there is so much about the kind of person that he wanted to be that he got right. Jay worked hard, he was a respectful young man, he didn't start a lot of drama, he was non-violent in how he handled the conflicts and the challenges that he encountered. He was a man who was positively striving to figure out his way in

L. Michael Gipson
LMG Consulting Partnerships, Ltd., Washington, DC

S. Loue (ed.), *Health Issues Confronting Minority Men Who Have Sex with Men.*
© Springer 2008

this world. He mentored those who came behind him and tried to help them avoid the pitfalls and dangers of this life. As young as he was, Jay was always serving as a guide to others about what to look out for, and people to watch out for and telling those willing to listen about how things really are out here. Given the horrific circumstances surrounding his death, I can't help but wish that Jay had listened more carefully to the elders in his life who tried to do for him, what Jay has done for so many of you. That is to teach people how to survive and help make it through this life with a minimum of unnecessary pain and suffering.

Like most young people raised right by a moral and loving family, Jay tried to live by the rules and expectations he'd seen modeled for him at home and here at the Center. Sometimes in his life, he struggled with doing what he knew in his heart was right. At times, the call of friends and the lure of good times in bad, but exciting places proved stronger than the call to do right. Among youth, Jay was not unique in that way, he may have been a young man who believed that these are the years in your life that you're supposed to take chances and experience all the things this world has to offer, both its good and the bad.

Society often tells its young that during these years of your lives that you are supposed to take risks and to rebel against your elder's rules and authority. That tasting everything on life's buffet is the hot thing to do. I'm here to tell the young among you that society is lying to you, that there are some items on that menu, some risk taking in this life that you may never recover from. That some of the fun and exciting times that some seek can also put you in harm's way, and the cost is more than you can afford to give. More than we as a Black people, as a gay or youth community, as a family can afford to give. We cannot afford to lose you, not one more of you; we need you to survive. You need one another to survive. It's not only you who pays the cost for believing the lie; it's all of us. We cannot afford to lose any more of our Black and Brown children, gay, straight, or transgender. I personally can't take losing any more of the young people that I love in this community.

Jay didn't ask to be targeted, nor did he ask to be robbed and killed. He asked to be loved and accepted for who he is and to be allowed to just be. To just be who he is. Unfortunately, we don't live in a world that allows many of us to just be. We don't live in a world that always recognizes our value or our worth as human beings. And so, it's important that we recognize and value ourselves. It's crucial that we value our lives and make choices that reflect just how much we value our own lives. It's equally important that we value one another's lives and support each other in making positive healthy decisions. It has and always will be necessary that we learn how to love one another instead of hate or hate on one another; before we lose another light, like Jay.

We need to start doing it today. There used to be a time during the civil rights movement, where we told those in power, why we couldn't wait anymore for our rights. I think today we as a people need a different kind of movement, a love movement. We cannot afford to wait any longer to love ourselves and to love one another. I think those of us who loved Jay understand, perhaps more today, than ever before how precious each day is and how important it is for each of us to love, honor, and respect each other in words and in deeds. For tomorrow isn't promised, and the person standing next to you today, may not be here tomorrow. I think in Jay's death we have an opportunity to reflect on how we are, what we do, the choices we make, how we can be better to ourselves and to one another.

How do you not make Jay's death not be in vain? Work to stop the violence and the hate in your community and in yourselves. Do good works in honor of him and his memory. Don't just say you want to do something good, do it. Be it. Take care of those coming behind you and each other. Be a light, like Jay. But also learn from his example, before it's too late. We cannot afford to lose any one of you, the pain and the price is just too high. Be blessed and thank you for listening.

Portrait Seven
Rage of Betrayal

Erik Bradford

A heart whole

full of life & know

is full of rage

A brother stabbed, betrayed and the damsel not sowed

Because of ones faults

& the revenge or blood for another

Cause you cared for that person,

Your Special Brother

To find out there's a new seed in the picture

makes you question that person

When their face is all you can see in the mirror

because of rage and betrayal brought across one's self

Has the gun loaded and shot, but there's no help

A life taken 'cause of self affliction and jealousy

Another life taken because that person messed over me

Jealousy, hate, rage, betrayal

Because of all these things we bid a life farewell

A child at heart, affectionate, and full of hope

that cared and loved but at the end could not cope

No guidance, misled, and not understood

Our mirror image suddenly face first in mud

Know locked up

Erik Bradford
Cleveland, OH

S. Loue (ed.), *Health Issues Confronting Minority Men Who Have Sex with Men.*   249
© Springer 2008

without anyway of bail

Because a lie was told and he believed that tall tale

Now face to face with the ghost of his victim

but not scared or frightened because the way he thinks

is sickening.

Our brother stabbed and shot because of ones rage

A life taken, stripped, from one of young age

A friend that can't talk, gone but stills sends

ghost mail

To the one who fell into the rage of

Betrayal.

Portrait Eight
Community Commitment

Various

S. Loue (ed.), *Health Issues Confronting Minority Men Who Have Sex with Men.*   251
© Springer 2008

"Community Comment" : In Loving Memory of Donathyn J. Rodgers

Querida Jayla:

Te echo mucho de menos. Yo te quería como a un hermano, lo que sucedió me hizo enojar y sentirme triste, no sabía que hacer. Sentí como si hubiera perdido a un miembro de mi familia. Yo te admiraba sabes, eras mi modelo a seguir. Tus sueños eran mis sueños. Podrías sin lugar a equivocarte decir que yo quería ser como tu. Las personas que te hicieron eso, serán capturadas y encarceladas. Sigue mirando por mí desde donde estés y espero que tu espíritu danzante se pose sobre mí.

Con amor,
Extrañándote
Johnboy.

Dear Jayla,

I miss you so much. Only if you knew that I love you like a brother, what happened made me so mad and angry that I knew what not to do. I felt like I lost a family member. I looked up to you like you were my role model. Your dreams were my dreams. You might as well say that I wanted to be just like you. The persons that did it will be captured and put away. So keep watch over me and let your spirit of voguing stay with me.

Love you.
Miss you.
Johnboy

This issue is dedicated to the memory of Donythyn J. Rodgers. The following are letters from his friends and family. We are honored to share their thoughts.

Donathyn J. Rodgers

I swear to the Lord

I still can't see

Why Democracy means

Everybody but me.

Langston Hughes

The Black Man Speaks

Jay era un amigo muy cercano y a otros de BIC (Beyond Identities Community Center.-Centro Más allá de las identidades-). El siempre será recordado por todos; por su manera de bailar Vogue, su estilo y su sonrisa. Otra cosa que quiero decir es que siempre lo mantendré en mis plegarias y lo querré.

Nunca serás olvidado
Tierra Coleman
FAB

Jay was a very close friend to me and other BICC (Beyond Identities Community Center). He will always be remembered to me and others for voguing, fashion, and his smile. One thing will and want to say is he will always be kept in my prayers and love him.

Never forgotten.
Tierra Coleman
FAB

Jay was special in his own certain way. Everybody loved Jay. Nobody really knew if Jay's feelings were really for them, but everybody loved Jay. Jay was caring, loving, and joyful. Everybody loved Jay. Jay was the one who you could go to if you wasn't feelin well or sad. Everybody loved Jay. Jay was the one for everyone. Everybody loved Jay. He would make you laugh and smile. That's why everybody loved Jay. He will always be missed.

Taesha

Jay era especial en su propia manera. Todo el mundo quería a Jay. Nadie nunca supo realmente cuales eran los sentimientos de Jay para los demás, pero todos le querían. Jay era cariñoso, tierno y lleno de alegría. Todo el mundo quería a Jay. Jay era esa persona a la que podías acudir cuando te sentías triste o mal. Todo el mundo quería a Jay. Jay era la persona para todos. Todos querían a Jay. El te hacía reír a carcajadas y sonreír. Por eso todos querían a Jay. El siempre será echado de menos.

Taesha.

La justicia es el pan del pueblo: siempre está hambriento de ella.

Chateaubriand

Fig. P8.1

Comentarios de la Comunidad": Recordando con cariño a Donathyn J. Rodgers

Este ejemplar está dedicado a la memoria de Donathyn J. Rodgers. Afectuosamente conocido como Jay/Jayla. Las siguientes cartas son de sus amigos y familiares. Nosotros nos sentimos honrados al compartir sus pensamientos.

Every human life is a reflection of divinity, and . . . Every act of injustice mars and defaces the image of God in man.

Martin Luther King

Where Do We Go from Here: Chaos or Community

A la comunidad:

Estoy escribiendo esto porque quiero investigar como fue que Jay murió y además quiero saber exactamente por qué lo mataron. Yo siento que fue una equivocación y algo muy bajo. Yo no puedo seguir culpando a Jay por la manera en que fue asesinado ni por como murió. Sucedió sin importar lo que le dijera, de estar por ahí en la calle. También creo que estuvo mal hecho de que alguien estuviera allí con él, y lo de dejarlo solo por una hora y 45 minutos. Esto debería de ser una llamada de alerta a todos aquellos que están por ahí vendiendo sus cuerpos, ya que nunca sabes lo que te pueda suceder. No digo directamente que dejes de hacerlo, pero toma esto en consideración.

La'Shante

To the Community:

I am writing this because I am dedicated to finding out how Jay was killed and I want to know exactly why they killed him. I feel as though it was wrong and it was lowdown. I can't stay mad at the fact that he got killed or he died. It did happen regardless of what I said to him about being out there. I also feel that it was wrong for whoever he was with to leave him there by himself for an hour and 45 minutes. It should be a wake-up call for those who still go out there and sell their body because you never know what could happen to you. I am not saying you should stop, but take heed to it.

La'Shante

"I still hear people say that I should not be talking about the rights of lesbian and gay people and I should stick to the issue of racial justice. ... But I hasten to remind them that Martin Luther King Jr. said, 'Injustice anywhere is a threat to justice everywhere."

-Coretta Scott King

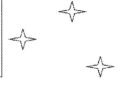

Donathyn J. Rodgers, mejor conocido como Jay era una persona muy alegre. No había un solo momento en el que pudieras decir que estaba enojado. Yo me acuerdo del primer día que lo conocí, inmediatamente congeniamos. Para mí, él era un ángel de verdad en la tierra, y Dios solo permite que sus ángeles estén aquí por un corto periodo de tiempo. Cuando recibí la llamada de que Jay había sido asesinado, mi corazón comenzó a latir rápidamente. Yo soy de los que creo que todo sucede por un motivo. Pero el motivo por el cual Jay fue alejado de nosotros, no te lo podría decir. Pero él esta ahora en un lugar mejor. Yo estoy bien triste porque se ha marchado aunque su espíritu continuara entre nosotros. Finalizando me gustaría decir que el tiempo que tenemos aquí es tan corto para desperdiciarlo, así que cualquiera que fue tocado por su luz lo tome como una lección.

Donathyn J. Rodgers aka "Jay" was a very happy individual. There was never a time you would see him mad. I remember the first day O met him, we immediately clicked. To me, he was truly an angel here on earth, and god only allows his angels to be here for a short period of time. When I received the cal that Jay had been killed, my heart started beating rapidly. I believe everything happens for a reason. His reason for taking Jay away I couldn't tell you. But he is in a better place. I am truly sad that he is gone but his spirit is still within all of us. In closing, I would like to say, time is to short to waste and also, take this and let it be a lesson for any and everybody who has been touched by his light.

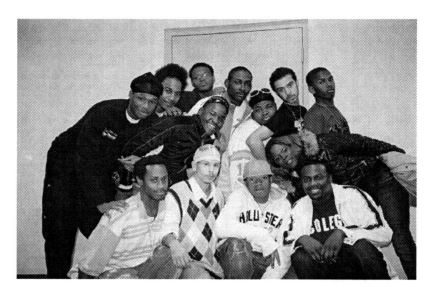

Fig. P8.2

Index

Acquired immunodeficiency syndrome, *see* HIV/AIDS
Activos, 16
Adolescence, 44, 57, 63, 76, 112, 116, 126
Adolescent Medicine Program, 168
Advancing HIV Prevention, 169
Affect management, 141
African Americans, 11, 16, 42, 93, 96, 110, 158, 159, 160, 162, 165, 166, 172, 177, 178, 179, 180, 181, 182, 183, 184, 186, 198
AIDS Taskforce of Greater Cleveland, 71, 235, 237, 239
Alaska, 159
Alaskan Native, 11, 96, 125, 128, 150, 158, 198
Alcohol, 44, 87, 88, 93, 94, 96, 97, 98, 111, 116–117, 120, 126, 130, 131, 133, 134, 135, 138, 140, 145, 146, 149, 150, 163, 164, 172
Alcoholics Anonymous, 100
American Indian, 11, 96, 125, 128, 141, 198
American Psychiatric Association, 14, 78
Amphetamines, 96, 117, 163
Amyl nitrate, 97
Anal sex, 11, 13, 42, 44, 46, 95, 160, 162
Anorexia nervosa, 68, 69, 78
Antiretroviral therapy, 161, 162, 185
Asians, 167, 197, 203, 206, 209, 211

Beck Depression Inventory, 225
Berdache, 15
Betances Health Center, 165, 171
Beyond Identities Community Center (BICC), 233–243
Bias, 44, 69, 70, 166, 179, 185, 186
Bipolar disorder, 18, 35, 36
Bisexuality, 7, 8, 184, 209
    concurrent, 9
    historical, 9

sequential, 9
transitional, 9
Body dysmorphic disorder, 77, 78, 79
Body image, 60, 61, 71–79, 94
    dissatisfaction, 68–69
    disturbance, 67, 70
    female, 75–77
    and HIV risk behavior, 72–73
    male, 69–70
Boriquen Family Health Center, 170
Brief Symptom Inventory, 120
Bulimia nervosa, 68, 70

California, 29, 115, 117, 159, 220
California Bridge Project, 172
Caregiver, 111, 119, 137, 138, 138, 148, 149
Case management, 150, 167, 171
Caucasian, 68, 70, 71, 74, 75, 76, 143, 158, 159, 160, 165, 166
Centers for Disease Control and Prevention, 96, 169, 181, 235
Centers for Epidemiologic Studies Depression Scale (CESD), 129, 134
Chicago, 45, 59, 60, 160, 168, 172, 173
Childhood sexual abuse, 41, 43–52, 88, 119, 130, 132, 161
    definition of, 43–44
    and HIV risk, 41, 46
    model of, 50–52
    prevalence of, 45
Childhood Trauma Questionnaire, 129
Chlamydia, 161, 180, 181, 182, 188
Church, 29, 30, 31, 32, 36, 58, 59, 100, 146, 164, 186
Cleveland Department of Public Health, 177, 180, 236
Cocaine, 94, 96, 97, 116, 117, 118, 172
Cognitive impairment, 68

Colorado, 29
Communication, 4, 121, 161
Community, 13, 16, 17, 32, 57, 60, 63, 94,
    100, 101, 109, 110, 112, 114, 117,
    118, 119, 120, 121, 122, 127, 128,
    135, 136, 137, 138, 140, 141, 145,
    147, 150, 151, 162, 164, 165, 168,
    169, 171, 172, 177, 181, 186, 188,
    190, 197, 200, 201, 202, 208, 209,
    210, 211, 219, 233–243, 245, 246,
    247, 251, 252
Comprehensive HIV Center, 172
Condom use, 72, 160, 162, 163
Coping skills, 92, 100
CORE Center, 168, 172, 173
Correctional facilities, 168
    See also Prison
Crack cocaine, 88, 98, 115, 116, 117, 118
Cross-dressing, 5
Cutting, 83–85, 136
Cuyahoga County, 177, 178, 179, 180, 181,
    182, 183, 185, 186, 187
Cybersex, 9

Depression, 35, 36, 48, 50, 51, 62, 68, 72,
    92, 93, 94, 115, 120, 126, 129, 132,
    134, 146, 147, 149, 150, 161, 169,
    223, 226, 228
Depressive mood, 129, 131, 132
Dignity, 31
Discrimination, 16, 47, 48, 76, 87, 91, 92, 93,
    100, 101, 121, 126, 137, 142, 143, 144,
    166, 179, 199, 201, 211, 230
Dissociation, 49–52, 93, 101
Domestic violence, 130–131, 133, 161, 241
    See also Childhood sexual abuse;
        Rape
"Down-low", 16

Eating Attitudes Test, 71
Eating disorder, 69, 70, 71
Education, 62, 91, 115, 122, 129, 133, 134,
    149, 166, 167, 170, 173, 180, 181,
    182, 183, 186, 188, 204, 206, 207,
    225, 227, 228, 234, 235, 236, 238,
    240, 241
Europe, 77, 118
Experience with Battering Scale, 130
Exploitation, 60, 92, 121

Families, v, vi, vii, 92, 111, 113, 150, 165,
    168, 172, 179
Familismo, 165

Fellatio, 15
Femininity, 16, 71, 75, 76, 77, 89
Filipino Americans, 163
Florida, 75, 76, 77, 170
Foreclosure, 179, 235
Friendship, vii, 30

Gay Liberation Movement, 17
Gay-Related Immune Disorder, 32
Gender expression, 5, 60, 128
Gender identity, 3, 4, 5, 16, 76, 88, 89, 120,
    128, 129, 131, 132, 241
Gender role, 4, 74
George Washington University Hospital, 219
God, 25, 29, 30, 31, 32, 60, 85, 100, 139,
    143, 146
Gonorrhea, 118, 160, 161, 180, 182
Greenwich Village, 35, 172
Guilt, 30, 31, 47, 51, 60, 94

Hate crime, 93, 243
Health Professional Shortage Area, 180
Hepatitis, 118, 171
Hermaphrodites, 15
Heroin, 31, 33, 70, 96, 97, 98, 116, 117
Heterosexuality, 7, 8, 9, 14, 17, 146
Hijras, 15, 16
HIV/AIDS
    Cleveland, 177–190
    community, 32
    diagnosis, 97, 158, 205
    national trends, 157–174, 198
    reduction efforts, 118, 121
    serostatus disclosure, 197–214
    services, 171, 172, 186, 235
    stigma, 197–214
    surveillance, 157–158, 177, 180–181,
        184–187
HIV Cost and Services Utilization
    Study, 166
HIV testing, 97, 169, 172, 181, 187, 188,
    239, 240
    barriers, 164, 168, 198
Homelessness, 3, 7, 87, 93, 109–122, 168,
    236, 239
Homophobia, 47, 48, 50, 51, 52, 60, 87, 89,
    90, 92, 93, 94, 99, 100, 125, 126, 146,
    209, 233
Homosexuality, 7, 9, 14, 15, 16, 31, 58, 60,
    70, 71, 75, 99, 164, 165, 170, 197, 201,
    202, 209, 220, 223
    defined, 7, 8, 14
HONOR Project, 127, 128, 135

Housing, 107–151, 235–236, 237, 239, 240
Human immunodeficiency virus, *see* HIV/AIDS

Identity, 3–18, 25–34, 35–37, 47, 58, 76, 90, 92, 94, 135, 136, 141, 145, 149, 162, 164, 199, 208, 211, 233, 234, 237, 239, 101, 127
    development of, 3, 6, 88, 99, 101
    ethnic, 200
    female, 75, 76
    gender, 3–5, 16, 76, 88, 89, 120, 128, 129, 131, 132, 241
    masculine, 13, 88–90
    positional, 59–90
    self, 3, 8, 9, 18, 101, 118, 147
    sexual, 3, 5, 9, 10, 13, 14, 17, 18, 31, 60, 110, 114, 122, 144, 145, 165, 169, 197, 199, 200, 206, 234
Identity conflict, 8
Immigration, 200, 201, 202, 204, 208, 210, 211
Impersonators, 5, 75
Index of Partner Physical Abuse, 130
India, 15
Intercourse, 15, 17, 42, 46, 72, 95, 160, 162, 163, 164, 180
Internet, 9, 160, 161, 235, 241
Interventions, 52, 121, 150, 165, 235
    body image disturbance, 79
    HIV, 46, 96, 113, 121, 161, 162, 169, 171, 174, 187, 188, 189, 208, 210, 229, 233–243
    substance use, 113, 120

Ketamine, 116, 163
Kinsey Scale of Sexual Orientation, 6
Korean American, 77

Language, 91, 166, 167, 173, 186, 198, 204, 205, 225
Latino Gay Men's Sexuality Study, 47, 49, 51
Latinos, 11, 13, 41–52, 70, 96, 158, 159, 160, 161, 162, 167, 172, 219–230
Lesbian, 14, 31, 57, 60, 71, 87, 88, 99, 125, 126, 128, 181, 243
Listening Guide, 136
Los Angeles, 13, 32, 36, 45, 96, 98, 114, 127, 159

Maleness, 14, 16
Manhood, 89, 90, 223

Marginalization, 202, 208, 211
Marijuana, 88, 94, 96, 97, 98, 111, 115, 117, 180
Marriage, 11, 16, 29, 31, 58
Masculinity, 14, 59, 71, 74, 75, 165, 202
    development of identity, 4, 14, 16, 88, 89, 90
Masturbation, 15
May-December relationships, 57–63
Media, 61, 69, 74, 75, 242
Mental illness, 14, 91, 234, 239
Methamphetamine, 88, 94, 96, 98, 115, 117, 118, 121, 163
Mexico, 29
Miami, 76, 98, 170
MINI International Neuropsychiatric Interview, 130
Minneapolis, 127
Minority Collaborative Research Program, 220
Misclassification, 159
Muscle mass, 78

Narrative analysis, 136
National Eating Disorders Screening Program, 70
Native American Housing Assistance and Self-Determination Act, 150
Native Americans, 15, 125–151, 159, 161, 163, 167, 168
Neill, John, 184
New York, 32, 35, 45, 98, 110, 114, 115, 116, 117, 127, 159, 160, 162, 165, 171, 172, 197, 211, 224
Non-Hispanic whites, 11, 96, 97, 160, 161, 172

Ohio Health Coalition, 183
Oklahoma, 127, 143
Oklahoma City, 127
Oppression, 47, 48, 136, 147, 148

Pacific Islanders, 158, 167, 178, 211
Pain, 31, 32, 33, 34, 83, 145, 222, 246, 247
Panama, 219, 220
Pasivo, 16
Peer advocates, 170
Philadelphia, 187
Pills, 57, 72, 85
Plastic surgery, 76, 78, 94, 95
Pornography, 69, 112
Posttraumatic stress, 119, 120, 126, 130–131, 133, 134, 169
Posttraumatic Stress Diagnostic Scale, 130

Poverty, 109, 115, 119, 120, 121, 126,
    164, 166, 167, 179, 233, 234, 235,
    236, 239
    See also Socioeconomic status
Predators, 62, 92
Priesthood, 30, 31
Prison, 7, 17, 33, 61
    See also Correctional facilities
Prostitution, 33, 114
    See also Sex trade
Puerto Rico, 10, 96, 99, 170

Quality of Social Support Scale, 225

Rape, 60, 143, 144
Religiosity, 16, 127
Reservation, 126, 138, 139, 141, 143, 150
Resiliency, 49–51, 100, 127, 148
Role model, 33, 75
Rupaul, 75

Safer sex, 42, 43, 95, 131, 160, 161, 162, 169,
    239, 240
St Paul, 127
St Vincent's Hospital and Medical
    Center, 172
San Diego, 31, 32, 117
San Francisco, 32, 45, 47, 88, 97, 98, 110,
    114, 117, 118, 127, 160, 162, 163,
    198, 220
Santa Barbara, 35
Seattle, 98, 116, 127, 128, 160
Self-esteem, 67, 68, 72, 87, 91, 93, 94, 100,
    122, 226, 227, 237
Sex
    biological, 4, 5, 128, 129
    oral, 11, 162, 165
    unprotected, 57, 72, 160, 169, 198–199
Sex toys, 17
Sex trade, 129, 132, 140, 163
Sexual desire, 15, 95
Sexual impotence, 15
Sexually transmitted diseases, 62, 112,
    160, 163, 170, 173, 180, 182, 184,
    188, 190
Sexual orientation, 16, 58, 60, 69, 70,
    72, 73, 118, 126, 128, 164, 165,
    168, 174, 200, 202, 204, 205,
    208, 210, 211, 223, 224, 225,
    229, 236
    behavioral view, 6
    conflict theory, 8
    determination of, 6–7

flexibility theory, 8
    formation of, 3, 6, 14
    Kinsey scale of, 6, 7, 11
    self-identification view, 6, 16, 58
Sexual reassignment surgery, 5
Sexual silence, 47, 50, 51
Shame, 16, 47, 50, 51, 90, 94, 146, 200, 208,
    210, 211, 223
Simpatia, 165
Single-Item Self-Esteem Scale, 225
Smoking, 16, 96, 180
Social exclusion, 202
Social marketing, 238–239, 240, 242
Social oppression, 47
Social support, 126, 149, 173, 199,
    205, 208, 209, 210, 225, 226,
    227, 236
Socioeconomic status, 90, 112, 169
    See also Poverty
Somatization, 93, 120
Steroid use, 69, 73, 78, 79
Stigma, 91, 92, 94, 101, 157, 164–166, 168,
    169, 170, 174, 187, 197–214
    management of, 141
Street competencies, 112–113, 137–142
Substance use
    incidence of, 57, 62, 73, 92, 97, 99, 111
    treatment of, 49, 100, 101, 116, 117, 119,
        126, 170, 171, 172, 234, 239
Suicidal behavior, 94
Suicidal ideation, 48, 120, 146
Suicide, 60, 85, 113, 115, 119, 120, 125, 126,
    129, 131, 132, 146
Survival sex, 112, 114–116, 118, 137,
    139, 150
Sweden, 9
Syphilis, 117, 160, 161, 180

Tacoma, 127
Testimonios, 136
Toronto, 35
Transfusion, 117
Transgenderism, 5, 35
Transsexuality, 5
Trauma, 49, 50, 60, 88, 92–94, 99, 100, 112,
    115, 119–121, 126, 129, 137, 138, 143,
    148, 149, 150
Tulsa, 127
Two-spirit persons, 125–151

Vaginal sex, 13, 118
Viagra, 163
Village People, 74, 75

Violence, 17, 90, 92, 99, 119, 125, 126, 127,
    130, 131, 133, 136, 142, 143, 144, 148,
    149, 150, 151, 161, 233, 234, 237, 241,
    242, 247
Viral load, 161, 163, 185, 204, 205, 211

Wahlberg, Mark, 74
Washington, DC, 171, 220
Whitman-Walker Clinic, 165, 171
Women, 5, 8, 9, 10, 11, 12, 13, 15, 16, 26, 31,
    44, 46, 48, 49, 60, 62, 67, 68, 69, 70, 71,
    73, 78, 79, 89, 90, 92, 128, 164, 173,
    202, 205, 209, 210, 223, 236

Young Men's Survey, 42, 158
Youth, 12, 13, 52, 57–58, 60–63, 73, 92,
    93, 100, 101, 110–116, 122, 126,
    137, 149, 168, 172, 173, 179–181,
    187, 190, 234, 236–243, 245–246
    GLBT, LGBT, 50, 57, 60, 61, 62, 63, 99,
    116, 120, 234
    HIV-positive, 12, 168, 172, 173
    homeless, 93, 110, 111, 113, 114, 115,
    119, 126
    sexual minority, 111, 119, 137, 187
    street, 114, 116, 119
Youth Risk Behavioral Survey, 180

Printed in the United States
96730LV00003B/1-60/A